Candida Albicans

D0542474

Candida Albicans

Could yeast be your problem?

Leon Chaitow
N.D., D.O.

Thorsons
An Imprint of HarperCollins*Publishers*

Thorsons
An Imprint of HarperCollins*Publishers*
77–85 Fulham Palace Road,
Hammersmith, London W6 8JB.

First published 1985
This revised edition 1991
10 9 8 7 6 5 4

© Leon Chaitow 1991

Len Chaitow asserts the moral right to
be identified as the author of this work

A CIP catalogue record for this book
is available from the British Library

ISBN 0 7225 2452 8

Typeset by Harper Phototypesetters Limited, Northampton
Printed in Great Britain by
HarperCollins Book Manufacturing, Glasgow

All rights reserved. No part of this publication may be
reproduced, stored in a retrieval system, or transmitted,
in any form or by any means, electronic, mechanical,
photocopying, recording or otherwise, without the prior
permission of the publishers.

Acknowledgements

The pioneering research of Dr C. Orion Truss in the uncovering of Candida's involvement in a wide range of diseases and conditions deserves recognition. I would respectfully dedicate this book to him. Others who have made major contributions to this knowledge, and to whom I owe a debt, include Dr William G. Crook, and Dr Jeffrey Bland. I have quoted from all three of these respected scientists, and thank them on behalf of all those who will benefit from their original work. The books of Dr Truss and Dr Crook (*The Missing Diagnosis* and *The Yeast Connection*, respectively) are worthy of study by anyone who wishes to have a deeper knowledge of this subject.

Contents

1

Candida Yeast and Common Health Problems

In the very recent past it has become clear that a great many common health problems, both physical and mental in expression, might have a common cause — namely, the spread in the body of a yeast that lives in each and every one of us. Its name is *Candida Albicans*, and we will call it Candida for short.

Since the first edition of this book was published in 1985 the major emphasis in my practice has involved people with Candida overgrowth and its associated health problems such as chronic allergy and chronic fatigue (M.E.). The degree of the problem world-wide has become increasingly apparent to me, as a result of the mail which continually arrives from readers of the book. Many contain phrases such as 'this book has changed my life', and often come with touching stories of desperate health situations which have been positively transformed (but not overnight) by the application of its principles. While receiving such letters is truly humbling, the real credit should go to pioneers of research such as Dr C. Orion Truss of Alabama, USA, who first noticed what no one else seemed able to see, although it was staring them in the face.

Because it is present in all people from about the age of six months onwards, Candida tends to become neglected in the eyes of doctors seeking the causes of particular diseases or conditions. Since it is in everyone, it seems that Candida cannot be causing particular symptoms in only some. This reasoning has prevented attention being given to Candida, except in rare conditions in which it proliferates to such an extent as to become life-threatening. This, interestingly enough, often happens in people whose defence mechanism (immune system) has become weakened by disease or drugs (in therapy or in abuse). This gives a clue as to why a great many people may indeed be suffering from a less pronounced spread of Candida, which, whilst not sufficient to endanger life, is certainly enough to produce a wide array of debilitating symptoms. These can include: depression; anxiety; unnatural irritability; digestive symptoms such as diarrhoea, constipation, bloating and heartburn; tiredness and a sense of hopelessness; allergies; acne; migraine; cystitis; vaginitis; thrush; menstrual problems and pre-menstrul tension.

The key to understanding the way in which this vast array of symptoms could possibly result from the effects of a yeast that lives in all of us, lies in an appreciation of those factors which can encourage a spread of yeast. In most people there is an uneasy truce between their body and the yeast that lives inside it. Over many thousands of years an equilibrium has been struck. The yeast can live, and thrive, and present no problems to its host, the body, as long as it confines itself to specific sites. Should it go beyond these sites, the defence capability of the body, as represented by its immune system in general and its white blood cells in particular, attacks and destroys the yeast. There are also actual physical barriers, such as the mucous lining of the digestive tract, which prevents intrusion through it by yeast or any other undesirable elements. All mucous membranes contain further protective substances which can destroy invading particles of yeast. We will consider these defences later, in our search for an understanding of this problem.

At this stage we should simply have an appreciation of the efficient defence capability, on the part of the body, which deals with toxins, bacteria and yeast, should any of them intrude upon areas in which they present a danger to the body. The problem arises when, because of one of a variety of causes, the defence capability becomes deficient or weakens. Should this happen, the controls which keep Candida in check would be removed, and it would be able to spread to other areas normally out of bounds. If at the same time the foods the yeast thrives on happen to be in plentiful supply, we have the recipe for an explosion of Candida activity. This is precisely the combination of factors that has been identified as having become widespread in Western society over the past twenty-five to thirty years.

We will look at the dietary aspect in detail, and also at those changes in medical care which have, inadvertently, allowed Candida's new-found freedom from adequate surveillance.

The introduction of broad-spectrum antibiotics, the use of the contraceptive pill, and the widespread use of steroids, have all played their part in Candida's growth. In addition the increase in the use of sugar and sugar-rich foods has provided the yeast with just the sustenance it loves. This is the unfortunate combination of factors that is the root cause of the problem for many people.

A careful look at the nature of the enemy is necessary, together with consideration of those factors and circumstances which allow it to proliferate, and what the consequences of such a proliferation might be. We will then be in a position to consider methods of controlling Candida. Fortunately this is the brighter side of the sorry mess. For it seems unlikely that the causative elements of the picture are going to be removed from the population at large, and so the fact that control is possible, in the majority of cases, is a blessing indeed.

It should be clearly understood that it is not being suggested that in all cases the conditions listed above are the result of Candida infection. It is certainly true that all of these *might* be such a result, but equally there can be other causes. It is the view of those practitioners now aware of the possibility of Candida's involvement in common disease problems of this sort that when a combination of such symptoms appears in a person, with no other obvious causes apparent, then Candida should be the prime suspect. Unlike most infection and infestations, it is not really possible to test for the presence of Candida to prove or disprove such an assumption. This is because, as has already been stated, Candida is present to some extent in all of us. This would make looking for it as pointless as looking for mice in a granary; they are always present, but in what number? Candida can be cultured in most people's blood, and it is so ubiquitous in stool cultures that it is usually ignored by microbiologists when they do come across it. A group of doctors recently wrote to a leading medical journal (*Lancet* No. 8527, Jan 1987) highlighting the difficulty of assessing, purely from tests, whether Candida is active even when in an advanced stage of overgrowth.

They report of one group of 48 patients with acute myeloid leukaemia that there was such widespread Candida infiltration in the lungs and other organs that 'entire microscopic fields were filled with mycelia', and yet the diagnosis could have been assumed from signs without waiting for the time-consuming proof positive from the laboratory. Half these patients died from Candidiasis and the doctors assert that had they been able to aggressively attack the yeast earlier this may have been averted.

The signs they suggest looking for all have drawbacks in terms of giving false negatives (showing all clear when this is not so) but they suggest that in advanced Candidiasis any two of these signs should alert the practitioner to start attacking yeast. They suggest the following:

1. Faecal culturing of Candida (although they admit this gives 25 per cent false negatives, ie people assumed from this test not to have Candida overgrowth even when it is rampantly present).
2. Looking for any rise in the bloodstream of Candida antibodies even within supposedly 'normal' levels (10 per cent false negatives).
3. Pain behind the sternum (breastbone) or thrush in the mouth. These signs are absent in 50 per cent and 30 per cent of patients who die of Candidiasis, respectively, showing that their absence proves nothing in terms of whether or not Candida is active. If present, together with other general signs (see pages 40-1) they are a strong indication of systemic Candidiasis.
4. A low continuous fever for four days or more which fails to respond to antibiotic therapy. In 16 patients with this sign, treated for Candidiasis, 11 became free of fever rapidly.

While these criteria may be useful in a hospital setting, in private practice or in self-assessment of Candidiasis it is generally recognized that the history and present symptoms (as outlined in

Chapter 4) give an accurate guide as to whether or not Candida is presently active. The way to prove that a condition (or a cluster of conditions occurring together) is the result of Candida, is to treat it, and if the symptoms then disappear the proof is then irrefutable.

This is one of the very few instances where the treatment is in fact the main means of diagnosis. The initial suspicions that result in the treatment being applied, rely upon recognition of the sort of symptoms that might be implicated by the presence of Candida, as well as an awareness of those factors that influence Candida's development and behaviour. This knowledge, combined with a careful background history which looks at previous and current medical treatment and drug usage, as well as at diet and stress factors, will give clear indications as to the likelihood, or otherwise, of Candida being a possible culprit.

It is these areas that we are going to explore, in order to formulate a series of recommendations for the control of Candida, and for the prevention of its accompanying complications.

This exaggeration of a previously fairly harmless interaction between ourselves and a yeast is one of the complications of civilization, and as such is rapidly becoming so widespread as to constitute an epidemic. The failure, thus far, by all but a handful of doctors to recognize the situation is tragic, for the degree of human suffering involved is enormous. Prevention is not difficult, and control, whilst a slow process, is not beyond the limits of any intelligent individual to institute.

The major credit for the unravelling of this mystery belongs to one man, who recognized that what he was seeing in his own patients had a worldwide import. He first set about diligently assembling his evidence, which he presented in a scientific journal (the *Journal of Orthomolecular Psychiatry*). He then went back to his task of investigation. Over a period of years his results, in an enormous range of diseases, from acne to schizophrenia, and what appeared to be multiple sclerosis, were so impressive that in true fashion the world beat a path to his door. Dr. C. Orion Truss, of Birmingham, Alabama, will be remembered for his work in this field by tens of thousands of grateful people. His masterly investigation and research, conducted in a normal medical practice, shows how important simple observation is in the quest for knowledge and the understanding of man's ills. Dr Truss has written his own history of this quest, and of the whole story of Candida, in his book, *The Missing Diagnosis*.

That book, and the excellent book on the same subject by another renowned American practitioner, Dr William Crook, entitled *The Yeast Connection*, both suggest for their attack on yeast, the use of an antifungal drug called nystatin. They also suggest other methods, including nutrition and desensitization. This book, however, will not attempt to echo the drug approach suggested by these two practitioners, but will present non-drug alternatives to the use of nystatin. This is not to say that this drug should never be used — only that in most cases there are ways of restoring the competence of the body to fight the yeast itself. There are also naturally occurring nutrients which enhance the controlling of the wildly proliferating yeast. This is the only reason this book has needed to be written, for in every other way the two books mentioned above are excellent, and are valuable contributions to the literature of health.

Our task is now to look at the nature of the enemy, what makes it active, and what we must look for to recognize such activity. After that we will begin to learn how to deal with it.

2

Candida and Your Defence System

The object of our interest is a member of the yeast family. Strictly speaking it is a member of a sub-group of that family of plants known as fungi (or moulds). Yeasts live practically everywhere on the planet. They can derive their nutrients from most organic sources. This means anything that is alive, or has been alive, can support yeasts. Rather than having roots like other plants, yeasts can derive their nutrients via the use of enzymes. Given the right conditions for growth and replication, yeast is capable of almost explosive growth, as anyone who has made bread will testify.

Roger Williams,[1] a world-renowned research scientist, states that if a single yeast cell is given a highly favourable environment, with a good assortment of nutrients, and the correct temperature, it can, within twenty-four hours, produce a colony of over a hundred yeast cells. At this rate of reproduction, Williams calculates, within one week, one cell could turn into a yeast colony weighing one billion tons. The fact that this has not happened, and that it is not likely to happen, is solely because the environment is seldom ideal for any creature on earth, least of all for yeast. It does, however, highlight a very pertinent point in our understanding of the Candida problem. Candida is a yeast which lives inside you and me, and, as far as is known, every other adult on earth, and most children as well. It seldom takes over our entire body, but when it does the consequences are horrific. It can only achieve such a state if the environment for it is excellent, and if the defence mechanisms that the body has with which to control its spread are weakened or absent.

As Williams points out, in nature, yeast cells are almost always hampered by imperfect or inadequate environmental conditions. Were it not so, they would have engulfed the earth long ago. Just the same fact controls the colonies of Candida (and other yeasts) that live in and on you.

Candida is usually a resident of your digestive system, largely in the intestines. It also tends to occupy sites in the vaginal regions and on the skin.

Research has shown that almost everyone has antibodies to Candida. This indicates that the individual's defence system has been challenged to respond to Candida's presence by producing antibodies. Truss states that by the age of six months, at the latest, Candida is living in or on at least 90 per cent of people, as evidenced by a positive skin test reaction when extracts of Candida are injected just under the skin.[2] This reaction shows that there has been a previous presence of the yeast to which the body has developed antibodies.

The fact that it is in all of us, and yet many people sail through life with no apparent ill effects, indicates that we have learned to cope with our passengers. Unlike certain other minute creatures that live in our digestive tract, and which serve a useful purpose, such as *Lactobacillus acidophilus,* which helps with the breakdown of our foodstuff and helps in the synthesis of some of the B vitamins, there is no symbiotic relationship with Candida. There is no 'trade-off' whereby houseroom is given in exchange for some useful function. So Candida is a pure and simple parasite — a freeloading parasite. This is perhaps inevitable, in terms of the multitude of opportunistic microscopic creatures, of both the animal and vegetable kingdom. Most, if not all, plants and animals 'enjoy' similar relationships with bacteria and fungi. Some of these relationships are mutually beneficial and some are distinctly one-sided. So Candida, for all the musicality of its name, is an unwelcome boarder and a potential danger throughout life. Once we know just what sort of situations will remove our natural controls of it, and what will give it that extra ability to proliferate by virtue of an environment conducive to its growth, we will have the beginnings of a picture as to what needs to be done to contain it.

Part of this picture is indeed an understanding of the ways in which the body has learned to take care of the threat of parasites. It may be that we cannot actually stop it from taking up squatters' rights in our body, but we can certainly confine its activities to a small and relatively safe part of the premises.

We should try to understand some aspects of our body's amazing defensive capability. It has long been observed that people who survive certain infections seldom suffer from that same disease again. They develop antibodies to the infecting organism. Apart from conferring such specific resistance to various disease-causing micro-organisms, the immune system plays a vital role in other biological reactions. We have, in essence, two systems, which together make up the immune system. One is based on the thymus gland (which lies just below your breast bone), which produces what are called T-cells. The other part of the immune system is made up of different types of white blood cells, called B-cells. These protect you from most bacterial invaders, and some viral infections. By producing molecules called antibodies, the B-cells neutralize many potential enemies. The two systems, together making up the surveillance and protection agency of the body, work in harmony, with, it is thought, the thymus taking the leading role.[3]

The white blood cells, which act as the soldiers in the front line of the battle, are manufactured mainly in the marrow of the long bones of the body. Some of these actually are turned into T-cells, by the influence of hormones from the thymus gland. Other white blood cells are turned into what are called lymphocytes. Anything that tries to get into the bloodstream, or the interior of the body, has to contend with the T- and B-cells, and their powerful ability to neutralize foreign substances or organisms. If a B-cell senses a foreign organism it produces antibodies that are specific against the invader. At the same time other B-cells are alerted to the alien presence, which causes them to manufacture antibodies to destroy the enemy.

It is believed that there are in excess of a million different kinds of antibodies in the bloodstream. As they are manufactured and deployed against the intruder, the lymphocytes go into action, with other white blood cells, to dispose of the debris and waste products of the battle between the intruder and the body. Thus a condition such as influenza is self-limiting, in that the fever and the symptoms of aching represent the intense body activity that is going on to deal with the invading virus, as well as the effects of the resulting degree of toxicity from the breakdown products of the battle.

When T-cells come across an invading organism, whether this be a virus or a fungus such as Candida (or even a mutant cancer cell), they produce what are called lymphokines which can kill micro-organisms (or cancer cells). One such lymphokine which has received much attention is interferon. Lymphokines can also call up assistance from a powerful ally in this battle called macrophage, which can eliminate micro-organisms and tumour cells by literally swallowing them whole. Sometimes the T-cells act as 'helper' cells to the B-cells in their production of antibodies to fight the invader, and they can also act as what are called 'suppressor' cells, to stop a defensive process from getting out of hand, when there may be a danger of B- or T-cells actually attacking friendly tissues in the body.

When for any one of a number of reasons (which we will consider in a later chapter) the immune system becomes weakened, we talk of the person being immuno-deficient, or of having a poor immune response. It is when these valiant soldiers, the T- and B-cells, and the macrophages and their various assistants are put into a weakened state, that silent squatters in our body can become free of the constraints that the defence system normally imposes, and spread to areas beyond their normal territory. At that point a vast array of problems and symptoms can arise.

This system of defence, with its checks and balances, may become disrupted to such an extent that the condition now known simply by its initials, AIDS, may occur. The initials stand for Acquired Immuno-Deficiency Syndrome, and in this condition it is the T-cells (from the thymus gland) that function inadequately. In fact the ratio between the helper and suppressor cells alters so that there is an excess of suppressor cells, in contrast with the opposite situation in normal health. One research effort in the AIDS battle involves the use of thymosin, a hormone produced by the thymus. It is obviously desirable to enhance the function of the thymus gland so that it can produce adequate, active T-cells and the desired amount of hormone. Among the nutrient factors which we can use to this end are vitamin C and the amino acid arginine. The amounts used in treating conditions, such as AIDS, where the immune system is severely disrupted are very large indeed (upwards of 20g of vitamin C daily, and 3-5g of arginine).

When the immune system is in a weakened state, not only do infections become more frequent but severe consequences arise, such as greater likelihood of cancer developing, because of the reduced surveillance by the B- and T-cells. In such a condition of inadequate protection it is no wonder that the ever-present opportunistic yeast may slip through the defence barrier and advance to areas previously closed to it. This is a simplistic picture of what happens, but it contains the essential facts. It is known that before it becomes invasive, the yeast (Candida) alters to a different form, known as its mycelial fungal form, in which it has characteristics which make it more dangerous, such as a root structure enabling it to penetrate through the mucosal barriers, with a variety of harmful consequences (see Chapter 4).

Recent research by Dr Truss[35] indicates that many of the toxic effects noted with Candida activity result from its ability to manufacture, under appropriate conditions, the substance acetaldehyde. He points out that this well-known toxin could produce both the clinical and the laboratory characteristics of Candida infection. He has analysed the amino acid profiles of the affected individuals in order to arrive at his finding and maintains that this theory appeals because it defines the symptoms of chronic yeast infection in terms of a toxin which common strains of Candida can be shown to produce in laboratory conditions. This provides the chemical link between normal yeast fermentation and the metabolic abnormalities found in susceptible patients. He stresses that no conclusive proof yet exists that Candida can ferment sugar into acetaldehyde in the body, but that this is highly probable, based on the evidence thus far. There are now tests which take advantage of yeast's apparent ability to turn sugar into alcohol (acetaldehyde). These tests measure any rise in blood alcohol levels after a 'sugar loading' and thus identify active yeasts in the bloodstream. However this test is not foolproof as yeast may be active in tissues other than blood.

Incidentally, some laboratory technicians performing these tests (and many practitioners involved in treating chronic Candidiasis) report being able to smell the alcohol resulting from eating sugar in people who never drink alcohol at all. In my personal practice I have treated individuals for Candidiasis who have been breathalyzed and found to be over the legal limit of alcohol in their bloodstreams, despite their not having consumed any alcohol.

There is also evidence from a variety of sources[36, 37, 38] that there is a degree of immune system depression which results from mercury toxicity reaching the body via amalgam fillings in the teeth. A number of researchers have shown there are several ways in which this highly toxic metal is able to penetrate into the body, and that this has a specific harmful effect on the immune system. There is evidence that this can be linked with the spread of Candida activity. A number of dentists are now helping affected individuals by removing mercury amalgams and replacing them with either a composite or gold filling. It should be stressed that research into the relationship between mercury, derived from amalgam fillings, and health problems in general and Candida involvement in particular, is as yet incomplete. That there is a link seems probable, however, and it is worth considering alternative choices for the filling of teeth, other than amalgams which contain mercury. The replacement of existing fillings may be required in cases where a link can be demonstrated between the health status and measurable mercury toxicity resulting from amalgams. The use of amino acid compounds, such as Glutathione, and of vitamin C, can help to ease mercury deposits from the body. Tests can be done to measure the sensitivity of the body to mercury, and also to measure the levels of mercury in the mouth (escaping as a gas), as well as the electrical activity in the teeth, set up by the combinations of metals in the mouth. These methods, as well as measuring mercury levels via hair analysis, can all indicate just how active this problem is in any particular individual.

A further dental hazard related to Candidiasis was discovered in a study which looked at 50 consecutive patients with respiratory disease who had all developed Candidiasis in the mouth and pharynx. Dentures were found to be worn by 32 of those in the study and this was thought to be a major predisposing factor in their Candida onset (among the others were use of cortisone, antibiotics and immune suppressing sedatives). The researchers stated, 'Dentures cause tissue trauma, provide sites for (yeast) colonisation and diminish salivary flow. Saliva is necessary for normal oral immune defence.' (Thompson P, 'Assessment of oral candidiasis.' BMJ, 292, June 1986).

It was found that if dentures were treated with antifungal chemicals this helped prevent this hazard. Regular sterilizing of dentures is suggested as a safe preventive measure along with oral rinsing with dilute aloe vera juice (an antifungal substance, see pages 71-2).

Our ultimate attempt to neutralize and control the spread and effects of Candida (for we can seldom get rid of it completely) depends upon the use of whatever safe methods we have at our disposal, to deprive it of its ideal nutrients, whilst at the same time building up, and enhancing, the embarrassed and depleted immune system. This can then get on with the job of keeping Candida in check. It is this double thrust of activity which we must undertake if we are to do more than temporarily suppress Candida. The use of an antifungal drug will, it is true, in time destroy a great deal of Candida's potency and reduce its resultant symptoms. However, this will stop happening the moment the drug is stopped. The answer to controlling Candida in the long term lies in a two-pronged attack which deprives the yeast of its optimum nutrient environment, as well as the reinstitution of normal controls, via the immune system and healthy intestinal flora. As we will see, there are other methods which, it is thought, can help by altering the ability of the yeast to multiply, and we will consider these natural, safe alternatives to the use of drugs later.

It must, however, be stated that there are conditions in which the use of antifungal drugs are to be advocated, especially if the condition is such as to indicate that the process of recovery is going to be a very long one. In the main, however, once we can learn to recognize those symptoms that indicate Candida getting out of hand, the natural, non-drug methods that I am suggesting will work, and work well. Nystatin is the main such antifungal drug now in use. Whilst effective against certain Candida strains, others are resistant to it. Not being a broad spectrum antifungal agent it allows proliferation of other fungi, such as trichophyton, when Candida is attacked.[39] An alternative exists in caprylic acid, an extract of coconuts (see page 75).

We will now go on to consider just what can happen to weaken your wonderful defence mechanism, the immune system, as well as additional ways in which Candida is sometimes allowed to go on the rampage, and so begin to infest other areas of your body.

3

How Candida Gets
Out of Hand

There are a number of predisposing factors which will allow Candida to get wildly out of control. To a greater or lesser extent these same factors may be involved in the more subtle spread of Candida which represents what happens in the majority of people affected by the sort of symptoms outlined in Chapter 1. There is a degree of overlap of course, for seldom will only one factor be involved. Among the main ones are:

1. An underlying inherited or acquired deficiency of the immune system.
2. The aftermath of steroids (hormones) in food or as medication.
3. The aftermath of antibiotics in food or as medication.
4. Diabetes.

As we shall see, these factors are also vitally interconnected with the diet of the individual, which 'feeds' the yeast. We will look at each of these and see how they transform Candida from its relatively docile state into that of a predator. First let us consider ways in which the immune system can be weakened.

Immune System Deficiency

As we have seen in the previous chapter, part of the response of the body to an intruder such as Candida is the production of antibodies to meet the particular antigen (a substance which stimulates a response on the part of the immune system) that is present in the foreign substance or organism. Candida has many antigens, and the efficiency with which the defensive operation is carried out, against any particular one of these antigens, can to some extent be inborn (i.e. genetic). There is a great variation in the degree of response in any one person to the different antigens. This can lead to a situation in which the immune system, unable to adequately counteract and expel the Candida invasion, tolerates it in increasing amounts.

It has been demonstrated by research, that we are all biochemically individual.[4,5] This means that there are wide variations in the particular requirements for any of the over forty nutrients that we require for survival and health. Many of these individual needs are determined before birth, and this has led to the genetotrophic theory of disease causation. This, put simply, says that because a person has individual inborn requirements, which may vary greatly from a mythical 'average' or 'normal' amount, there is a good chance of one or other of these needs not being met by the normal dietary intake. This leads at best to a lowered degree of function, and at worst to a deficiency disease.

To a large extent this individual inborn (genetic) factor also applies to our ability to handle one or other of the pathogens, or micro-organisms, capable of infecting us. This is the case in our ability to handle Candida efficiently. It seems that since infestation by this yeast is almost universal, we are incapable of totally controlling its presence in our bodies. Some people will be more able than others to keep it under control, and limit its spread. Thus some people will, without the involvement of such factors as antibiotics and steroid drugs (see below), become 'tolerant' of a degree of spread of the yeast.

The commonest areas for this spread to occur are in the mouth, the throat and in the vaginal areas. If this initially produces a degree of reaction and activity on behalf of the immune system, then we would see manifestations of the condition called thrush. This would flare up periodically when, perhaps, there were factors which lowered the general vitality. Eventually, in many cases, the condition might no longer evoke an acute flare-up, but would remain in a semi-permanent, chronic state. This happens when the body becomes 'tolerant' of the yeast's 'foothold', and is no longer able to mount attacks on it. This is an indication of impaired or deficient immune function. Among the many aspects of our environment which can influence this are stress factors, nutritional inadequacy and pollution, as well as the use of specific drugs which weaken the immune system further.

We are all nowadays familiar with the concept of tissue and organ transplantation. This involves the use of powerful drugs which are designed to prevent the body of the recipient from rejecting the new foreign tissue or organ. These are called immuno-suppressive drugs, simply because it is their prime task to stop the natural defences from working adequately — in other words, to suppress the immune system. The risk of infection and of other diseases resulting from this is all too familiar to patients who have gone through such treatment. Drugs such as steroids (hormones) have this effect, and these are employed in a variety of conditions ranging from rheumatic disorders to asthma and hormonal imbalances. The most widespread use of steroids, however, is not in the treatment of disease but in the contraceptive pill. One of the most devastating effects of the long-term use of this type of medication is on the immune system in general, and on the ability of Candida to proliferate wildly, in particular. The contraceptive pill is dealt with more fully below.

There are now known to be a variety of nutrient substances which are absolutely vital for the adequate functioning of the immune system.[6,7] These include a number of vitamin and mineral substances which have antioxidant properties. This means that they are able to slow down, or stop, a process in which substances known as 'free radicals' can cause tissue damage. The major free-radical scavengers are vitamin C, vitamin E (acting in conjunction with a substance called selenium) as well as certain amino acids (parts of the protein chain) such as methionine, cysteine and glutathione (which is itself a combination of three amino acids — cysteine, glutamic acid and glycine). Vitamin B6 (pyridoxine), zinc, manganese and other important nutrients have been shown to be involved in compromising the immune system when deficient.[8]

It should be realized that apart from the nutrients mentioned in this section, it is possible for any of the forty-plus nutrients vital to life to be required in extraordinary amounts by a particular person to meet idiosyncratic inborn needs. These needs may also vary markedly under different conditions (infection, stress, pregnancy, etc.) in the same person, and so any vitamin, mineral or other nutrient, is capable of upsetting the chain of complex biochemical interactions which allow the immune function to operate efficiently. The ones cited above just happen to have a more dramatic impact than some of the others. Assessment of personal needs is a task requiring patience. Some personal detective work can be useful, and books such as *Your Personal Health Programme* by Jeffrey Bland (Thorsons) and *Your Personal Vitamin Profile* by Michael Colgan (Blond & Briggs) enable this to be successfully achieved by using questionnaires aimed at providing specific indications as to nutrient requirements.

Stress, which involves repeated, or constant, states of anxiety, and all that this entails in terms of depletion of vital nutrient reserves, as well as imbalances of internal secretions and functions, is a major cause of immune incompetence. One of the ways in which this can be most dramatically demonstrated is that during periods of stress people become far more prone to infection. This indicates the lowered efficiency of their immune system, as well as the increased usage by the body of vital nutrients such as zinc and vitamin C at such times.

The interaction between anxiety/stress conditions and nutritional incompetence leads to the immune system being deprived of the ability to operate efficiently. If at the same time there is increased demand on the effective functioning of the immune system, to meet environmental or nutritional toxicity (pollution of air, cigarette smoke, alcohol, caffeine-rich drinks such as coffee, chocolate and tea) then a complex picture emerges in which excessive demands, inadequate nutrition (with associated deficiencies) and perhaps drug usage, such as the contraceptive pill, all interact to deplete the immune function. Let us examine the manner in which drugs in common use can further complicate the situation.

Antibiotics, 'the Pill' and Steroids

It is clear from many years of research that the use of antibiotics removes from the scene biological controls over the yeast that lives in us. As has been mentioned, one of the major sites for this to take place is the long, dark, warm and moist (ideal environment for yeast) digestive tract, which it should be noted is also inhabited by upwards of 5lb of other micro-organisms, most of which are friendly and helpful to the body. One such friend is *Lactobacillus acidophilus,* which by its presence helps to keep a check on the spread of yeast. When antibiotics are used to destroy pathogenic (harmful) micro-organisms which might be harming the body (as in treating an infection), the friendly bacteria in the bowel are also destroyed, or severely damaged. When this occurs, the yeast, which is totally unaffected by the antibiotic (being a yeast and not a bacteria), will find room for expansion. This becomes even more likely as the resistance of the immune system will at that time be compromised. In a variety of ways the same thing happens with the use of steroid drugs, such as cortisone (even cortisone ointments, so commonly prescribed for skin problems cause a yeast increase, by being absorbed into the system). All steroids, including those used in the contraceptive pill, will have a depressing effect on the immune system.

It is worth noting at this point that there is another, almost totally ignored source of antibiotics and hormonal residues, to which all but the vegetarian sector of the population are exposed. This is of course commercially reared meat and poultry (with the exception of lamb). Antibiotics and hormones are fed to animals in order to speed their growth as well as to control the heightened susceptibility to disease that their unnatural existence generates.

Anyone who has been regularly eating beef, pork, veal and chicken (and many people eat one or more of these daily) will have absorbed prodigious amounts of antibiotic and hormone residues (unless the source of the meat was from a farm which did not employ the addition of such drugs).

Low-level intake of these substances over many years may have a devastating effect on the ability to control Candida, as would the regular employment of these drugs in the form of medications. This area is yet to be adequately researched, but it does provide one more argument in favour of adopting a vegetarian diet.

It has also been noted that, because of the hormonal changes that take place during pregnancy, a degree of control over Candida is lost.

Yeast therefore finds this a good time to expand its activities.

Imagine then, if you will, a young lady who has grown up in this era characterized by common usage of these drugs. She has had antibiotics prescribed to her over the years for minor problems such as tonsillitis and ear infection. She may have then developed cystitis from time to time, and also have had a broad-spectrum antibiotic for this. Her skin may have had a good deal of acne, and again this would commonly have been attacked with antibiotics. Should she have had cause, she may have had steroids for asthma or some other condition. Going on 'the Pill', and subsequently coming off it and becoming pregnant, would also have enhanced the chances of yeast spreading, and causing problems (the acne and cystitis are frequent examples of Candida activity). Thus the child in her womb would be exposed to a variety of antigens (up to 790) from the Candida activity in her body, all the while inheriting the possibility of a weak immune response (not all children inherit a weak response), and so the pattern will be set to repeat itself. We have still left out of this picture all the other variables, such as nutritional imbalances, which are common in modern society: pollution; excessive use of sugar-rich foods (which yeast loves), and stress factors in general. The picture emerges of a person who is doing just about all that is possible to bring about the ideal conditions for yeast to thrive in. And the result, in terms of the general population, of this typical scenario? An explosion of Candida-caused problems, over the past thirty years or so, which is now reaching epidemic proportions.

We will discuss later a very important aspect of Candida's spread, which is the diet of the individual, not in the sense of helping to create a situation in which the immune system is less efficient, but as adding actual supporting nutrients to Candida. The two main areas in which this occurs are the use of sugar-rich foods, which all yeasts love, as well as foods that are themselves associated with yeasts or fungi. In the meantime it should be evident that many aspects of life in civilized society are working towards the disadvantage of our defensive ability, and to the advantage of prospective enemies, such as Candida.

Dr Truss, who has done so much to research and publicize the Candida problem, is scathing in his attack on the use of certain drugs which have compounded the problem. Antibiotics are often used inadvisedly, in cases in which they have no role to play at all.

Incorrectly diagnosed viral and fungal conditions may be uselessly treated by antibiotics, for example. This actually increases the likelihood of the condition worsening. The treatment of acne with tetracycline is another major cause of Candida spreading, and Truss insists that there is no way anyone suffering from Candida problems can control their condition if they continue with tetracycline. In many cases acne is actually the direct result of Candida infection, and will worsen rather than improve on such treatment.

In the use of the contraceptive hormone, too, Truss sees great harm. Fully 35 per cent of women using the Pill have, associated with it, acute vaginal Candidiasis. There are undoubtedly many others who have less pronounced changes in this regard, as their immune competence is gradually compromised by the hormonal onslaught. As Truss points out, 'Chronic yeast vaginitis tends to be at its worst when progesterone levels are high, as in pregnancy, and the luteal phase of the menstrual cycle. Therefore the progesterone component of contraceptive hormones may well be responsible for their effect.' It is clear that the association between Candida vaginitis and emotional problems such as irritability and depression frequently appears soon after the first use of the contraceptive pill. It is worth reflecting on the fact that the degree of biological individuality which we display in our individual reactions to any harmful factor such as Candida must play a large part in deciding just who will, and who will not, succumb to a spread of Candida. Since 35 per cent of women do not control the vaginal Candida when on the Pill, we must assume that the other 65 per cent do. This highlights the fact that for many people there is an inborn genetic weakness in their ability to meet such a challenge. For some this will have been acquired via the very factors we have been discussing in this chapter — antibiotics, immune system weakened by stress, nutritional factors, etc. We shall see that the approach to controlling Candida must include methods that deal both with the building up of the immune system, as well as reducing as many factors as possible which help to sustain the yeast in its advance. Among the most important of these is the eliminating of the use (unless absolutely vital) of antibiotics, hormone preparations and contraceptive pills, as well as the making of alterations in the diet to avoid actually feeding the yeast.

Since yeast loves sugar, it is clear that if a person has additional levels of sugar in the bloodstream, as in a diabetic condition, this will fuel the spread of Candida. For this reason diabetic individuals are more prone than average to Candida problems, and they must be even more rigorous in their efforts to control it.

The possible involvement of mercury toxicity in harming immune system control of Candida has been mentioned (see page 20) and deserves re-emphasis.

Foods that Help to Spread Candida

Yeast loves carbohydrate-rich foods. This in effect means that we must attempt to deprive it of its sustenance by limiting, or cutting out all together, all sugar-rich foods and refined carbohydrates. Details of this will be outlined in the nutritional programme (Chapter 5). It is also considered to be important that the intake of any foods that contain fermented products, moulds or fungi be limited.[2,9] This means things such as vinegar, alcoholic beverages, yeast extracts and spreads, mushrooms, blue cheeses. This aspect of the programme to control Candida should be carefully observed at the outset. Once the yeast is controlled, there is no reason to keep to a strict prohibition, but the return of classic symptoms of Candida activity, such as abdominal bloating after eating one of the offending foods, will tell you if it is time to return for a period to the avoidance strategy. Just as foods which contain moulds or fungi are considered undesirable, so will it be found that symptoms will always be worse in humid, damp environments, which are conducive to mould and fungus spores being present in the atmosphere. Thus, it is important to eliminate from the home any areas of damp on walls, etc., as many moulds can reinforce the effects of Candida by their presence. For this reason, inhaled spores of any mould or fungus should be avoided during the active phase of Candida infection.

Candida gets out of hand because we allow it to. We may well do so in ignorance, but it is folly to blame the yeast when we have the power to control it, as millions of people have done before. Once you begin to suspect that your many and varied symptoms (see next chapter) may be the result of Candida activity, it is time to grasp the problem firmly and take responsibility for the situation. Candida will not go away. Its current spree may be the result of any combination of factors which have released it from our normal efficient control. To get it back where it belongs (or at least to where it can do least harm) we must restore our defence capacity to its optimum, and we must stop doing those things that are helping the yeast to thrive. It's as simple as that. You can do this by your own efforts, by the reform of your dietary pattern, by the use of particular nutrient substances, and by overall stress and pollution reduction. Once you have put Candida in its place, you can relax your vigilance to a great extent, in the sense of allowing your diet to contain certain of the 'undesirable' substances from time to time, but you should be aware of the factors which allow Candida to advance in the first place, and avoid these as stringently as possible.

We will now look at the sort of problems that Candida can cause when it gets out of control. Be prepared for some surprises.

4

Candida and its Consequences to Your Health

The actual list of conditions in which Candida has been implicated as a major causative factor is very long indeed.

As has been mentioned, it is necessary to deduce the involvement of Candida from the history of the patient. (Were antibiotics used? Is, or was, the contraceptive pill in use? Have cortisones or other steroids, e.g. prednisone, been employed? etc.) The range and type of symptoms also give indications of its involvement. This is because it is useless asking a microbiology lab to look for Candida's presence, since we already know it to be present in practically all adults. So what would an analysis prove? We must deduce from the history and the symptoms that Candida seems to be involved. The proof of its involvement is obtained by carrying out an anti-Candida programme and finding out whether or not this gets rid of most of the list of symptoms usually present.

Before considering them all (or at least the major ones) one by one, let us look at a list of the sort of conditions that are now known to be the possible result of Candida's activity.

Vaginitis; thrush (oral or vaginal); endometriosis; athlete's foot;

headaches (migraine type); fatigue; constipation; bloating; allergy; sensitivity to perfumes, fumes, chemical odours and tobacco smoke; poor memory, feelings of unreality, irritability, inability to concentrate; depression; numbness, tingling and weak muscles; heartburn; abdominal pain; diarrhoea; recurrent sore throats and nasal congestion; swelling and discomfort in joints; blurred vision, and so on — and on. The diagnosis becomes more clear if symptoms are aggravated during damp weather (or places) or when in an environment with a lot of mould or fungus. Also, if the symptoms are worse after eating sugar-rich or fungus-containing foods, the evidence for Candida's involvement becomes stronger.

After we have looked at these conditions more closely, we will try to pull all this together in the form of a questionnaire, which should enable you to assess the chances of Candida being involved in your health make-up. Truss draws a picture of a typical case of chronic Candida infection in his article 'Restoration of Immunological Competence to Candida Albicans'.[10] He states, after pointing to the influence of multiple pregnancies, birth control pills, antibiotics and cortisone, as well as other factors that depress the immune system:

> The onset of local symptoms of yeast infection, in relation to the use of these drugs, is especially significant and usually precedes the systemic response. Repeated courses of antibiotics and birth-control pills, often punctuated with multiple pregnancies, lead to ever increasing symptoms of mucosal infections in the vagina and gastro-intestinal tract. Accompanying these are manifestations of tissue injury, based on immunological and possibly toxic responses to yeast products released into the systemic circulation. Many infections are secondary to allergic responses of the mucous membranes of the respiratory tract, urethra and bladder, necessitating increasingly frequent antibiotic therapy that simultaneously aggravates, and perpetuates, the underlying cause of the allergic membrane, that allowed the infection. Depression is common, often associated with difficulty in memory, reasoning and concentration. These symptoms are especially severe in women, who in addition have great difficulty with the explosive irritability, crying and loss of self-confidence that are so characteristic of abnormal function of the ovarian hormones.

Truss then points out that accompanying this sad catalogue are what he calls 'poor end-organ response' resulting in acne; loss of libido (disinterest in sex); menstrual bleeding and cramps; intolerance to foods and chemicals, etc. The commonest (but by no means only) type of individual suffering from Candida infection, is seen to be a woman somewhere between puberty and the menopause, who has undergone some, or all, of the predisposing factors described previously, and who has some, or all, of the symptoms outlined in Truss's picture above. A mixture of unaccountable vaginal and bowel symptoms, ranging from discharge and itching, to bloating, discomfort, diarrhoea and/or constipation; as well as an array of mental-emotional symptoms are typical. Classically such women are labelled as neurotic, and this must be the crowning insult to an individual who has literally begun to feel her body and mind giving way in all directions.

The vaginal and intestinal tracts are the most usual areas for Candida to inhabit, since they provide the damp atmosphere, and the nutrients it thrives on. If circumstances allow, Candida has been known to spread along the entire length of the digestive tract, from the anus to the mouth. The tongue may be coated, and there may be yeast deposits on the insides of the cheeks, the corners of the mouth and gums. White spots and a coating on the tongue are the obvious signs, accompanied by a soreness and tingling of the gums. When the oesophagus is affected it can result in symptoms commonly assigned to 'heartburn'; indigestion and acid stomach are symptoms which can be the result of Candida activity in the stomach region. If the infestation is prolific in the small or large intestine, then diarrhoea may be the result. This may be chronic, and may be accompanied by mucus and/or blood. There may be cramp-like pains ('spastic colon') and colicky pains, often associated with difficulty in passing normal bowel motions. Bloating and distension of the abdomen is a frequent occurrence with Candida, and there may be a variety of abdominal noises as a result. If constipation is indeed a factor, then haemorrhoids are a likely consequence, as is the possibility of rectal discomfort and itching.

The very nature of Candida changes under certain conditions. It can turn into what is called its 'mycelial fungal' form, from its simple yeast form. Candida is what is known as a dimorphic organism. This means that it has two quite separate identities. In the yeast form it has no root, but in its fungal form it produces what are called rhizoids. These are long structures, similar to roots. The complication that this presents is that these 'roots' can actually penetrate through the mucosa of the tissue in which they are growing. One of the key controls which prevents this change is the abundant presence of the B vitamin, biotin. In good health, biotin is manufactured in the intestines by friendly bacteria. After antibiotic treatment (or anything else which upsets their function) these are severely depleted and unable to manufacture biotin. Thus control is removed from the yeast and the aggressive fungal form emerges to start its onslaught on new territories in your body. Supplementation with biotin helps to control this as does restoration of normal bowel flora ecology, via supplementation of potent, viable strains of these friendly bacteria. These are important and usually successful strategies in the campaign against Candida. Until this control occurs, the change from yeast to fungus allows a breach by fungal roots of the boundary between the body proper and the self-contained world of the digestive tract. This allows substances to enter the bloodstream of the individual which would otherwise have been kept out by this boundary. The fungal form of the Candida organism is invasive, and it can use this avenue to enter the body proper. The main result of the breaking of the intestinal barrier is that undigested proteins from the food eaten, as well as toxic wastes from the Candida infestation, may begin to circulate in the bloodstream. These are frequently the cause of a wide variety of disseminated symptoms, often of an allergic type. If these substances reach the brain, there is a chance for the production of what have been termed 'brain allergies'.[11] These can result in a wide variety of mood and personality problems, ranging from depression, irritability and mood swings, to conditions which look for all the world like the symptoms of schizophrenia.

These substances, which enter the brain and act upon the receptors there, to produce these mental and personality symptoms, have been given the label *exorphins*.[12] This differentiates them from *endorphins*, which are substances produced in the body which have roles to play in the control of many aspects of the biochemistry of life, including pain control. The externally originating substances (proteins from incompletely digested food) which slip into the bloodstream through the gates opened by fungal 'roots' of Candida are able to cause havoc in whatever tissues with which they come into contact. They will be seen as 'foreign' by the immune system, which will attempt to neutralize them. If such a process is long continued, and this sort of thing can run on for many years, then this in itself is a factor contributing to the ultimate depletion of the immune function of the body. It simply becomes overwhelmed by the constant onslaught. The defensive reaction by the immune system to such substances may result in a wide range of what are seen as allergic symptoms, including asthmatic attacks, nasal and respiratory conditions, skin reactions, palpitations, aches and swellings, etc.

The female reproductive organs are a major site for Candida activity. If it irritates the urethra it can be a common cause of cystitis. If, for any of a number of reasons, the acidity of the region alters, then the relatively benign yeast form can alter into the fungal form, and become actively invasive and spread to other regions, accessible from the vagina. This can lead to inflammatory conditions in the womb, Fallopian tubes and ovaries themselves (see Chapter 7, 'Case Histories'). A wide variety of consequences can be envisaged, including the tragic possibility of infertility or sterility. The symptoms related to Candida involvement in this region can range from frequency of urination, coupled with a burning sensation, to chronic discharge, as well as pre-menstrual and menstrual problems, and the whole gamut of inflammatory and infectious involvements of the reproductive system.

An American hospital study (reported in *Female Patient* July 1987) strongly supported a link between much PMT and Candida activity. Thirty-two women with severe symptoms of premenstrual syndrome, as well as vaginal Candidiasis, were treated with a diet low in yeast and sugars (see Chapter 5) together with antifungal medication. They were compared with an equal number of women with similar problems who did not receive the anti-Candida approach. All these patients had previously failed to respond to treatment of their PMT using vitamin treatment and psychotherapy.

The results? Two thirds of the women receiving anti-Candida therapy showed significant PMT relief while none of those not having this approach improved. The study clearly showed that if PMT and thrush co-exist, dealing with the yeast will often clear the other symptoms as well, thus implicating yeast's activities in much PMT.

The concurrence of mild, or major, emotional and mental

symptoms with any such pattern of ill health should alert you to the strong possibility of Candida activity. Often mental symptoms are no more than a general feeling of inability to concentrate, accompanied by memory lapses, and feelings of lethargy and exhaustion. They may, however, be far more dramatic, as Truss and others have proved. The first articles on the subject, by Truss, discussed the fact that many conditions are given names or 'labels' simply because they fit into a pattern which is more or less recognizable as being similar to a particular known illness. That is to say, a combination of symptoms which may have no obvious cause, is somehow more 'manageable' medically if it is labelled.

Truss initially reported on six cases. Two of these women had been repeatedly diagnosed as 'schizophrenic'. Another woman in this original report was diagnosed previously as having 'multiple sclerosis'. Pointing out that they all recovered on anti-yeast treatment, and that they were all in good health up to seventeen years after recovery, he asks the pertinent question, 'Were two of these women really schizophrenic, or was it just that *Candida albicans* was responsible for brain function so abnormal that highly competent specialists never doubted the diagnosis of schizophrenia?'. He further asks, 'In the third woman, did *Candida albicans* induce neurological abnormalities sufficiently typical of multiple sclerosis that a competent neurologist would mistakenly diagnose the disease?' He answers by saying that either the treatment dealt with a yeast infection, which can produce symptoms which mimic these diseases (and many others) or that yeast can actually cause the diseases which are labelled with these names. The indication, after many years of work by Truss and others, is that this is not just a case of remission (which is not uncommon in either schizophrenia or multiple sclerosis) but that Candida induces symptoms *similar* to those of other illnesses, which may then be wrongly diagnosed and labelled.

Candida and Chronic Fatigue (M.E.)

Most people with Chronic Fatigue Syndrome (also known as M.E. — myalgic-encephelomyelitis, as well as Post Viral Fatigue Syndrome) are affected with yeast overgrowth, and in many instances this is the major cause of their condition. It was reading about the way the first edition of this book had changed someone's life that first drew my attention to this fact, for it was following the anti-Candida advice contained in it that was credited, by Sue Finlay (in the *Observer*, June 1 1986), with having made all the difference in her recovery from M.E.

She tells of how her doctor, at her insistence, had already prescribed nystatin and that this had taken her from being 'confined to bed, hardly able to stand, tears all day and suicidal' to a point where 'the feeling of being poisoned left me, a little energy returned.' She then states that after some months of variable but gradual improvement, 'I came on the book *Candida Albicans — Could Yeast be Your Problem?* by Leon Chaitow. I changed my diet radically. I cut out sugars and refined carbohydrates. All bread, mushrooms, tea, alcohol, vinegar, coffee, chocolate were dropped. All these foods feed the yeast (see note below). I used vitamin supplements to enhance my immune system, olive oil and garlic to attack the yeast and acidophilus powder to replace the Candida with healthy intestinal flora. I ate vegetables, salads, whole cereals and fruit in abundance. At present I am able to walk nearly half a mile without total collapse, I am beginning to work in the garden a little, I still have to rest every day and be careful not to overdo things and cause a relapse, but I have had eight months of improvement and am steadily reducing the nystatin.'

Sue Finlay has continued to improve, and her message is the one I want people with M.E. to listen to. It is not all in the mind. M.E. is more likely to cause depression than to be caused by it, and is often largely the result of a faulty immune system, weakened by Candida.

It is clear that the ramifications of Candida infection are not yet fully understood, and that much clarification and research remains to be done. In the meantime, since it is not difficult to identify reasons to suspect its possible involvement, it seems reasonable that a Candida control approach should be adopted in cases where the history and symptoms approximate any of the patterns touched on above, whatever previous diagnosis has been made. The treatment

Note: Only one thing needs correcting in Sue's story. The stopping of yeast-based foods is not because this 'feeds the yeast' but rather because the system of the person thus affected will usually have become sensitized to yeasts, and eating foods based on yeast, or containing moulds, will further irritate and aggravate this situation.

is, after all, harmless and indeed health-promoting. Other conditions which are sometimes confused with Candida involvement are frequently labelled as psychosomatic. This can be a way for the doctor to avoid having to say that he cannot find the cause. Calling conditions such as this 'functional' or 'psychosomatic' may, if repeated, result in patients beginning to believe that they really *are* not quite balanced. The terms 'neurotic' and 'nervous' are often ascribed to such individuals, with devastating effects on morale and self-esteem. The yeast or fungal cause may remain unsuspected, or, if noted as part of the problem (if thrush is a part of the 'psychosomatic' symptom picture for example), be simply ignored as a minor piece of the puzzle, unworthy of therapeutic effort.

There is reason to believe that Candida infection is a rampant problem in modern society. It has been let loose by the use of drugs, used in good faith to help in other directions, as well as by a dietary pattern which is ideal for the sustenance of the yeast, rather than the host. The number and variety of possible consequences is mind-boggling and deserves the attention of every individual involved in the healing professions.

The alertness of one man has brought about the current increase in awareness of the significance of Candida. He may not be totally right in his concept, but the results he has so far obtained in thousands of cases bearing a range of symptoms such as those already discussed — simply by paying attention to the yeast component of the problem — are proof of the validity of this method of treatment.

There is no area of health more amenable to self-assessment and self-help, and the information which will be provided in subsequent chapters should enable improvement in most cases in which Candida is the culprit.

The questionnaires on the following pages will give you the chance to assess the possibility of Candida being a major part of your current health picture. It is possible for most of the symptoms described to be the result of causes other than Candida. If, however, you have more than one of the indications on List 2, as well as some of the lesser symptoms listed at the end of the questionnaire, then the possibility increases to a probability, especially if you can identify a possible causative link with at least one of the factors in List 1.

Candida Albicans Checklist

The completion of this questionnaire will give clues as to whether Candida is an active agent in your current health spectrum. It is not possible to make a diagnosis by these means alone, but a strong indication, as evidenced by positive answers in all sections of the questionnaire, is possible and can be used to assist in deciding upon the undertaking of the Candida control programme.

List 1 — History of Drug Usage, etc.

1. Have you ever taken a course of antibiotics for an infectious condition which lasted for either eight weeks or longer, or for short periods four or more times in one year?

2. Have you ever taken a course of antibiotics for the treatment of acne for a month or more continuously?

3. Have you ever had a course of steroid treatment such as predisone, cortisone or ACTH?

4. Have you ever taken contraceptive medication for a year or more?

5. Have you ever been treated with immuno-suppressant drugs?

6. Have you been pregnant more than once?

List 2 — Major Symptom History (Candida Implicated)

1. Have you in the past had recurrent or persistent cystitis, vaginitis or prostatis?

2. Have you a history of endometriosis?

3. Have you had thrush (oral or vaginal) more than once?

4. Have you ever had athlete's foot or a fungal infection of the nails or skin?

5. Are you severely affected by exposure to chemical fumes, perfumes, tobacco smoke, etc.? Or are your symptoms worse

after taking yeasty or sugary foods or drinks?

6. Do you suffer from a variety of allergies?

7. Do you commonly suffer from abdominal distension, 'bloating', diarrhoea or constipation?

8. Do you suffer from pre-menstrual syndrome (fluid retention, irritability, etc)?

9. Do you suffer from depression, fatigue, lethargy, poor memory, feelings of 'unreality'?

10. Do you crave for sweet foods, bread or alcohol?

11. Do you suffer from unaccountable muscle aches, tingling, numbness or burning?

12. Do you suffer from unaccountable aches and swelling in joints?

13. Do you have vaginal discharge or irritation, or menstrual cramp or pain?

14. Do you have erratic vision or spots before the eyes?

15. Do you suffer from impotence or lack of sexual desire?

If there are one or more positive answers to the first section, and two or more in the second section, as well as some of the following being present, then Candida is probably involved in your symptoms causation. Symptoms usually worse on damp days; persistent drowsiness; lack of co-ordination; headaches; mood swings; loss of balance; rashes; mucus in stools; belching and 'wind'; bad breath; dry mouth; post-natal drip; nasal itch and/or congestion; nervous irritability; tightness in chest; dry mouth or throat; ear sensitivity or fluid in ears; heartburn and indigestion.

Life-threatening Implications of Candida

We have looked at some of the common, sometimes serious — sometimes merely nuisance — results of Candida overgrowth. We should take note though that life itself may be threatened by specific combinations of infection which can result when our immune function is low, and Candida is active. Before we discuss research evidence of a terrible symbiosis between *Staphylococcus aureus* and *Candida albicans* (both of which, incidentally, can be controlled naturally by friendly bacteria such as acidophilus) we should briefly examine some of the known disease states which *Staphylococcus aureus* is known to produce.

Toxic Shock Syndrome (TSS)

This is typically found in young women (95 per cent of cases). Those affected by TSS begin to notice symptoms on about the fifth day of their period (tampons are usually being used). Symptoms include a widespread rash, fever, watery diarrhoea, vomiting, sore throat, headaches and aching muscles. The skin may begin to peel off, kidney failure may ensue and both respiratory and cardiac complications are common. One or two out of every ten people affected by TSS die.

The cause is rampant infestation with *Staphylococcus aureus*, with the symptoms being largely the result of toxins which this bacteria produces.

Scalded Skin Syndrome (SSS)

This condition affects infants, young children and immune-suppressed adults, and usually follows a spread of *Staphylococcus aureus* from a primary infection somewhere else in the body such as conjunctivitis. SSS is characterized by fever and profound weakness and a bright red, very tender, skin rash involving large blisters which slough off in sheets of skin, leaving large areas of the body without skin at all. Even normal looking skin shears away with light pressure. Complications occur relating to the body's temperature control and fluid balance mechanisms being disrupted in this way. As with TSS, this is caused by a toxin secreted by the bacteria.

Between 80 and 90 per cent of *Staphylococcus aureus* infections which are found in hospital settings are 'superinfections', resistant to penicillin treatment. Other conditions associated with *Staphylococcus aureus* include gastroenteritis, bone and joint infections (osteomyelitis) and septic arthritis, pneumonia, meningitis, inflammatory heart disease, etc.

The Candida connection with TSS and SSS

In a series of experiments Dr Eunice Carlson, of Michigan University, established that when there was a combined infection of *Staphylococcus aureus* (or *Streptococcus faecalis* or *Serratia marcescens*) and *Candida albicans* there was an enormous potentiation of the infection caused by the bacteria. She tells us, 'Although these studies show that Candida has a strong amplifying effect on the virulence of other organisms (*Staphylococcus aureus, Streptococcus faecalis*) how this is achieved is a mystery.' She continues: 'One possibility is that the candidal infection progress causes physical damage to the organ walls which makes them 'leaky' allowing other microbes or chemicals (perhaps toxins), or both, to penetrate more easily: it is also possible that Candida directly stimulates the growth of *Staphylococcus aureus.*' We know now of Candida's ability to make tissues 'leaky', as in the digestive tract, when it changes from its yeast form to its aggressive fungal stage.

Dr Carlson looks at the almost inexplicable fact that Candida is seldom automatically dealt with by doctors, and gives the example of Candida infection related to denture wearing. 'This is now believed to be very common and to occur in 60 per cent of all denture wearers. Biopsies of inflamed areas however consistently fail to demonstrate tissue invasion (with Candida). We can speculate that an equivalent infection of the small intestine would be virtually undetectable.' So because Candida's presence is not obvious it is ignored!

One of the most important messages this book can give is that we have to assume Candida's active presence on the basis of the person's symptoms and history, not on expensive, time-consuming scientific tests, which are commonly inconclusive.

Dr Carlson continues, 'Physicians have reported therapeutic cures for a variety of diverse disease conditions using anti-candidal drugs. It now appears possible that this fungus may play a key role in many disease conditions, not by its own toxic or invasive growth, but rather by enhancing secondary infection.'

The methods outlined in the following chapters are suitable for preventing the sort of ailments which Candida produces on its own, and also for the disasters which are possible (TSS and SSS for example) when other infections occur alongside it.

5

Controlling Candida Naturally (Including Supplement Programme and Diet)

If it has been possible to come to a position where it looks as though Candida is a likely suspect in your condition, then it is necessary to prove this by means of adopting an anti-Candida programme. If this succeeds in making a major impact upon your condition, by virtue of its controlling Candida and improving your symptom picture, then you will have proved the assumption to be correct. Dr W. M. Crook calls this a 'therapeutic trial'.[9] It is really the only way of being sure, since there is as yet no way of discovering whether Candida is involved by any laboratory tests.

This is a stumbling block for many people. They want cast-iron 'proof' that Candida is the culprit. None the less all we can do is look at the picture that is currently present in your particular condition and add to this a review of your past history. If that looks like a 'Candida picture', then there really is no other choice but to introduce anti-Candida measures, apart from going on as you are. If a culture were made of your fluid discharges, tissues or excreta, it would inevitably display Candida's presence, somewhere in your body. This would not prove or disprove anything, as far as your symptoms are concerned, since a positive test result could also be obtained from almost every adult in the land. Only by looking at the known and suspected pattern of symptom production that has been built up around Candida's activity can we guess its active presence (as opposed to its benign presence if your immune system and intestinal flora are keeping it under control). The only real proof is in the treatment results. If you are better after controlling Candida, then you will know that what you assumed was accurate, and that your programme was the correct one. The very least that you will achieve is that you will have reformed your dietary pattern, and will have swallowed some harmless vitamins and other supplements, as well as building up your immune system's ability to combat its adversaries.

It would be quite reasonable to question whether it is really necessary to attack Candida which may be obviously active in a local region (oral or vaginal thrush for example) by an approach which is aimed at the intestinal tract as well. Fortunately there is now clear evidence that this is the right way to tackle the problem.

Researchers writing in the *American Journal of Obstetrics and Gynecology* (15, 1986) detailed their findings in which they treated women with serious vulvo-vaginal Candidiasis. These people were also assessed for intestinal Candida activity and in all 258 women involved this was shown to be evident. The patients were divided into two groups, one of which received antifungal medication both by mouth (for the intestines) and vaginally. The other group had antifungal medication locally for the vagina but took a dummy tablet (placebo). The medication was used for just one week and the women were reassessed after one week, three weeks and seven weeks.

The results showed that 88 per cent of those receiving both the digestive tract and local antifungal approach clear of Candida overgrowth as against 75 per cent of those who had intravaginal therapy. While this shows a significant, although not massive, benefit, when both the local (vaginal) and the intestinal Candida are treated simultaneously, there is an even more important result when both are attacked, a reduction in recurrence which is far higher amongst women not also aggressively treated for digestive yeast overgrowth. (see page 76 for details of local treatment for vaginitis).

The controlling of Candida falls into three different segments. First there are a number of nutrient supplements which, for several reasons, can help to control Candida. Secondly there is a pattern of eating which reduces the intake of yeast-conducive foods and so deprives it of its growth potential. Finally there are specialized methods and substances, including antifungal drugs, which can be employed only by a health professional. These will be described to complete the picture of anti-Candida methods, although, as has been stressed, it is in the self-help field that the greatest long-term results will be found, and the first two segments of the programme, special supplements and diet, will prove to be worthy of adoption by anyone suspicious of Candida's role in their current health picture.

There are also a number of general tips which can be useful in coming to terms with the condition, and these will be found at the end of this chapter.

Specialized Supplemental Anti-Candida Methods

When antibiotics are used they destroy a number of 'friendly' bacteria which inhabit the digestive tract, and which, as well as providing other valuable symbiotic (mutually beneficial) contributions to the body's economy, also act as a controlling element, in stopping Candida from spreading. One of the major bacterial 'friends' which we have is *Lactobacillus acidophilus*. If sufficient of this bacteria can be encouraged to re-establish residence in the bowel, it will push back the yeast, which may have crowded into the vacant space left when antibiotics destroyed acidophilus colonies. *Lactobacillus acidophilus* is obtainable in a number of forms. It comes in capsules, and also in its active state in some yogurt cultures. Cultured milk products containing acidophilus should therefore play a part in the anti-Candida programme. The taking of acidophilus is also an important element in this programme.

There are variations on the source and type of acidophilus which are worth mentioning. A recent development in the USA is the introduction of 'Megadophilus' (marketed in the UK as 'Superdophilus'). There are over 200 strains of *Lactobacillus acidophilus* and one in particular has been identified by a research authority in the field of cultured dairy produce, Natasha Trenev, as being infinitely more potent in its ability to destroy other bacteria, than others. This has been incorporated into 'Megadophilus', which contains at least one billion active organisms, per gram. This is over a hundred times more potent than comparable commercial acidophilus preparations, and, in some cases, many thousands of times more potent. This and another similar product, 'Vital Dophilus', should be the first choices in acidophilus supplementation. Dosage of Superdophilus or Vital Dophilus, if as dry powder or as a capsule, is 2g (or 1 teaspoonful) three times daily between meals. If available as a powder the acidophilus should be kept refrigerated, and never exposed to temperatures above 80°F/27°C. Dosages of up to 10g daily are in order (5 teaspoonsful of powder) with no toxic level known. When consumed as a powder, it should be stirred into non-chilled water, and drunk. This is best done well away from mealtimes. The acidophilus culture will become active in the small intestine, where it produces a number of nutritional compounds, including lactic acid, B-vitamins and enzymes, as well as natural antibiotic compounds.[13,14,15]

It may not be realized, but in the average bowel there exist colonies of micro-organisms which in total weight come to between 3 and 5 lb. These are not all helpful or friendly, and in order to repopulate the bowel with such helpful residents as acidophilus, large amounts are required. In re-establishing their territorial claim, the intruders such as Candida will be pushed back and often eliminated from the area.

Dr Khem Shahani, one of the world's leading researchers into probiotics (therapeutic use of friendly bacteria) and their medicinal properties, is quite clear on the usefulness of the *lactobacilli* against yeast infections. 'Continuing research has revealed that supplementing the diet with friendly bacteria, like acidophilus and other compatible organisms such as *Bifidobacteria bifidum* . . . should help in curing Candidiasis.'[42] This viewpoint is confirmed by Japanese research (in 1984) which examined the degree of overgrowth of Candida as ascertained by the levels found in the faeces of patients with leukaemia who were receiving drug therapy. The Candida counts were very high indeed, before treatment with bifidobacteria (this is another family of friendly bacteria which inhabits the large intestine unlike acidophilus which lives mainly in the small intestine). Bifidobacteria supplementation had the effect of reducing the levels of Candida in the faeces of some patients from a high of 10,000,000 per gram to a mere 10,000 per gram, after treatment. The effectiveness of bifidobacteria in achieving this was seen in all sixteen patients treated, whereas eleven 'control' patients not receiving bifidobacteria supplementation showed no change at all in their Candida levels.

Many researchers report that *Lactobacillus acidophilus* (and bifidobacteria) seems to actually manufacture substances which retard the growth of Candida, and this is borne out when *Lactobacillus acidophilus* is added to culture dishes in which Candida is growing, where an ability is seen to slow and even stop its growth.

An additional bonus is received when bifidobacteria are supplemented against Candida, as this has a uniquely powerful ability to enhance detoxification via the liver, as well as its extremely useful detoxifying role in the intestinal tract itself.

For these many reasons I can only echo the words of leading American nutrition expert, Dr Jeffrey Bland, when he states.

We have been very excited about an alternative therapy for the management of Candida infection, which avoids the use of anti-yeast medication (nystatin, etc). It is well recognized that a disturbed flora of the GI tract can establish a proper environment for yeast proliferation. By reinocculating the bowel with the proper symbiotic acid producing bacteria (*Lactobacillus acidophilus* and bifidobacteria) there is a reduction in the compatibility of the intestinal environment for the yeast proliferation. We have recently used an oral supplement of *Lactobacillus acidophilus* . . . this has been extremely successful in reducing *Candida albicans* in the intestinal tract. The *Lactobacillus acidophilus* is given as a dry culture.

This approach of using friendly bacteria to repopulate the digestive tract will be seen to play a major part in the strategy which I outline below. This is suitable for anyone with active Candida overgrowth.

These (*Lactobacillus acidophilus* and bifidobacteria) are therefore the first of the anti-Candida supplements you should introduce, together with acidophilus-cultured yogurt and/or sour milk with meals. A remarkable new milk derivative, a concentrate of whey, has been found to dramatically improve the way in which friendly bacteria recolonize their territories (and so drive out yeasts). This probiotic (enhancer of life) substance which was described in the *New England Journal of Medicine* (May 1988) is marketed in the UK as Ig-Plex and is known to contain massive amounts of active immunoglobulins (part of the immune system's defence capability) which help in both this task of repopulation by friendly bacteria, as well as in increasing local immunc activity in the intestine against hostile micro-organisms. The next major nutrient employed against Candida is the B-vitamin biotin. Research in Japan has indicated a fascinating way in which Candida can be deterred from altering from its relatively harmless yeast form, into its invasive and dangerously mycelial form.[17] This alteration of form is found to occur more rapidly in a medium in which there is a relative biotin deficiency. Biotin, which has also been called vitamin H, produces a number of skin conditions when known deficiency occurs in humans. These include a dermatitis which is characterized by a greyish, dry, flaky appearance. This is accompanied by a lack of appetite, nausea, lassitude and muscular pains. It is interesting that all of these symptoms are common when Candida is proliferating, and it is worth questioning whether the supposed symptoms of biotin deficiency are not at least in part the result of Candida activity brought about by that deficiency.

Egg-white contains a substance called avidin, which is capable of combining with biotin, thus neutralizing its usefulness in the body. For this reason raw egg should not be included in the anti-Candida diet (avidin is destroyed by cooking).

Biotin should be taken as a supplement, three times daily, in doses of between 350 and 500mcg in association with acidophilus (i.e. between meals).

Other Bacterial Aids

A number of other useful bacterial cultures are available which assist in controlling Candida. These include 'Vitalplex' and a new Scandinavian product 'Probion'. Much research indicates that by combining the cultures found in one, or both, of these, with acidophilus culture, a better degree of control is achieved, in a shorter space of time. (See caution pages 55-6.)

Aloe Vera Juice

The juice of the desert plant Aloe Vera is a powerful antifungal agent. Two or three spoonfuls of pure Aloe Vera juice taken twice daily in a tumbler of pure water is recommended. (See page 76 for local use against topical or vaginal Candida.)

Garlic as an Anti-Candida Agent

Garlic has been the subject of research worldwide. Russian scientists have proved the reality of its long-reputed antibacterial quality by the introduction of garlic extract into colonies of bacteria, which ceased to function within minutes. Fresh garlic juice was employed in these tests. Reports in Western medical and scientific journals confirm such claims,[18] in this case against *Salmonella typhimurium* and *Escherichia coli,* two extremely active micro-organisms. Garlic is also active against yeast and fungi. This was confirmed in recent reports showing it to be more active against human ringworm (a fungal infection) than currently used drugs.[19] *The Book of Garlic* quotes researchers as stating, 'garlic in the form of juice is a very potent anti-microbial agent, both to bacteria, and *Pathogenic yeasts*. We can thus suppose at least staphylococcal and fungal skin and alimentary tract disease can be effectively cured by the juice of garlic.[20]

Research at the University of Indiana suggests the value of garlic against fungal infections is very great. 'An aqueous extract of garlic bulbs inhibits growth of many aspects of zoopathogenic fungi', the first reported stated.[21] The second concluded, 'Allicin [the active sulphur-rich compound in garlic] may provide the model system for chemotherapy of *Candida albicans* infections.'[22]

The aesthetic aspect of garlic's employment is of course a factor to consider. Whilst there are many who can happily eat whole cloves of garlic, there are others who find the taste and odour unpleasant. The recent development of a completely odourless garlic (High Potency Garlic) is a boon to such as these.

Part of the anti-Candida campaign should include the daily intake of either fresh garlic or deodorized garlic in capsule form. The former is preferred; the latter is an acceptable compromise. Take 2-3 garlic capsules, morning and evening, after meals, or eat as much raw garlic as you can learn to enjoy. Slice it finely on cooked vegetables, or crush it on to salads, or simply eat it, clove by clove, with fish or poultry, as many Greeks do.

A further aid in the prevention of the transformation of Candida to its mycelial form is the use of olive oil.[16] This contains a substance called *oleic acid*, which also acts upon the yeast in a similar way to biotin. The recommended amount of olive oil is 6 teaspoonsful of olive oil daily, divided into three doses. This can be included in the meal or taken before or after, as desired.

Immune-System Enhancement by Supplementation

In order to strengthen the immune system it is suggested that a number of nutrients be included in the programme.

The primary nutrient in this regard is vitamin C. We have discussed this vitamin's importance in the economy of the body and its defensive T-cells. These contain a very high level of vitamin C. It has been noted that the lower the vitamin C content of these vital cells the less efficient is their performance in defending the body against intruding organisms or materials.[6,7] Any stress factor, pollutant or infection puts demands upon the vitamin C in the body. This is a water-soluble vitamin, and the body has no stores of it, so a constant supply is needed. Research has shown a fascinating adaptation which takes place when requirements increase because of such factors as those described above. Under normal conditions, if a person takes more vitamin C than they actually require, they are likely to develop a degree of diarrhoea. This is well known, and it is a way of assessing just how much vitamin C a person needs. If someone takes 5g daily, with no diarrhoea resulting, then they can be assumed to need that amount, at that time. If under normal conditions, however, someone develops diarrhoea after ingesting only 2g daily, it can be shown that should circumstances alter, and the need for vitamin C becomes apparent (owing to infection, stress, etc.) then that same person could increase vitamin C intake by many times the previous tolerance level, without any bowel symptoms at all. Dr Robert Cathcart has shown that if necessary the intake of vitamin C can be as high as 100g a day (never try this without supervision), with no bowel sensitivity apparent.[23] When the crisis passes, however, such doses would produce diarrhoea, as previously. Thus the body, in its wisdom, seems to be able to alter its function to meet particular requirements in this way. In order to assist a deficient immune system, such as might accompany a Candida spread, the recommended amount for this purpose (in the absence of any bowel reaction) is 1-3g daily, with food.

The effect of vitamin C on the T-cells depends of course on the T-cells being there to do their work. The thymus gland, which lies below the breastbone, can become relatively inactive, and one of the main nutrients which can enhance its production of T-cells, is the amino acid arginine.[24] A dose of 3g daily for a short period (say a month) will boost the thymus activity at the outset of the programme, when it is most needed. Note: If there is a history of herpes simplex infection, then do not take arginine supplementally, for it has also been found to enhance herpes activity (this is countered by another amino acid, lysine).[25]

Take the arginine before retiring, on an empty stomach, with water. A long-term use of arginine at these levels is not suggested, although there are no known side-effects in doses lower than 20g daily. Rough, thickened skin may develop on the elbows, for example, in doses of above 20g daily, though this will disappear when the supplementation is stopped. The reason for suggesting a time limit to the use of arginine is that the thymus may come to depend upon such nutritional supplementation, whereas it should be encouraged to return to normal activity by the total programme of Candida suppression. Therefore take the 3g daily for only the first month of this programme.

It is a further aid to the immune system to increase the intake of certain of the B-vitamins.[6] It is important to the programme that these are not derived from yeast sources.[29] All the B-vitamins are available in synthetic forms, and these rather than yeast-derived vitamins, are suggested in cases involving Candida. Between 20 and 50 mg of vitamin B6 (pyridoxine); between 20 and 50 mcg of vitamin B12, and the same quantity of folic acid, should be taken daily. An excellent non-yeast source B-complex capsule is available in the UK.

An additional B-vitamin (B5), should also be taken to assist in the enhancement of the B-lymphocytes, especially if there is any evidence of allergic reactions, or digestive involvement. This should be taken in the form of pantothenate, at a dose of 500mg daily.

The minerals zinc, selenium and magnesium are all also commonly implicated in deficient immune response conditions,[5,6,11] and should ideally be added to the programme. Just as in the selection of B-vitamins, it is important, in obtaining selenium, that a non-yeast source is found. This may prove difficult, but if sufficient demand is forthcoming then such problems will diminish and supply will become more plentiful. Doses required of these minerals are as follows: zinc (in the form of zinc-orotate), 50mg daily; selenium, 50mcg daily; and magnesium, 250-500mg daily. All should be taken with food.

Finally, a supply of some of the fat-soluble vitamins is called for in our effort to resuscitate the immune response. This calls for a moderate intake of vitamin E (make sure that you are buying natural vitamin E, which can be identified by the name *d*-alpha tocopherol, rather than *dl*-alpha tocopherol, which indicates a synthetic form), at a dose of around 200i.u. daily, vitamin A in the form of beta-carotene, in a dose of around 10,000i.u. daily, and finally the oil of Evening Primrose (vitamin F), in a 500mg capsule twice daily.

Supplement List

Anti-Candida:
Lactobacillus acidophilus, 2g one to three times daily, between meals (Superdophilus or Vital Dophilus for preference).

Bifidobacteria 1g three times daily ideally at a different time to acidophilus.

Biotin (vitamin H) 350-500mcg with acidophilus, three times daily.

Garlic capsules (if fresh garlic is not being eaten prolifically). Three capsules, twice daily (morning and evening), after meals.

Oleic acid (as virgin, first-pressing, olive oil), 2 teaspoonsful three times daily. Can be taken with meals or separately.

To Enhance Immune System:
Vitamin C, 1g three times daily with meals.

Arginine, 3g (with water), on an empty stomach, before retiring. Take for one month only.

Vitamin B6 (pyridoxine), 20-50mg daily ⎫ Or one vitamin B-
Vitamin B12, 20-50mcg daily.   ⎬ complex capsule
Folic acid, 20-50mcg daily.   ⎭ daily (yeast-free)

Calcium pantothenate (B5), 500mg daily (especially if allergy symptoms present).

Selenium, 50mcg daily.

Zinc, 50mg daily.

Magnesium, 250-500mg daily.

Vitamin E (d-alpha tocopherol), 200i.u. daily.

Vitamin A (as beta-carotene), 10,000i.u. daily.

Vitamin F (as oil of Evening Primrose), one to two 500mg capsules daily.

Note: Ensure vitamin C is 'with bioflavonoids'; ensure that B-vitamins and selenium are not from yeast source; ensure that zinc and magnesium are orotate form (or picolinate).

In order to obtain a suitable acidophilus supplement it should be one of guaranteed high potency. This should be a viable, active form (which would therefore require refrigeration at all times) and should be taken as part of a programme which also includes other lacto-bacillus such as a bifidobacteria (or *L. bulgaricus*) supplementation.

Dosage of acidophilus, for someone with Candida, is as outlined above. It should be taken in filtered or spring water, two or three times daily, *away from meal times*; bifidobacteria powder and a quarter to a half teaspoonful of *L.bulgaricus* should be taken together in water at a separate time from the acidophilus, two or three times daily.

Important Caution: A large number of 'copy-cat' products, often called 'something'-dophilus or containing multiple mixtures of bacteria are being marketed for treatment of Candida and other forms of bowel dysbiosis. Many respected researchers feel that such 'cocktails' (more than one friendly bacteria together in any container) may not be as potent as claimed due to interaction between organisms, and may in some instances have the potential for actually being harmful. This is most likely with some strains (such as *S. faecium* or *E. Coli*) should they alter genetically, a not unknown phenomenon. *For these reasons I urge that only pure, single strain, friendly bacteria, of known safe strain, and of guaranteed potency, with an expiry date clearly shown on the label, be taken. Ideally such products should be contained in dark glass, not plastic; should state that they were not centrifuged in their production, and should require refrigeration to maintain the organisms in a quiescent state until they are taken. The products recommended in this book fulfil all these requirements.* (For further reading on probiotics see Recommended Reading).

It will be clear from the above that we are using the supplements in two directions at the same time.

Firstly we are using acidophilus and biotin (as well as oleic acid) as substances which directly inhibit the alteration of Candida to its dangerous fungal form, or which resist its spread. The other nutrients are employed to build up the immune function (B- and T-cells) so that the body can better cope with the invading micro-organism. This two-pronged attack requires that you take this large number of supplements at the same time. This is both moderately expensive, and off-putting. Let it be clear, however, that what is at stake is your health. For this reason there should be no hesitation in grasping this opportunity to fight off the cause of your ill health by whatever safe methods are at hand. The methods that are being advocated are safe. They are also effective in most cases. It can take time to control Candida once it is rampant, and six months should be seen as the minimum length of time to maintain this programme.

Important Note: During periods of rapid yeast destruction, as the supplementation and dietary programme get underway, the body's organs of elimination, such as the liver, will be called on to detoxify the breakdown products of this process, and this can lead to your feeling particularly seedy, nauseated and off-colour. The reaction is known as yeast 'die-off' or 'burn-off' and can last for some days, or even weeks. The use of proven strains of high potency bifidobacteria, together with the general dietary strategies discussed above, should minimize this. In any case don't be tempted to stop the anti-Candida programme if this process becomes evident as this does not indicate that 'it is not working', quite the contrary.

This is a critical stage of the treatment which, if stopped suddenly, can lead to a rebound of the Candida activity and even greater feelings of ill-health. 'Burn-off' should not last for more than a week or ten days, by which time, if you stick to the guidelines given, gradual improvement should be noticed. A total control of the fungus, and therefore an eradication of symptoms, can however take many months.

Our next consideration is the importance of combining the supplemental attack on Candida, and the enhancement of the immune system, with a dietary programme which deprives the yeast of its main sources of food.

Anti-Candida Diet

There are two major areas of consideration in the dietary pattern necessary to reduce the spread and activity of Candida. These are the elimination of all foods derived from, or containing, yeasts or fungi; the second is the reduction, as far as possible, of all carbohydrate-rich foods, in order to deprive Candida of its favourite nourishment, which as anyone who has made beer or wine will testify, is sugar.

Foods Derived from or Containing Fungi and Yeast

The following list of foods and substances contain yeast or yeast-like substances, and so should be avoided as much as possible during the initial stages of dealing with Candida infection. It is probably wise to maintain vigilance for these foods for at least three months, after which time a degree of relaxation can be exercised, with the proviso that if such foods are reintroduced, and symptoms which had become quiescent begin to become active again, a return to a stricter mode of eating for a time is called for. The rationale behind such avoidance is that in practice these foods seem to aggravate a Candida-induced condition, especially if allergic symptoms are part of the picture, as well as if there are symptoms such as bloating and intestinal gas.[2,9] In a letter Dr Truss states:

> If someone has no symptoms, I see no reason to have him avoid these yeast promoting foods, although I will say that in excess, and combined with a high-carbohydrate intake [sugars, etc.], these may actually induce this condition [Candida infection] even without the stimulatory effects of antibiotics, birth control pills, cortisone, etc.

Yeast-Promoting Foods and Substances

The following foods contain yeast as an added ingredient in their preparations,[26] and are therefore undesirable, especially in the early stages of an anti-Candida programme.

Breads (non-yeasted whole wheat or corn bread is acceptable).
Cakes and cake mixes.
Biscuits and crackers.
Enriched flour.
Buns, rolls and pastries.
Anything fried in breadcrumbs (fish fingers, etc.)

The following contain yeast, or yeast-like substances, because of the nature of their manufacture, or of their own nature.

Mushrooms.
Truffles.
Soya sauce.
Buttermilk and sour cream.
Black tea.
All cheeses, including cottage cheese.
Citric acid (almost always a yeast derivative).
Citrus drinks if canned or frozen.
All dried fruits.
All fermented beverages, such as beer, spirits, wine, cider, ginger ale.

All malted products (cereals, sweets or dairy products which have
  been malted).
All foods containing monosodium glutamate (which is often a yeast
  derivative).
All vinegars, whether grape, malt, cider or anything else. These are
  frequently used in sauces and relishes, as well as salad dressings,
  sauerkraut, olives and pickled foods.

The following are either derived from yeast, or contain elements that
are.

Antibiotics.
Multivitamin tablets (unless specifically stating that they are from a
  non-yeast source).
B-complex vitamins (unless specifically stating that they are from a
  non-yeast source).
Selenium (as above).
Individual B-vitamins (as above).

Dr Truss singles out some foods from this long list as the main
culprits in his eyes. He states: 'It is my belief that there are several
foods that are primarily to be avoided. These include all fermented
drinks, as well as vinegar, mushrooms, and mouldy cheeses. I allow
my patients to have cottage cheese, as well as yogurt.' He goes on
further to say, 'It is rational to remove all of these foods from the diet,
only if there is an indication that patients are having trouble with
yeast [Candida]'.[27]
    In this light it should be clear that the elimination of all alcoholic
beverages and vinegar (and its by-products, as listed) as well as the
foregoing of the joys of blue cheeses, and the eating of mushrooms,
are the major areas of alteration for some months to come, apart, that
is, from the reduction in refined carbohydrates and foods rich in
sugar, which we will now consider.

Sugar-Rich Foods

Sugar (sucrose) itself, in whatever guise, is to be strictly avoided
during the battle to control Candida. This means white sugar, brown
sugar, black sugar, and any shades in between. There is no such thing

as a healthy sugar. We do not need sugar, as such, for health, and its sole claim for our attention is its taste, which it is quite easy to do without. All sugar will aid the growth and proliferation of yeast. This includes syrups, honey (yes, I'm afraid so) and other forms of sugar, such as fructose, maltose, glucose, sorbitol, etc. It includes molasses, date sugar, maple sugar and in fact all of that range of non-foods with which our real foods and beverages have been sweetened. Sweets, chocolates and all soft drinks should also be totally avoided. Honey may come as a surprise to you in this context. I myself had assumed that honey was relatively safe, in that it did not seem, to my knowledge, to become mouldy. I was corrected by Dr Truss who communicated the fact that honey does indeed contain yeast spores. He pointed out, 'Species of Zygosaccharomyces [a yeast] have been found particularly active in causing yeast spoilage of honey.' It is known that honey is indeed hygroscopic (it absorbs water) and that at a certain degree of moisture content there will be sufficient water at the surface to lower the concentration of sugars to a point that the yeasts and bacteria which might be present, can grow. Thus yeasts and other micro-organisms capable of surviving in concentrated sugar solutions (in which no yeast will grow) at a certain point in the dilution of that medium, become able to thrive. In order to prevent this from happening, honey is heated, and often has additives mixed with it, such as sodium benzoate, which inhibit the growth of fermenting yeasts. Truss and Crook both insist that honey be added to the list of banned foods during the anti-Candida campaign, and this is also my view. The length of time that this will be necessary will depend upon the speed of recovery. It should not be anticipated to be less than three months, and is more likely to be six.

The most important single dietary alteration that the Candida sufferer can make is the removal from the diet of sugar-rich foods.

As has already been discussed, the undesirability of eating yeast-containing foods at this time removes from the scene bread, pastry, biscuits and cakes, etc. This is doubly necessary, since these are in the main undesirable because of their high carbohydrate content (unless totally wholegrain).

Any carbohydrate which has been refined beyond the simple grinding stage is undesirable. Whole wheat, or oats as employed in making porridge, or millet, or brown rice, are all highly desirable foods, rich in what are known as complex carbohydrates. These can, and indeed should (especially oats) be a part of the diet. Once these are broken down into fine flours, and are refined further, they become less desirable, and actually become food for the yeast, rather than for you.

So even in the middle stages of the programme when, hopefully, symptoms are on the wane, and you might justifiably feel that a little relaxation of the stricter aspects of the diet are allowable, please remember that refined carbohydrates are the natural food of yeast, and Candida will thank you for the delivery of such foods by a rapid expansion of its activity. As Truss puts it, 'Decreased availability of carbohydrates slows the rate of multiplication of yeast cells, and thus should reduce the amount of yeast products entering the bloodstream.' The converse is true as well: the more of these foods there are in the diet, the greater will the chances be of further spread of Candida. So out of the diet goes pasta, pastry, flour products of all sorts, biscuits, cakes, buns, rolls, bread (unless any of these are made with whole grains, and without yeast or sugar).

Many foods have 'hidden sugar', in that there is sugar added in the processing or preparation. These are often foods with which sugar is not usually associated. Frozen peas, most canned foods, and many packaged and processed foods, all contain either refined flour products, or sugar, or both. For this reason, as well as for the general undesirability of many such foods from a nutritional viewpoint, these should be avoided. Not only are you actually providing the favourite foods of the yeasts within your body when you eat sugar, you are also causing a degree of metabolic and physiological mayhem.

It should be recalled that until about 100 years ago, the average annual intake of sugar in Western countries was in the region of 20lb per head. Even this was a part of the dietary pattern which included far more 'natural' vitamin- and mineral-rich foods than is currently the case. The present annual intake of sugar in the UK and USA is over 100lb per head of the population. The human body is most adaptable, but it takes more than a century to get used to such a change in nutritional intake.

Organs such as the pancreas (the source of insulin and essential protein digesting enzymes) are grossly overworked when sugar plays a large part in the diet. The pancreas, when faced with sugar, pumps out insulin. This has the job of maintaining the proper level of sugar in the bloodstream. Insulin is also released in response to stimulant drinks, such as coffee and tea, which initially cause a release by the liver of stored sugar (as does stress). Thus a diet rich in sugar, and which contains the usual pattern of tea, coffee and alcohol (as well as cola drinks and chocolates, which also contain caffeine to stimulate this cycle) will produce a situation in which a major organ is grossly overworked. In this sort of pattern, the fluctuations in blood-sugar levels, boosted by dietary and liver-stored sugar, and then depressed and controlled by the pancreatic insulin, have a profound effect upon health and personality of the individual. At the same time it is noted that because of the sugar-rich diet, it is less likely that the individual will eat enough foods containing vitamins and minerals to allow him to meet the minimum standards of nutrition. Thus other systems in the body become deficient, including the immune system. This whole process may of course take years, all the while accompanied by declining well-being and an unseen rise in Candida activity. Sugar has been well described as pure, white and deadly.

It is suggested that in the first few weeks of the programme (say three weeks for safety) even fresh fruit should be avoided, because of its high content of natural fruit sugars. Even when fruit is resumed after the three-week break, it should not include the very sweet melons, which are too high in sugar for the Candida sufferer (and often contain mould).

Milk contains its own form of sugar, and this too is thought to be undesirable throughout the programme. Pasteurized milk encourages Candida.[9] The exception to this is yogurt — if it is natural and 'live', which will be clearly stated on its container. There are many 'dead' yogurts about, and a good many that have sugar added. These are quite unsuitable to the programme. Yogurt itself is helpful since it contains (when 'live') bacteria which inhibit Candida, and which assist in the repopulation of the bowel (along with acidophilus, which is often used in yogurt culture).

Other Foods to Avoid

It is best to avoid smoked meats and fish, sausages, corned beef, hot dogs and hamburgers because of the substances added to them, some of which derive from yeasts. Nuts, other than freshly cracked ones, should also be avoided, because of the degree of mould that these attract as they become rancid. Any foods which have been kept for a while, other than in a frozen state, are liable to be slightly mouldy, and these should be avoided too.

You now have a picture of the type of foods not to eat: mainly the yeast- and fungus-related foods, as well as the refined carbohydrates, and anything containing them.

The degree of adherence to such a programme that is possible, depends upon many factors, but none less than motivation. Just how much do you want to get better, and just how much effort are you prepared to make in that quest? It is really not up to anyone but you. Certainly the taking of the supplements, as described, will go a long way towards that end. So will avoidance of yeasts and foods derived from them. But by putting the whole programme together, including the sugar-free aspect of the diet, you really give the whole system a chance to work quickly, and work well.

What you can still eat is varied and exciting. Below I have outlined a pattern of eating which is nutritious, tasty and above all 'anti-Candida' in its format.

Once you have tried to follow this type of pattern for a while, it is unlikely that you will ever want to reintroduce most of the 'undesirables', even when Candida is back under control.

Dietary Pattern

Breakfast: It has been found that a high-fibre diet is the best suited to the resolution of the Candida problem. In Professor Jeffrey Bland's words, 'The diet should be higher than normal in fibre, using oat bran fibre to increase the absorptive surface of the faecal material and also hasten the elimination of metabolic by-products.'[16] Choose therefore from the following, for a wholesome and non-Candida-supporting breakfast. In passing, it is suggested that three meals are eaten daily, and that meals are not skipped unless you are off-colour and really have no appetite.

Choose one or more of the following for breakfast:

1. Oatmeal porridge. Add a little cinnamon and some ground cashew nuts for additional flavour. Use no sugar or honey. Make with water, not milk.

2. Mixed seed and nut breakfast (combine sunflower, pumpkin, sesame and linseed together, with oatmeal or flaked millet). These can be eaten as they are, or soaked overnight in a little water to make a softer texture, or moistened with natural live yogurt. Add wheatgerm and freshly milled nuts if desired.

3. Alternate days: two eggs, any style except raw.

4. Bread or toast (made without yeast or sugar) and butter.

5. Brown rice kedgeree (rice and fish).

6. Wholewheat or rice and oat pancakes (no sweetening).

7. Natural live yogurt (add wheatgerm if desired).

8. After the first three weeks or so of the programme, fresh fruit can be added to the menu; for example, item 1 or 2 could be complemented by sliced banana or grated apple, or item 7 could have fresh fruit added, or fruit could be eaten as a major part of the meal, with a handful of nuts (fresh), and/or seeds (sunflower, pumpkin, etc.) Continue to avoid fruit juices however.

9. Fish (not smoked) or meat (not cured or salted).

10. Wholewheat, or whole rice, flakes and yogurt (ensure no sugar in cereals). The use of muesli-type breakfast mixtures is in order if they are homemade. If shop-bought they will contain dried fruit and nuts of almost certain rancidity, and frequently sugar or honey as well. By the simple mixing of oat flakes, or millet flakes, with fresh nuts or seeds, as mentioned in item 2 above, it is possible to have a high-fibre, nutritious and tasty meal.

If items 1 or 2 are eaten, then a high fibre content will be ensured, and these are suggested as the most desirable. If any of the other choices are eaten, then add a heaped teaspoonful of linseed and bran (50:50), mixed together, to the meal or swallow at the end of the meal with a little water.

Remember to chew all food, especially carbohydrates, thoroughly. There is no way in which half-chewed carbohydrates can be digested, since the enzymes present in saliva are essential to the breakdown of these foods. For this reason it is undesirable to drink with meals, as the liquid is frequently used as a moistening agent to facilitate swallowing, which reduces efficient chewing as a result. A high-fibre meal is ideal for the provision of the type of food needed for the anti-Candida programme. It also ensures a steady release of natural sugars into the bloodstream, rather than the rapid rise produced by most refined sugar-rich foods. This helps to keep blood-sugar levels even, and avoids ups and downs in available energy (and mood) which can be a major cause of the craving for a quick 'sugar fix'.

Drinks at breakfast time should consist of either green tea, china tea, herb tea (such as Rooibos or camomile), all unsweetened, or a mineral water, such as Perrier — not fruit juices, however, unless diluted 50:50 with water.

Main Meals

There should be no great problem in eating quite splendid food, during the strict avoidance period of the dietary programme. One area of contention exists in the choice of animal proteins. It is important to realize that most commercial meat and poultry now contains residues of antibiotics and hormonal substances, which are fed to the animals in the process of rearing them for market. This means that regular eating of beef, pork or chicken, unless it is from a source known to avoid such methods, is a potential danger to the success of the whole programme (and a health hazard at all times). Indeed it is not improbable that this very factor is a major, if as yet unrecognized, element in the whole Candida scenario. Whilst the use of antibiotics and steroids in medication can be relatively easily remembered and identified in the medical history, it is impossible to know just how much of these same substances are entering people on a daily basis through their food.

For this reason it is suggested that efforts be made to track down non-steroid-fed meat and poultry, in which antibiotics have not been employed. In major cities this is probably possible. Such shops as 'Wholefood' in Paddington Street, London, will guarantee such supplies. In California there is a chain of supermarkets ('Mrs Gooch's Ranch Markets') which provide a complete range of meats and poultry, guaranteed free of all contamination. Lamb and mutton is less likely to be affected by this sort of additive, as is rabbit and any other game meat, or poultry. Fish is safe, apart from other sources of pollution, which do not concern Candida directly. For the duration of the diet, therefore, it is suggested that unless the source of meat or poultry can be certainly identified as free of hormones or antibiotics, meat should be limited to game, rabbit (unless 'farmed'), mutton or lamb. Fish of course can be eaten regularly as well.

Ideally, in order to maintain the high-fibre type of meal that is so desirable when Candida is active, the two main meals of the day should include as wide a variety of fresh vegetables as is possible. These should be eaten both raw and cooked, and an excellent pattern to adopt is as follows. One of the main meals (say lunch) each day, is a source of protein such as fish, poultry, lamb, egg or fresh nuts, together with as large a mixed salad as imagination can conjure and appetite can cope with. The other main meal should also contain protein, in addition to cooked vegetables. The source of protein at each meal does not of course have to be based on animals. The combining of a cereal and a pulse (say brown rice and lentils, or millet and chick-peas) at the same meal, ensures that adequate protein is available to the body.

What is essential is that adequate protein be eaten daily, whether from a 'safe' animal source, or from the judicious mixing of complementary vegetable proteins. What is adequate for one person is not necessarily so for another. For example, people of oriental origin require, for good health, less protein than people of northern European stock. The difference lies in the efficiency with which the orientals digest and absorb what they do eat in the protein line. Thus 50g a day of first-class protein is adequate for an oriental, and 75g (or more depending upon activity, etc.) may be required by a European.[5]

Since natural live yogurt (a source of protein) is going to play a part in the diet, it is unlikely that the eating of protein at both of the main meals, in addition to this, is necessary. It should be possible to have, for example, a mixed salad, together with a jacket potato or savoury rice dish, and additional nuts and seeds, for one meal, whilst having a 'safe' animal protein and a variety of cooked vegetables at the other. In any case the tastes and preferences of individuals will differ markedly, and the variations that are available as to what to eat are so great that no more than broad guidelines can be given.

The essentials are to ensure the following:

● Avoid all yeast-based, or yeast-containing foods.

- Avoid all sugar and refined cereal products, and foods containing them.
- Avoid all foods and drinks based upon fermentation.
- Avoid meats containing residues of antibiotics and steroids.
- Do eat three meals daily.
- Do ensure adequate protein intake.
- Do ensure that a high dietary fibre content is maintained.
- Avoid fruit for the first three or four weeks of the programme.

Once symptoms begin to abate, and you find that you would like to increase the range of foods slightly, it is of course permissible to experiment a bit. This should not be before the end of the second month on the programme, and then only if there has been a marked improvement. If you then introduce one food which has been on the 'no-go' list, observe the consequences carefully. If these are non-existent, you might extend your experiment to another food after a week or so. If symptoms return, go back to basic avoidance, as specified above, until they calm down again. I am not saying that you *must* experiment in this way, only that if you must, or if you feel constrained by the limitation imposed by the programme, then at least do it carefully, with the knowledge that it might (only might) upset things. If it does, it just means being patient for a little longer. There are many excellent books available which explain the principles of rotation diets which can help in formulating a strategy for eating certain foods only periodically in a systematic way.[28] It is not suggested that the reintroduction of sugar-containing foods be started at this stage, other than in the very minimal sense or perhaps introducing something such as pasta or honey.

Other Essential Information Regarding Food

Moulds are present on most fruits and vegetables, and these should be kept well washed and eaten fresh, for obviously the longer they are kept, the more the mould development will be encouraged.

Yeasts also grow on grains of all sorts, and the fresher these are the better. A good many people with Candida problems are allergic to grains. This allergy may well diminish during the programme of Candida control, and a little experimentation is in order after two or three months if symptoms generally have declined. A reminder is called for regarding nuts. Peanuts and pistachios, in particular, are subject to mould development (in the case of peanuts this is a highly toxic, potentially cancer-causing agent). All nuts, unless freshly opened by you, will contain some degree of mould, and certainly a degree of rancidity of the natural oils. Eat current season nuts, freshly opened by yourself, or else avoid them.

Apart from a little butter, and natural live yogurt, it is suggested that all milk products be avoided (Dr Truss does allow cottage cheese).

If you are forced to eat at a restaurant, or if friends invite you for a meal, then make sure that you stick to basics. Avoid sauces and gravy; avoid desserts; avoid stuffing, or any obvious undesirables, such as mushrooms. A meat, poultry or fish dish, with salad or vegetables, is the safest bet, and stick to water instead of wine.

What about sugar substitutes for those who cannot keep away from sweet things? These are open to question, as far as long-term safety is concerned, but in small amounts, for the duration of the programme (at least six months) they at least do not encourage Candida. Aspartame and saccharin fall into this category, but not fructose, corn syrup or any other sugar-rich substitute for the real thing.

Remember that all commercial breakfast foods, such as cornflakes, are undesirable. They are processed, and most contain yeast and/or sugar products.

Water from the tap should be filtered before drinking if possible. There are many inexpensive water filters available, and this will remove a variety of organic substances which otherwise find their way into food, or directly into you. Most bottled water is acceptable, but ensure this is not carbonated if you have problems with bloating and gas. As for coffee and tea, this is a sticking point for many. They are undesirable, not only as sources of mould, but because they stimulate sugar release from the liver, and consequently (a) pancreatic activity, which exhausts this vital organ further, and (b) the feeding of Candida by this sugar. There are other good reasons for not using tea, as it reduces the efficiency of both protein and iron absorption by the body; and coffee is suspected of involvement in certain forms of cancer. Herb teas are often better, and some have been found to help in the control of Candida, and related problems (Rooibos, a South African tea, used as a tea substitute, and by allergic subjects) and taheebo (helpful in catarrhal problems caused by Candida), etc., are worth trying, if you can find them (try a health food store).

The steaming of vegetables is the best way to help to retain the vital minerals so often destroyed and lost in boiling. Dressing a salad with lemon juice, olive oil and a little natural yogurt can replace the vinegar or other dressings not compatible with the programme. As the programme produces its results, and symptoms become tolerable, or disappear, so can a limited quantity of foods based on or containing mould or yeast be reintroduced. Wine, or real ale, in limited amounts, or tea, etc., may be taken occasionally. However, the need for vigilance must continue, because it is not the aim of the programme to remove Candida from the scene altogether, nor would this be possible. Even if the problem is attacked vigorously, with the use of antifungal drugs as well as the programme outlined above, the yeast will remain in the body.

The long-term answer, after initially controlling the yeast by these means, is to maintain a high level of immune function, by respect for what the diet should contain, in terms of nutrient value, as well as avoidance in the main of those factors which you now know can reduce its optimum ability to defend you. This does not mean that the programme is a life-sentence. It is hoped that after a while you will come to regard sweet tastes as unpleasant, and no longer crave, or even enjoy sweet foods. It is also to be hoped that your new sense of well-being will help to motivate you towards following the pattern of eating suggested more or less permanently, because you will actually enjoy it, as well as because it is good for you.

Other Factors

It is important not only to avoid foods and beverages containing fungal or yeast substances, but also to avoid inhaling these organisms or their spores. This is the reason for keeping well away from damp, dank places and for dealing with the presence of any mould and wet or dry rot that might be present in your environment. If there is any danger of damp in rooms, cupboards, cellars or lofts, do something positive about dealing with this, or, if absolutely necessary, move to a new, dry place of residence. *Your home might be making you ill.*

This advice is especially applicable to anyone who notices a worsening of symptoms in weather that is damp or muggy, or who is obviously affected by contact with mouldy or dank environments.

The availability to you of full-spectrum light is another important element which can improve immune and general function.[29] It is known that the eyes contain photo-receptors which carry impulses directly to the pituitary gland, which lies in the head. This is the 'master' gland of the body and is vital for normal health and function. If light is denied the eyes (not artificial light, but the full spectrum from the sun) then demonstrable imbalances occur in the hormonal system as a direct result. Behavioural and physical symptoms can occur in consequence. The immune system is affected, and this is the reason for our interest. The advice to all who wear glasses, or who spend most of their days indoors behind glass, is that they should get outside for at least half an hour a day, with nothing between natural light and their eyes. If going out is not possible, then spend the time by an open window, without glasses or contact lenses. In a polluted city the light getting through is distorted to a degree, and so more exposure is required. This does not mean looking at the sun, even on an overcast day; just being outdoors is enough if the eyes are not shielded.

There are now available full-spectrum fluorescent lighting units and it has been found that health and productivity improve dramatically when such lighting is introduced into the workplace. As one of the additional supports for the immune system, the implementation of access to unpolluted, unfiltered, pure light is a positive step.

The immune system also benefits from adequate exercise. This means trying to apply the ideals set out in Dr Kenneth Cooper's book *Aerobics*.[30] At least every other day there should be a form of physical exercise sufficient to stimulate the circulation and respiration. A brisk walk of one or two miles is the safest and easiest form of exercise that can produce such results. The book mentioned should be read, and its graded advice followed. Its beauty lies in the way in which it is made applicable to anyone, at any stage of fitness, or otherwise, so that the reader can gradually lift himself to his own level of optimum fitness in slow stages.

The avoidance of stress and anxiety is a fundamental need, as is the requirement we all have for what has been called TLC (tender loving care). These ingredients for a healthy life have been well described in many popular and readily available books. The requirement of the immune system for such inputs should encourage the study of relaxation and meditation and general stress-reducing methods. I have outlined a programme of stress-reduction in my book on the subject,[31] and this should be helpful in both assessing and dealing with those stress factors which affect life. In considering the overall importance of the immune system, it is worth commenting upon an area of medical research which tends to be ignored, because of its unpopular message. There is abundant proof that women who are promiscuous, or who have relations with a large number of men, are more prone to cancer of the womb than those who have relations with only one or a few partners.[5] Early sexual experience is also shown to predispose the individual towards diseases which should be prevented by an intact immune system.

AIDS is more common among homosexuals who have multiple partners, rather than those who have steady relationships with a single partner. It would seem therefore that what is happening is that in close physical contact of a sexual nature there is a role for the immune system. It is assumed that if this is called upon to cope with antigens from a wide variety of different sources (remember that sperm is a foreign protein to the body) then it could well be a factor in depleting the immune response of an individual (along with a great number of other factors).

This viewpoint has been expressed in numerous medical journals since the AIDS epidemic began.[32] It points to a necessary return to relative fidelity, in sexual terms, as being desirable for anyone who wishes to maintain an intact immune system. This does not mean that celibacy is called for, but that frequent changes in sexual partners are to be avoided. This is desirable both in heterosexual and homosexual relationships, at the very least during the carrying out of the programme against Candida.

Aloe Vera Juice and Candida

The amazing healing qualities of the desert plant, Aloe vera, have been known since Phoenecian times. In recent years attention has been drawn to its usefulness in a range of digestive conditions.

Professor Jeffrey Bland has demonstrated that the activity of the fresh juice, on Candida, can be very useful to sufferers. He writes (*Jnl. of Alternative Medicine,* June 1985): 'In a study of ten subjects, six had markedly altered stool cultures in microbiological assays. Four of these had indications of yeast overgrowth in their stools, before taking Aloe vera, and had reduction in yeast abundance after Aloe vera supplementation. Aloe vera has an antifungal action as well as improving overall bowel flora condition and improving the local acidity balance.' As Bland says, 'It promotes a favourable balance of gastro-intestinal symbolic bacteria.'

It has a similar effect on bacterial and fungal infection on the skin, and can be applied to such conditions locally.

One or two teaspoonful of Aloe vera juice in water, should be taken twice daily, by anyone with Candida problems. (*Note*: Once opened, Aloe vera juice bottles should be kept refrigerated. The optimum shelf-life thereafter is about one month.)

We will briefly consider other methods by which some practitioners attempt to control Candida.

Note: It should be clear from the earlier discussions that there should be no intake of antibiotics, steroids or the contraceptive pill during the course of the anti-Candida programme unless absolutely vital.

6

Additional Methods of Candida Control

Nystatin

The treatment of fungal infection, such as Candida, by drug methods, involves the use of antifungal antibiotics, such as nystatin. This is active against a wide range of yeasts, and yeast-like fungi, including Candida. This drug comes in a variety of forms: as a liquid, for use in the mouth; as tablets, for use in treating Candida in the intestinal tract; as suppositories, for use in the vagina; and as creams, ointments and powders, for the treatment of surface areas, nails, etc.

Nystatin is lethal to yeast cells on contact. Getting them into contact is not always easy, especially if the area involved is deep in the bowel. The nystatin, passing through, will kill surface yeasts, but any that are embedded deeper into the wall of the intestine will remain untouched. There is poor absorption of nystatin, so little reaches the bloodstream.

There is general consensus that nystatin is well tolerated, and causes few side-effects.[2,9] The major reason for not opting for its use is that it deals only with the short-term situation. If a condition such as Candida has become so widespread as to cause a problem, then it is vital that the immune system and bowel flora which should be controlling the situation are revitalized. Reliance on nystatin will leave the immune system in the same state, except that there will, over a period, be fewer yeast by-products entering the bloodstream to challenge the immune system. This, it is thought (Truss, Crook, etc.), allows the immune system to revive gradually. There is certainly no objection to nystatin being employed if the condition is severe enough to warrant it, but this should only be done in combination with the sort of programme outlined in the previous chapters. Otherwise there will be but short-term gains and the condition will recur. It is important to realize that nystatin is itself derived from a mould source and can cause allergic symptoms in sensitive individuals. Some patients become dependent on nystatin and find difficulty in being weaned from it.

The dosage of nystatin is usually around 2 million units daily (4 tablets of half a million units each), but double this dosage is relatively safe. Side-effects are limited to nausea, vomiting and diarrhoea, which occur only with very high doses (over 4 million units daily).

The above information should not be taken as an explicit recommendation for the use of nystatin. The major recommendations given in this book regarding the control of Candida by natural rather than drug methods are effective in the majority of cases. Taking nystatin does not necessarily shorten the process of control, and indeed may result in the individual relying on the drug and thus allowing the supporting anti-Candida programme to lapse.

By relying on the dietary and supplementation programme it is not only possible to control Candida, but to improve general well-being dramatically. This is something no drug can achieve, however few side-effects it produces.

Anti-Candida Herbal Products

Plant extracts other than Aloe Vera (page 71) have been found to be useful against Candida, including:

Tea Tree Oil (*Maleluca Alternofolia*): An extract of this Australian plant has powerful antifungal properties. Douching daily with a 1 per cent solution in water (or once weekly soaking a tampon which is then inserted vaginally for no more than 24 hours) can be very useful for vaginitis or cervicitis. This approach is useful whether the cause is Candida or trichomoniasis.

Chamomile (*Matricaria Chamomilla*): Contains antifungal substances in its oily extracts. Used as a tea or topical application it has soothing qualities (as has taheebo (Pau D'Arco) (see page 69), which is derived from the South American plant *Tabebuia Avellanedae* which has strong anti-Candida (and anti-tumour) effects).

The most powerful anti-Candida herbs contain berberine, such as *Berberis vulgaris* (barberry), *Hydrastis canadensis* (goldenseal) and *Berberis aquifolium* (Oregon grape). Berberine's action against Candida prevents overgrowth after antibiotic use, where it also helps repopulation with friendly bacteria. Berberine is an anti-diarrhoea agent when chronic bowel infection is involved and also has immune system enhancing capabilities as it destroys bacteria, yeasts, viruses and cancer cells . . . quite a catalogue of benefits.

Dosage suggestions: 1 to 2 grams of dried bark or root of *Berberis vulgaris* or *Hydrastis canadensis* (powdered or as a tea) three times daily, or 1 to 1½ teaspoons (4 to 6ml) of tincture of either of these plants (diluted 1:5), three times daily, or a quarter to half a teaspoon of fluid extract of either of these plants, three times daily.

A new development has been the use of extracts of citrus (usually grapefruit) seeds as a safe, natural, anti-Candida and antiparasitic agent.

Caprystatin

The antifungal activity of certain fatty acids has been demonstrated by investigators such as Neuhauser[40] who has shown dilute (0.01) caprylic acid (coconut extract) to destroy Candida effectively. He has successfully treated patients with severe intestinal Candida by using caprylic acid in a form which allows a timed release as it passes through the bowel. If not in such a form the caprylic acid is ineffective, being absorbed in the upper intestinal region. Caprylic acid mimics the fatty acids produced by normal bowel flora, which are a major factor in the body's control over Candida. Caprylic acid is now widely available.

This fungus killer is recommended in preference to the commonly employed antifungal medical drug nystatin, because the latter is itself yeast based and research at the Washington University School of Medicine shows that ultimately, after a period of treatment, when nystatin is stopped, it often results in even more colonies of yeast developing than were present before its use. Caprylic acid has no such rebound effect when its use ceases, after Candida is controlled (we never actually get rid of the yeast remember, but only try to get it back under control).

Local Vaginal Treatment

Three approaches are suggested for soothing inflamed vaginal tissues during anti-candida treatment.

1. Using a special soft-tipped disposable applicator insert a solution of high potency acidophilus culture. This can be mixed with pure water or even, more usefully, mixed with a little dilute aloe vera juice.
2. Aloe vera juice alone, diluted (two teaspoonsful to half a pint of water) can be used as a douche to relieve itching and burning.
3. A cream derived from mountain ash berries (*Sorbus aucuparia*) has been shown to have powerful antifungal and soothing effects when applied locally into or onto the vagina (marketed in the UK as Cervagyn). The active constituent, potassium sorbate, is a common food preservative (antifungal agent) but in much higher concentrations prevents yeast proliferation by interfering with its ability to feed off carbohydrates (sugars). In studies of 37 women with Vulvo-vaginitis, using potassium sorbate in a 1 per cent strength, there were only 11 recurrences of Candidiasis over a three month period. When a 3 per cent solution was used there were no recurrences at all out of 32 women after 6 months.

There was also rapid symptomatic relief where yeast was the sole infecting agent. Where other micro-organisms were involved other methods were also needed. Results were uniformly better when the diets of the women involved were low in sugar of all sorts.

Colonics and Enemas

Colonic irrigation involves the administration of water into the bowel, sometimes combined with other substances, in order to clear debris from the region and to influence its health. Useful in this respect are garlic extract, oxygen and acidophilus (or as Crook suggests, nystatin). By making repeated applications of water, coupled with one of these additives, there is every chance of greatly influencing the condition of the bowel. Enemas are less effective, since they penetrate only a short distance, unlike the colonic which can pass water the length of the large bowel. The technique requires expert skills, and its use in Candida problems would require additional knowledge. In principle, however, such treatment is recommended, at least in the early stages of the programme. There is no reason why acidophilus should not itself be administered in this way rather than orally alone, to assist in the repopulation of the bowel and control of Candida.

Desensitization

Carefully controlled doses of Candida extract may be injected into the individual in the hope that this will produce a response on the part of the immune system. Antibodies thus produced by white blood cells are useful in assisting the defence against antigens entering the system because of the yeast. The use of yeast extracts as a 'vaccine' of this sort also appears to assist general immune function, by helping to balance or regulate aspects of the system relating to 'helper' and 'suppressor' cells, as discussed earlier (see Chapter 2).

The whole exercise is complicated in the extreme, because whilst *Candida albicans* is a strain of yeast which is clearly identifiable, it contains within its make-up, a large number of variables. Thus the Candida which is growing in one person is not exactly the same as that growing in another. This biological individuality applies to yeasts just as much as to every other living creature, including people. Thus the same extract of Candida, injected into two people, will not produce the same response. Not only is the yeast likely to prove different from that to which the individual is normally exposed, but his/her individuality, superimposed upon that fact, makes for a process of trial and error, in achieving a response which is going to help the individual's immune system to fight the particular strain of Candida present in his system. Hereditary factors may largely be responsible for the differences in response of individuals to such treatment, and this requires that whoever is employing anti-Candida desensitization treatment be expert in the field and be able to cope with the complex variables.

Even should such expertise be available, this approach, with all its possible pitfalls in terms of variable reactions, can at best deal with just one aspect of the problem. It may assist in bolstering the immune system against the by-products of Candida's infestation. This is especially desirable for those people who are suffering from the type of allergy symptoms mentioned earlier. But it will do little for the local symptoms currently active in the bowel or reproductive system. Only those aspects of Candida's harmful effects which are mediated by the bloodstream will be helped. Valuable as this may be, it would leave much of the underlying condition the same, and would still necessitate that the programme of anti-Candida diet and supplements be implemented, in order to control its spread and deny it its nutrients.

Truss points out that the use of this type of 'vaccination' programme is contra-indicated in patients suffering from what are called auto-immune conditions. These include rheumatoid arthritis. Stimulation of the immune response in someone who is being attacked by his own immune system would lead to aggravation of this condition. Truss has written:

> I obtain yeast from supply houses that have been made aware of the necessity of bio-assaying each new batch on humans. Prior to their being informed of this fact, they were putting out a number of batches that would not give a positive skin test on known reactors. The preparation as I order it, is simply Candida albicans 1:10. [34]

This indicates one more pitfall in this method: it is vital that the Candida extract used is actually active, and that this has been proven in each batch produced, otherwise the pitfalls desribed above are compounded.

These two major anti-Candida methods are the primary forms of treatment recommended by both Dr Truss and Dr Crook. They do of course strongly advocate the dietary approach, especially in the prevention of Candida spreading, as well as being supportive of these treatments.

The natural approach to the control of Candida has been outlined in previous chapters, and the reader must choose for himself the method that appeals the most.

The following case histories will give an indication of the way in which this 'natural' approach works.

7

Case Histories

Mr E. M., age 36

This young man, employed as a local government officer, consulted me in 1982 after seven years, during which his health had declined dramatically. His major symptoms (and there were others) included bloating of the abdomen, accompanied by nausea and flatulence, heartburn and indigestion. Constipation had become chronic. There was a tendency to light-headedness and dizziness. There were periodic attacks of shivering, followed by high temperature, which incapacitated him.

The onset of the condition, previous to which his health was unremarkable, came after an attack of gastro-enteritis whilst on holiday. Treatment had, naturally enough, been with a broad-spectrum antibiotic. In his own words,

> For the eighteen months following [the gastro-enteritis] I suffered all the symptoms daily, which were so severe it resulted in my being unable to attend work for six months continuously, and the

remaining twelve months I attended only with massive support from my colleagues, who shared my work load, and understanding superiors who allowed me to go home, or rest, when the attacks were extremely severe.

There had been a gradual improvement over the following years until some twelve months prior to my seeing him, when, after an acute attack, he was left with all the symptoms described above. At that time he wrote, 'At present I am struggling to cope with each day as it comes, and deal with this extremely debilitating and distressing illness as best I can.'

In these intervening years between the onset of his illness and consulting me, he had been seen by numerous medical practitioners. An endoscopy showed no disease of the bowel. He was checked for what is called a malabsorption problem, and again no abnormality was discerned. He went to the Royal Homoeopathic Hospital on two occasions, and consulted a herbalist, an osteopath and a medical specialist in allergies (a clinical ecologist). He had been placed on a rotation diet, which helped him to avoid repetitive contact with suspected food families, but which had little effect on his condition.

At the time I first saw him his diet was as follows. Breakfast: *Bacon* and tomato or *sausages. Rice cakes* and *marmalade.* Decaffeinated *coffee* and *fruit juice* (not freshly made). Mid-morning he had fresh fruit. Lunch was a salad and baked potato plus *ham* or cottage cheese. The evening meal was either *chicken* or *pork* or *sausages* or fish and vegetables. He had *rice cakes* and a hot *milk* drink before retiring. I have italicized those aspects of his eating pattern which are contra-indicated in an anti-Candida diet.

He appeared exhausted, but was a bright and intelligent patient who I felt would co-operate actively in any programme designed to assist recovery.

After tests including cytoxic tests to elicit specific foods to which he might be reacting as well as hair analysis (low in chromium, iron, manganese and selenium), he was prescribed the following:

1. An anti-yeast, anti-fungus pattern of eating, low in carbohydrates.

2. Supplements of vitamins A, E, B1, B2, B3, B6, calcium pantothenate (B5), calcium, magnesium and manganese. Vitamin C was also added. The vitamin A was in emulsified form for easy absorption.

3. The pattern of eating was to include a seed and yogurt breakfast, a salad lunch and an evening meal of 'safe' protein with vegetables.

At this time the knowledge regarding biotin and acidophilus was not current, and the above programme, which the reader will recognize as a modified version of that given in earlier chapters, had a remarkable effect. Improvement began soon after the institution of the programme. Two months later biotin and acidophilus were introduced. When seen six months after the first visit, the report was of at least a 50 per cent improvement in all symptoms; there were still some days of exhaustion, but overall an upwards trend in the health spectrum was noted, after seven years of decline. Confirmation of the involvement of Candida came with an attempt early in the programme to introduce an organic iron supplement, in a liquid yeast-based form. This was met with an immediate return of constipation, which had more or less resolved itself. A check-up six months later found a continued improvement, with lapses in the diet producing confirmatory flare-ups. There is no reason to doubt that the condition will be kept under control, and that the health of the patient will continue to improve. A letter just eighteen months after the start of the programme states, 'Please accept apologies for delay in contacting you. It is an indication of the progress we have made that I am well enough not to have to adhere so strictly. I am very much better overall.' (Letter dated 8 November 1984.)

Mrs E. V., age 50

This patient consulted me with a history of extreme itching and inflammation of the skin of the neck and scalp, of one year's duration. She had an earlier history of acne, which was treated by antibiotic therapy (unsuccessfully). She suffered from flatulence and had a history of colitis and a 'delicate' digestive system. She had consulted a herbalist, with little result, and a hypnotist who taught her relaxation and helped her to stop scratching the area. The condition remained as before. At the time of the consultation I was not yet aware of the work of Dr Truss on Candida and my approach was to use a nutrient supplementation, based on her general clinical picture, a nutritional questionnaire, a hair analysis and her current symptoms. Her dietary pattern was excellent (which, since this turned out to be a Candida problem, had probably saved her from far wider infestation).

She was placed on the following supplements, each taken orally: emulsified vitamin A, 60,000i.u.; zinc orotate, 200mg; calcium and magnesium orotates, 1g each; chromium orotate 10mg, and selenium 50mcg; as well as oil of Evening Primrose (vitamin F), 1g. I also suggested she take yeast tablets as a source of vitamin B. At this point she wrote to me (she lived a considerable distance from my practice) saying 'I am following your suggestions carefully, except for the brewer's yeast. Over the years I have tried a number of times to take it, but it creates gas and is most unpleasant.'

This set off alarm bells, for I had just read the first of Dr Truss's articles that week. I immediately revised the pattern of eating, which, whilst good under usual conditions, contained substances derived from yeast, and of course a certain amount of 'yeast food' such as honey and muesli bars. The patient cancelled her following appointment with the comment that, as her symptoms had disappeared, she felt the journey unnecessary. I quite agreed. A year later she remained symptom-free, including both skin and bowel condition.

Mrs D. B., age 31

I was consulted by this lady, a computer-programmer, with the following list of complaints.

Eyes bloodshot and irritating, for the past nine months. Odd aches, in joints and muscles. Fingers slightly swollen. Puffiness under eyes (and sometimes above) after sleep. Ten years since the onset of this she had had cosmetic surgery and diuretics, to no avail. She had been on a macrobiotic diet as well, with no improvement.

Periods were erratic and painful. Breasts swelled and became sensitive at this time.

She felt unnaturally tired a good deal of the time.
There was a history in the family of bronchial problems and depression, from which she too suffered.

Her current diet was:

Breakfast: shop-bought *muesli with added sugar* plus *milk* or apple juice (once a week she had eggs and *bacon* and *sausage* for breakfast).

Lunch: A cooked vegetarian savoury or *sandwiches.*

Evening meal: Fish and rice, occasional meat.

During the day she had the odd *sweet* and had three cups of *tea,* plus *sugar* and *biscuits.*

She had noticed a progressive inability to cope with alcohol. Her diet was reformed to remove the sugars and milk, and to increase complex carbohydrates. She was prescribed (after appropriate tests) vitamin B complex, kelp, oil of Evening Primrose, vitamin B2, glutamic acid (an amino acid), and the minerals chromium, iron, manganese and selenium. Also prescribed were biotin and acidophilus, after meals. Within two months she reported that her period had been on time for the first time in years, there had been a less overall tendency to swell (eyes or breasts), and she was able to cope with alcohol. (It was in fact proscribed from her diet, which raises the problem of patients complying with instructions — a major headache for practitioners.) Three months later her condition was vastly improved, and her tiredness, bloodshot eyes, aches in muscles and joints, had all diminished to a point where they no longer bothered her. A year later she was symptom-free.

Miss G. H., age 29

The tragic progression of ill health in this case is a clear indictment of the failure of many health professionals to recognize Candida when it is staring them in the face.

Before consulting me, the lady in question wrote to me as follows:

I have been suffering from Pelvic Inflammatory Disease (PID) for almost two years now. The problem started when I began to experience lower abdominal pain and feel generally unwell. I was, at the time, using the contraceptive IUD, which I had removed, believing this to be the cause of the pain. [Prior to this, it turned out, the young lady had been using the contraceptive pill, and had a history of recurrent thrush.] However, this [removal of the coil] had no effect and the pain became worse. Unfortunately my GP did not diagnose PID, and I therefore received no treatment in the early stages of the disease. Eventually I went to hospital, where the gynaecologist diagnosed PID through a laparoscopy. At that time there was some damage to the Fallopian tubes and adhesions in the pelvic area. I was put on to antibiotics, and for a time the condition seemed to improve. After a short time, however, I began to experience further attacks, and had to take larger doses of antibiotics regularly, and strong painkillers for much of the time. At times the pain was incredibly intense. In January 1983 I was admitted to a Women's Hospital in London for another laparoscopy. They found that both Fallopian tubes were blocked, and it sounded as though damage/adhesions in the pelvic area had progressed. Despite this I was told that the pain I was complaining of was psychological, and though they would be prepared to do tube reconstruction, for fertility purposes, there was nothing more they could do for me.

I visited a consultant, in Harley Street, in February 1983, who said that my symptoms and pain were classic PID, but there was nothing he could do to help . . .

My menstrual cycle had now gone from four to six weeks. Apart from the pain, other symptoms were active nausea, stomach upset, dizziness, slightly raised temperature. I also became very depressed. In July 1983 I had surgery after consulting a leading gynaecologist at Hammersmith Hospital. This consisted of removal of left Fallopian tube and reconstruction of the right; separation of adhesions to tubes, ovaries and uterus through microsurgery; presacral neurotomy (removal of nerve to uterus); steroid treatment to prevent regrowth of adhesions.

After this all was well until early November 1983, when symptoms began again. Although pain was not as severe, tests showed the infection was active again. I was put on heavy doses of antibiotics. It did not clear up, and I am now in my sixth week of antibiotics. The consultant told me that there was nothing more they can do surgically, and that I may have the condition for the rest of my life, and must learn to live with it. I have a very positive attitude towards getting better, and find it very difficult to believe that there is nothing else I can do to beat this disease, or at least fight it more effectively.

The patient's history indicated that she had commenced on this sad slide to ill health at the age of 12, when cystitis was first apparent, after which she soon began a thirteen-year history of vaginal thrush.

In late January of 1984, this patient was placed on the programme as outlined in earlier chapters: high fibre, low refined carbohydrate; no fungal foods; and supplements of biotin, acidophilus, olive oil, zinc, vitamin F and garlic. Two months later she reported that she was feeling quite a lot better, apart from a couple of bad spells from which she recovered more quickly than usual.

A letter dated 10 January 1985 reads as follows, 'I have been feeling considerably better. The pain problem is now limited to a few days a month (around period time). After my last laparoscopy the consultant said that it was the best result from that type of operation that he'd ever had. My remaining Fallopian tube was tested and is clear, so I am a lot happier in myself'. This is a clear and dramatic example of the tragedy that occurs when Candida becomes active in a young body, and of the effectiveness of the programme outlined in this book.

Miss S. R., age 35

This young actress suffered from a continuous form of facial acne, which was both unsightly and a disadvantage in her work, as well as being psychologically upsetting. This condition had been present since the age of 14. Her past history was unremarkable, apart from a highly stressed lifestyle, a surgical intervention (cryo-surgery) to deal with a cervical erosion, and a tendency not to ovulate regularly. When under stress in the past, the skin erupted into very large pustules. By following the anti-Candida programme (as outlined in earlier chapters) her skin was normal and she was ovulating regularly, after just three months. This has been maintained for the past year.

Candida is possibly the least understood, most widespread cause of ill health currently in our midst. Precisely because it is known to be everywhere, it is largely ignored, and not even considered, when diagnosis of conditions such as that of the young lady with PID is sought. The cases quoted by Dr Truss, which include similar pictures to those described above, as well as individuals who were diagnosed as schizophrenic, manic depressives, and as having multiple sclerosis, deserve to be emphasized. All of these were restored to normality with the application of the sort of nutritional programme we have been considering, together with anti-yeast drug treatment.

A wider awareness of this diagnosis as a possibility would perhaps lead to a marked reduction in human suffering. This is not just a minor health irritant. It can destroy the physical and mental cohesion of the individual in a very short space of time. Prevention is by the same means as those described for treatment. The knowledge that we now have as to what makes Candida spread is easy to understand and easily put into practical use.

Self-help is always necessary, and until the profession of medicine becomes aware of the import of this knowledge it is vital. Past experience in this regard is not comforting. It can take 50 years, or more, for the penetration of an idea such as this to permeate the profession as a whole. Let us hope that with modern communication, and the help of the media, this will be speeded up in the case of Candida. The name of Dr C. Orion Truss, of Birmingham, Alabama, will eventually become well known throughout medicine. He is deserving of the gratitude of us all for his research into *Candida albicans* and its role as a cause of so much ill health.

Recommended Reading

C. Orion Truss M.D., *The Missing Diagnosis,* obtainable from author, P.O. Box 26508, Birmingham, Alabama 35226, USA.

William G. Crook M.D., *The Yeast Connection,* Vintage Books, 1988.

John P. Trowbridge M.D. and Morton Walker, *The Yeast Syndrome,* Bantam Books, 1986.

Leon Chaitow, *Post Viral Fatigue Syndrome,* Dent, 1989.

Leon Chaitow, *Beat Fatigue Workbook,* Thorsons, 1989.

Leon Chaitow and Natasha Trenev, *Probiotics,* Thorsons, 1990.

References

1. Roger Williams, *Biochemical Individuality* (University of Texas Press, 1979).
2. C. Orion Truss M. D., *Missing Diagnosis* (see Recommended Reading for address).
3. Jay Stein (ed.), *Internal Medicine* (Little Brown, 1983).
4. R. Williams and G. Deason, *Proceedings of National Academy of Sciences* (USA, 57, p.1638, 1968).
5. J. Bland (ed.), *Medical Application of Clinical Nutrition* (Keats, 1983).
6. Jeffrey Bland Ph.D., *Nutraerobics* (Harper & Row, 1983).
7. Dr Michael Colgan, *Your Personal Vitamin Profile* (Blond & Briggs, 1983).
8. Roger Williams Ph.D., *Nutrition against Disease* (Bantam, 1981).
9. W. M. Crook M.D., *The Yeast Connection* (Professional Books).
10. *Journal of Orthomolecular Psychiatry,* Vol. 9, No. 4 (1980), pp.287-301.
11. W. Philpott and D. Kalita, *Brain Allergies* (Keats, 1980).
12. Dr W. Hemmings, *Food Antigens in the Gut* (Lancaster Press, London, 1980).

13. K. Shahani and A. Ayeno, 'Role of dietary lactobacilli in gastrointestinal microecology', in *American Journal of Clinical Nutrition* Vol. 33 (Nov. 1980), pp.2448-57.
14. M. Speck, 'Contributions of micro-organisms to foods and nutrition', in *Nutrition News* Vol. 38, No. 4 (1975) p.13.
15. G. Reddy *et al.*, 'Natural Antibiotic activity of *Lactobacillus acidophilus* and *bulgaricus*', in *Cultured Dairy Products Journal* Vol. 18, No. 2 (1983), p.15.
16. Dr Jeffrey Bland Ph.D., 'Candida Albicans — An Alternative Therapy for an Unexpected Problem', in *Journal of Alternative Medicine,* July 1983, pp.18-19.
17. *Medical Science Proceedings* (Yamaguchi, 1982).
18. *Applied Microbiology* June 1969; Lloyd Harris, *The Book of Garlic* (Aris Books, 1979).
19. *Medical Journal of Australia* Vol. 1, No. 60 (1982).
20. Tyarcke and Gos, 'Inhibitory Action of Garlic on Growth and Respiration of Micro-organisms' (1979).
21. *Mycologia* Vol. LXVII, No. 4 (1975).
22. *Mycologia* Vol. LXIX, No. 4 (1977).
23. Robert Cathcart M.D., 'Vitamin C-Titrating to Bowel Tolerance', *Medical Hypothesis* 7: 1359-76 (1981).
24. *American Journal of Clinical Nutrition* Vol. 37, No. 5, (1983), pp.786.
25. *Dermatologia* No. 156, (1978), pp.257-67.
26. Brown and Binkley, *Yeast: A Brief Description of Common Sources* (1980).
27. Personal Communication to Author, 1983.
28. Robert Forman Ph.D., *How to Control Your Allergies* (Larchmont Books, 1979).
29. John Ott, *Light Radiation and You* (Devin Adair, 1982).
30. Kenneth Cooper, *The New Aerobics* (Bantam, 1977).
31. Leon Chaitow, *Your Complete Stress-Proofing Programme* (Thorsons, 1984).
32. Editorial *New England Journal of Medicine,* 10 Dec. 1981; Editorial, *Lancet* 12 Dec. 1981.
33. Dr J. Sorenson 'Therapeutic and Medicinal Uses of Copper Aspirinate', in *Copper: Its Medicinal and Biological Effects* (Academic Press, 1979).
34. Personal Communication to author, 1984.
35. *Journal of Orthomolecular Psychiatry* Vol. 13, No. 2 (1984), pp.66-93.

36. Betsy Russel Manning, 'How Safe are Mercury Fillings?', Cancer Control Society, Los Angeles, 1984.
37. *Health Consciousness*, April 1984, pp.18-24.
38. *Holistic Medicine* (USA), June-July 1984, p.29.
39. Robert A. Da Prato M.D. *'Fatty acid ion exchange complexes in treatment of Candida Albicans.'* Report by Arteria Co., Concord, California.
40. I. Neuhauser, *Arch. Int. Med.* 93: 53-60.
41. Fernandes, C., Shehani, K., Amer M., 'Therapeutic role of lactobacilli', *FEMS Microbiology Reviews* 46, 1987.
42. Shehani, K., 'Nutritional and Therapeutic aspects of cultured dairy products.' Proc. XIX *Intern'l Dairy Cong.,* Vol. 1e 1974.
43. Carlson E., 'Enhancement by Candida of S.aureus, S.marcescens, S.faecalis in the establishment of infection.' *Infection and Immunity* 39:1 Jan. 1983.

Index

Nostradamus, born in Provence in 1503, showed a great interest in astrology from an early age. He studied medicine and healed many people stricken by the plague, which was at that time endemic in Southern France. His prophetic powers began to manifest themselves while he was still a young man. After 1550 he produced a yearly Almanac and by 1555 he had completed the first part of his book of Prophecies that were to contain predictions from his time to the end of the world.

In order to avoid prosecution as a magician, Nostradamus writes that he deliberately confused the time sequence of the Prophecies so that their secrets would not be revealed to the non-initiate. His fame spread rapidly. Queen Catherine de' Medici asked him to write horoscopes for her seven children, which caused him some problems, as he had already foretold their tragic fates in the Prophecies. Nostradamus died in 1566.

To Alexander and Jamie

Also by Erika Cheetham
THE FURTHER PROPHECIES OF NOSTRADAMUS
and published by Corgi Books

The Prophecies of
Nostradamus

Translated, Edited and Introduced by
Erika Cheetham

STIRLING
DISTRICT
LIBRARY

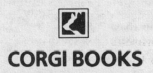

CORGI BOOKS

THE PROPHECIES OF NOSTRADAMUS
A CORGI BOOK 0 552 09828 0

Originally published in Great Britain
by Neville Spearman

PRINTING HISTORY
Spearman edition published 1973
Corgi edition published 1975
Corgi edition reprinted 1975 (twice)
Corgi edition reprinted 1976
Corgi edition reprinted 1978 (three times)
Corgi edition reprinted 1979
Corgi edition reprinted Australia 1979 (twice)
Corgi edition reprinted 1980
Revised Corgi edition published 1981
Revised Corgi edition reprinted 1981 (twice)
Revised Corgi edition reprinted 1982
Revised Corgi edition reprinted 1984
Revised Corgi edition reprinted 1986
Revised Corgi edition reprinted 1987
Revised Corgi edition reprinted 1988
Revised Corgi edition reprinted 1989
Revised Corgi edition reprinted 1990
Corgi edition reprinted 1991
Corgi edition reprinted 1992

133.3
NOS

00164 0387

Copyright © 1973 Erika Cheetham

Conditions of sale
1: This book is sold subject to the condition that it shall
not, by way of trade *or otherwise,* be lent, re-sold, hired out
or otherwise *circulated* without the publisher's prior consent
in any form of binding or cover other than that in which
it is published *and without a similar condition including this
condition being imposed on the subsequent purchaser.*

2: This book is sold subject to the Standard Conditions of
Sale of Net Books and may not be re-sold in the U.K.
below the net price fixed by the publishers for the book.

This book is set in Baskerville 9 on 10 point

Corgi Books are published by Transworld Publishers
Ltd., 61–63 Uxbridge Road, Ealing, London W5 5SA, in
Australia by Transworld Publishers (Australia) Pty. Ltd.,
15–23 Helles Avenue, Moorebank, NSW 2170, and in New
Zealand by Transworld Publishers (N.Z.) Ltd., 3 William
Pickering Drive, Albany, Auckland.

Printed and bound in Great Britain by
Cox & Wyman Ltd., Reading, Berks.

INTRODUCTION

In the autumn of 1939, soon after Germany had declared war on Europe, Frau Dr Goebbels was lying in bed reading an obscure book on occult literature. It contained some predictions made by a certain Nostradamus, printed in 1568. Her husband was asleep, but Frau Dr Goebbels was so excited by what she had read that she woke him and made him read the relevant passages. He was sufficiently impressed to arrange that his Propaganda Ministry hired the services of a Swiss astrologer named Ernst Krafft who was soon to be found reproducing material based on Nostradamus' Prophecies, using them to some effect psychologically in occupied Europe. How could an obscure medieval French doctor cause such consternation in both Goebbels' and Himmler's Departments? How could he also cause the British Secret Service to spend a reputed sum of £80,000 on retaliatory propaganda?

He was Michel de Nostredame, more commonly known by the Latinized form of his name, Nostradamus, born at noon on December 14, 1503 by the old calendar, in St Rémy de Provence. His family were not the illustrious line of Jewish-Italian doctors working at the Courts of King René of Anjou and of his son, as has commonly been claimed, but people of simple lineage from around Avignon. His grandfather was Peyrot or Pierre de Nostredame, an established grain-dealer, who married a Gentile girl named Blanche. Their son Jaume or Jacques, Nostradamus' father, moved to St Rémy in 1495 and gave up the family trade. Here he married Reyniere de St Rémy who was the grand-daughter of an ex-doctor, turned tax-collector. The family were converted from Judaism to the Catholic faith by the time Nostradamus was nine years old, as his parents are listed in 1512 as being part of the new Christian community. It is important to remember the Jewish element of Nostradamus' childhood when trying to decipher the Prophecies, as he was greatly influenced by occult Jewish literature. Nostradamus was the oldest son, and had four brothers; of the first three we know little; the youngest, Jean, wrote a great

5

many ribald Provençal songs and commentaries, and eventually became Procureur of the Parliament of Provence.

Nostradamus' great intellect became apparent while he was still very young, and his education was put into the hands of his grandfather, Jean, who taught him the rudiments of Latin, Greek, Hebrew, Mathematics and what Nostradamus calls celestial science, Astrology. When this grandparent died the boy returned to his parents' house in the rue de Barri and his other grandfather endeavoured to continue his education. Soon, however, Nostradamus was sent to Avignon to study, and probably stayed with some of the many cousins he had in the town.

He already showed a great interest in astrology and it became common talk among his fellow students. He upheld the Copernican theory that the world was round and circled around the sun more than 100 years before Galileo was prosecuted for the same belief. His parents were quite rightly worried by this attitude because theirs was the age of the Inquisition, and as ex-Jews they were more vulnerable than most. So they sent him off to study medicine at Montpellier in 1522. Nostradamus was now nineteen years old and had the advantage of some of the most progressive medical minds in Europe to stimulate him. He obtained his bachelor's degree (baccalauréat) after three years, with apparent ease, and once he had his licence to practise medicine he decided to leave the University and go out into the countryside and help the many victims of the plague.

Plague was endemic in Southern France during the 16th Century, in particular a very virulent form known locally as 'le charbon' because of the great black pustules that appeared on the body of the victim. Nostradamus had many detractors throughout his lifetime but not one has ever denied his courage in facing disease, his humanity, his kindness towards the sick, and his generosity towards the poor. It was at this early stage, 1525, that his reputation as a healer became known. Nostradamus went from town to stricken town dispensing his own cures, the prescriptions for some of which are found later in a book he published in 1552. He was very unsettled and went from Narbonne to Carcassonne where incidentally he prescribed an elixir of life for the local bishop, which if it did all the author claimed for it would be the salvation of every jaded man! Next we hear of him at Toulouse in the rue de la Triperie, again at Bordeaux where the plague was severe and then back to Avignon where he remained studying for some months. His interest in magic and the occult may spring from this period of his life, for the library at Avignon held many occult books. At the same time he managed to concoct a delicious recipe for quince jelly for the Papal Legate and the Grand Master of the Knights of Malta who were then in the town. It is a good recipe but with rather too much sugar for modern tastes.

After nearly four years of sporadic travelling he returned to Montpellier to complete his doctorate and re-enrolled on October 23, 1529. Nostradamus had some trouble in explaining his unorthodox remedies and treatments, for his success and renown had made him enemies among the faculty. Nevertheless his learning and ability could not be denied and he obtained his doctorate. He remained teaching at Montpellier for a year but by this time his new theories, for instance, his refusal to bleed patients, were causing trouble and he set off upon another spate of wandering, moving from place to place as his work and fancy took him. Throughout his life he was to suffer from this wanderlust. Dressed in his dark scholar's cap and gown he must have looked the epitome of the Wandering Jew.

While practising in Toulouse he received a letter from Julius Cesar Scaliger, the philosopher considered second only to Erasmus throughout Europe. Apparently Nostradamus' reply so pleased Scaliger that he invited him to stay at his home in Agen. This life suited Nostradamus admirably, and circa 1534 he married a young girl 'of high estate, very beautiful and admirable', whose name unfortunately has not come down to us. He had a son and a daughter by her and his life seemed complete. His practice was famous and profitable and he had the brilliant mind of Scaliger to help sharpen his wits. Then a series of tragedies struck. The plague came to Agen and, despite all his efforts, killed Nostradamus' wife and two children. The fact that he was unable to save his own family had a disastrous effect on his practice. Then he quarrelled with Scaliger and lost his friendship—a not unlikely happening, as Scaliger quarrelled with all his friends sooner or later. His late wife's family tried to sue him for the return of her dowry and as the final straw, in 1538, he was accused of heresy because of a chance remark made some years before, which had been reported to the authorities. To a workman casting a bronze statue of the Virgin, Nostradamus had commented that he was making devils. His plea that he was only describing the lack of aesthetic appeal inherent in the statue was ignored and the Inquisitors sent for him to go to Toulouse. Nostradamus, naturally having no wish to stand trial nor to suffer the rack or the stake, immediately set out on his wanderings again, keeping well clear of the Church authorities for the next six years.

We know very little about this period of his life. From references in his later books we know that he travelled in the Lorraine and went to Venice and Sicily, making a point of meeting the apothecaries of each place and noting down those who were efficient or bad for his book, the Traité des Fardmens.

It was probably around this period that he started to translate the Horapollo of Philippus from the Greek into French. It is nothing but a collection of treatises on ethics and philosophy and is of no great literary merit. Legends about Nostradamus' prophetic powers also start to appear at this time. Apparently when in Italy he saw a young monk who had been a swineherd pass by him in the street, and immediately knelt down and called him 'Your Holiness'. Felice Peretti became Sextus V in 1585, long after Nostradamus' death.

There is another amusing tale concerning a certain Seigneur de Florinville, who was discoursing with Nostradamus about prophecy and asked him to put his gift to the test by telling him the fates of the two suckling pigs in his yard. Nostradamus replied that the Seigneur would eat the black pig and a wolf the white one. Immediately de Florinville went to his cook and ordered the white pig to be killed for that night's dinner, which it duly was. Unfortunately a tame wolf-cub, belonging to the lord's men stole the meat. The terrified cook killed the black pig and served it for dinner. Seigneur de Florinville then told Nostradamus that they were now eating the white pig. When Nostradamus insisted that it was the black one, the cook was sent for and confessed to the whole incident.

By 1554 Nostradamus had settled in Marseilles. In November of that year, Provence experienced one of the worst floods of its history. The plague redoubled in virulence, spread by the waters and the polluted corpses. Nostradamus worked ceaselessly. Most doctors had fled with those people who were still well enough to move, thus carrying the infection farther. According to contemporary memoirs, the plague was particularly bad at Aix, the capital of Provence, and the city sent for his help on May 1. Nostradamus was alone throughout the epidemic, working among the sick, curing many, and insisting on fresh air and unpolluted water. The sense of hopelessness was so great when he first arrived in the city that he saw one sick woman sewing herself into her own shroud because she knew there would be no one to do it for her when she was dead.

Once the city recovered, Nostradamus moved on to Salon, which he found so pleasant a town that he determined to settle there for the rest of his life. But almost immediately the city of Lyons sent for him to cure a pestilence which may, in fact, have been an epidemic of whooping cough. Whatever it was, once over, Nostradamus returned home laden with yet more gifts from the grateful citizens. Characteristically, he gave many away to the poor of the town before leaving. It is difficult to separate truth from legend in these reports of his great generosity but they almost certainly have some foundation in fact.

Back home in Salon in November, he married Anne Ponsart Gemelle, a rich widow. The house in which he spent the remainder of his days can still be seen off the Place de la Poissonnerie. Now Nostradamus seems to have led a quieter existence. His interest in the occult was strong and presumably he was still experiencing odd flashes of prophetic insight. He does not seem to have practised much medicine at this period, and appears to have concentrated more upon his writings. After 1550 he produced a yearly Almanac and after 1554 the Prognostications—which seem to have been successful, and encouraged him to undertake the much more onerous task of the Prophecies.

Nostradamus converted the top room of his house at Salon into a study and as he tells us in the Prophecies, worked there at night with his occult books. He also mentions later that he burnt a lot of them once he had finished with them, but it is difficult to believe that a true scholar could possibly do this. It was more probably an attempt to mislead the Church authorities. The main source of his magical inspirations was a book called De Mysteriis Egyptorum, a copy of which was published at Lyons in 1547, and which Nostradamus almost certainly possessed, as he quotes from it line for line in some of his prophecies.

It was also about this time, 1554, that Jean-Aymes de Chavigny, a former mayor of Beaune, gave up his position in that city and came to Nostradamus as a pupil to study judicial astrology and astronomy. He wrote several books about Nostradamus after the prophet's death and certainly helped to edit the first complete edition of the Prophecies, but, like Nostradamus' son César, he seems to have exaggerated his own importance with regard to the prophet. The evidence for this lies in Nostradamus' will, a long and detailed document referring not only to his money but detailing all his possessions. There is no reference to Chavigny concerning Nostradamus' papers which he states specifically are to be left to whichever of his sons on reaching maturity 'has drunk the smoke of the lamp' i.e. is a true scholar. Chavigny did, however, edit a great many of Nostradamus' papers, probably with the consent of his widow.

By 1555 Nostradamus had completed the first part of his book of prophecies that were to contain predictions from his time to the end of the world. The word Century has nothing to do with one hundred years; it was so called because there were a hundred verses, or quatrains, in each book, of which Nostradamus intended to write ten, making one thousand quatrains in all. For some unknown reason, the Seventh Century was never completed, and there are indications among his papers that Nostradamus was considering adding an Eleventh and Twelfth Century, which were prevented by his death.

The verses are written in a crabbed, obscure style, with a polyglot vocabulary of French, Provençal, Italian, Greek and Latin. In order to avoid being prosecuted as a magician, Nostradamus writes that he deliberately confused the time sequence of the Prophecies so that their secrets would not be revealed to the non-initiate.

It is extraordinary how quickly the fame of Nostradamus spread across France and Europe on the strength of the Prophecies, published in their incomplete form in 1555. The book contained only the first three Centuries and part of the fourth. At this time books were an expensive luxury and were usually owned and read only by the rich, for most of the population were illiterate. The Prophecies became all the rage at Court, and one or two seemed to invoke a certain uneasiness among the courtiers, particularly the one which appeared to predict the king's death (I.35). Be that as it may, the Queen, Catherine de' Medici, sent for Nostradamus to come to Court, and he set out for Paris on July 14, 1556. The journey took only one month because the Queen had horses posted for him, instead of the more usual eight weeks. On August 15, Nostradamus booked a room at the Inn of St Michel, near Notre Dame. The Queen must have been very anxious to see him because she sent for him the next day and the Chief Constable took him to the Court at St. Germain en Laye.

One could only wish that there had been a witness to record

their meeting. Nostradamus and the Queen spoke together for two hours. She is reputed to have asked him about the quatrain concerning the king's death and to have been satisfied with Nostradamus' answer. Certainly she continued to believe Nostradamus' predictions until her death. The king, Henri II, granted Nostradamus only a brief audience and was not greatly interested, although he sent Nostradamus one hundred golden crowns, and Catherine sent another thirty. This seemed poor recompense to Nostradamus, who had expended one hundred crowns for his journey alone. However, his lodgings were exchanged for the grandeur of the palace of the Archbishop of Sens, where he remained for some two weeks seeing people who came for advice, drawing up horoscopes, and offering prophetic guidance. The Queen then sent for him a second time and now Nostradamus was faced with the delicate and difficult task of drawing up the horoscopes of seven Valois children, whose tragic fates he had already revealed in the Centuries. All he would tell Catherine was that all her sons would be kings, which is slightly inaccurate since one of them, François, died before he could inherit. If on the other hand what he actually said was that he saw four kings to come, then the prediction was accurate because Henri III was king of Poland before returning to be king of France.

Soon afterwards Nostradamus was warned that the Justices of Paris were enquiring about his magic practices, and he returned quickly to Salon. He was welcomed home as a person of importance. From this time on, suffering from gout and arthritis, he seems to have done little except draw up horoscopes for his many distinguished visitors and complete the writing of the Prophecies. Apparently he allowed a few manuscript copies to circulate before publication because many of the predictions were understood and quoted before the completed book came off the printing press in 1568, two years after his death.

The reason for this reticence was probably the king's death in 1559. Nostradamus had predicted it in I.35 and may have felt that it was too explicit for comfort and it would be advisable to wait a few more years until things had quietened down. But the following year, 1560, King Francis II, married to Mary, Queen of Scots, died, and this time the courtiers openly quoted quatrain 39 of Century X.

'The eldest son; a widow of an unfortunate marriage with no children; two islands in discord; before eighteen still a minor; for the other one the betrothal will take place when even younger'. Francis II was Henri II's eldest son. He died six weeks before reaching the age of eighteen leaving a widow, Mary, Queen of Scots, whose return to her country was to put two realms at discord. Francis' younger brother, Charles, had been betrothed at the early age of eleven to Elizabeth of Austria.

In 1564 Catherine, now Queen Regent, decided to make a Royal Progress through France with her second son Charles IX and the rest of her family. The progress was to take two years and the court entourage was reduced to a minimum of eight hundred people. While travelling through Provence Catherine naturally came to Salon to see Nostradamus. He dined with the King and Queen and she also visited him at his house and admired his children. This time Catherine gave Nostradamus three hundred gold crowns and the title Physician in Ordinary, which carried with it a salary and other fringe benefits, which doubtless pleased him.

Another interesting incident occurred during this visit to Salon, when Nostradamus asked to see the moles on the body of a young boy in the entourage. This was a common form of prediction but the child was shy and ran away. Nostradamus went to see him the next day while asleep and declared that he would one day be king of France, although Catherine still had two sons living. The boy was Henri of Navarre, who later became Henri IV.

By now the gout from which he suffered was turning to dropsy and Nostradamus, the doctor, realized that his end was near. He made his will on June 17, 1566 and left the large sum, for those days, of 3,444 crowns over and above his other possessions. On July 1, he sent for the local priest to give him the last rites, and when Chavigny took leave of him that night, told him that he would not see him alive again. His body was found the next morning, as he himself had predicted, 'trouvé tout mort pres du lit & du banc'. He was buried upright in one of the walls of the Church of the Cordeliers at Salon, and his wife Anne erected a splendid marble plaque to his memory. Nostradamus' grave was opened by superstitious soldiers during the Revolution but his remains were reburied in the other church at Salon, the Church of St. Laurent, where his grave and portrait can still be seen.

HISTORY OF THE CENTURIES SINCE PUBLICATION

In evaluating the works of anyone who claims to have prophetic powers it is essential to know which of those writings attributed to him are really his own, and which publication dates are genuine. Nostradamus in particular has been the victim of many forgeries over the centuries which may help to account for his undeservedly bad reputation.

There is great confusion about all the early editions of Nostradamus' works, including the Prophecies, because they were first printed in two parts, in 1555 and 1568. Several of the oldest editions are undated and there are several counterfeit 'first' editions which have altered texts and were printed more than one hundred years later than the date on their frontispiece.

There are so many editions of the Prophecies that it is impossible to list them here, but Nostradamus is probably the only author who could claim that his work has never been out of print for over four hundred years, apart from the Bible. The interest he generates is extraordinary. On an average about thirty books, either editions of the Prophecies, or cititical appreciations of them, have been published each century since his death. Of course, times of crisis, such as the French Revolution, and the First and Second World Wars, produce a spate of such books. Some are frankly bad, and make no attempt at impartiality of judgment and often change the text to suit themselves. Others are sceptical and critical, but none manage wholly to dismiss out of hand the small hard core of Nostradamus' accurate predictions.

Nostradamus was used as a propaganda machine as early as 1649 and as late as 1980. In 1649 the opponents of Cardinal Mazarin, who felt he had too great an influence in the French Court, published an edition of the Prophecies, dating it 1568, in which they planted two obvious quatrains against the Cardinal. When the Bastille was stormed on July 14, 1789, the Revolutionaries recognized themselves in the Preface to the Prophecies, for apparently a copy was laid open on a table in the prison, and for ten days the people filed past, to read confirmation of their achievements. Napoleon's attention was drawn to the Prophecies by the Empress Josephine, but he was also the victim of an unscrupulous forgery which was declared to have been written by Nostradamus, called the Prophecies of Olivarius. It was a fake and its true date is circa 1820. A later similar forgery appeared in 1839 called the Prophecy of Orval. Neither of these works have anything to do with Nostradamus.

His fame was not confined to France. Editions of the Prophecies appeared all over Europe within twenty-five years of their first publication. Again it is impossible to list them all here, but if one mentions that twenty-six known editions and four forged ones were published in Europe between 1555 and 1643, at a time when books were valuable, one is given some idea of the strength of Nostradamus' popularity, which has continued to the present day.

From 1860 onwards a provincial French curé, called the Abbé Torné to which he added the surname Chavigny after Nostradamus' pupil, produced a series of interpretations of Nostradamus' quatrains which shook France and affected many political decisions of the time. He was convinced that the Bourbon line would be restored to the French throne. Equally he was certain that in the next war France would be invaded by means of Switzerland, and it was because of this information that the then French Chief of Staff ordered the drawing up of the disastrous Maginot line on the strength of Quatrain 80 in Century VI. Incredible but true.

Hitler's interest in Nostradamus was first aroused by the notorious Hister quatrains discovered by Frau Dr Goebbels who, as I have mentioned, drew her husband's attention to them in 1936. By May 1940 onwards, the Germans were dropping from aircraft crude forgeries of various quatrains from the Prophecies which predicted that Hitler would be victorious and that the war would not affect South-eastern France. By this means the Germans hoped to clear the roads to Paris and the Channel ports. In retaliation, British Intelligence, 'inspired' by Louis de Wohl, who was probably as great a charlatan as any, spent an enormous sum on anti-German propaganda, carefully composing and imitating selected German Nostradamus quatrains which Allied pilots dropped over France and Belgium. This occurred as late as 1943. Books have continued to be written about Nostradamus ever since.

The final problem remaining with regard to Nostradamus is as to whether the man was prophet or fraud. He believed himself to possess certain powers, although there is reason to believe he could not draw on these to order. They certainly sometimes let him down in the Prophecies. The reader must decide whether it is possible to believe in prediction, whether a man who wrote over four hundred years ago could possibly glimpse incidents in the future, or whether it was just inspired guesswork. It is essential for thinking man to believe in free will, to believe that his future can be changed by thought and action. Prophecy denies this and declares that all futures are immutable and fixed, that nothing man strives towards is relevant, as it is already preordained by whatever governs his future, be it God or Destiny. I believe that mankind must have free will; but also I must admit the disturbing fact that although I can dismiss ninety-five per cent of Nostradamus' predictions as historical coincidence, there remain a few quatrains which are hard to reconcile with this. What about the one describing Louis XVI's flight to Varennes, the ones mentioning Napoleon and Hitler and the deposition of the Shah? What about the verses giving the actual month and year of any occurrence, such as that which describes the obscure treaty between the Persians and the Turks in October 1727, or another which gives the day and the month of the assassination of a Prince?(III.96) I find this type of quatrain difficult to explain away completely. They appear to me to be more than coincidence.

The modern disciples of Einstein recognize nothing but an eternal present which was also what the ancient mystics believed. If the future exists already then precognition is a fact. The whole trend of advanced knowledge is to place the laws of physics in a four dimensional continuum, that is, the eternal present. If this is so, then past, present and future exist simultaneously. Perhaps it is only our consciousness that moves? One day we may know and then precognition would become an accepted fact.

But, on the other hand, the answer may lie in Dunne's concept of alternative variable futures which run parallel to each other. Each man receives the future dependent upon his earlier actions. Nostradamus could have glimpsed these parallels of time which may or may not have occurred, depending upon the earlier freely determined actions of other men. No man can be in any sense an island; all our actions affect someone else. Thus if Louis XVI had done the sensible thing and stayed in Paris instead of fleeing in a panic to Varennes, there would have been another incomprehensible quatrain in this book. Equally, however appalling it may appear, if Hitler's attention had not been drawn to the Prophecies and the connection between Poland and Britain, would he gave gone to war at that time?

The reader can try to reconcile the concept of free will with the mathematical probability of chance. By means of E.S.P. or some similar faculty, possibly the future may be vaguely seen and grasped at—a future conditioned by the education of the man who receives it. Humanity does seem to repeat its mistakes, or as Dr Inge says, resemble itself to a remarkable degree. This is proven by the fact that some of the quatrains—the ones I call split quatrains—will quite accurately predict events separated by over a century in time. But it seems that if we wish to avoid the gloomy future that Nostradamus foresees for mankind, we must break away from our present behaviour pattern, conditioned over the last few hundred years, and grow outwards towards a new concept of worldwide peace and brotherhood, and away from Nostradamus' medieval concepts of famine, war and tragedy.

THE TEXT, TRANSLATION AND COMMENTARY

Throughout this edition I have used the text of the first edition, published by Benoit Rigaud in 1568. The concessions I have made to the reader are mainly in the realm of spelling. I have changed u to v when required, y to i, f to s, and added n or m when only indicated by an accent, e.g. côplaire = complaire. I have copied the same punctuation, accents and capital letters as the original.

Opposite each quatrain I have given a very literal translation, which may seem nonsensical at first sight because I have kept as closely as possible to the Latin style of the original. I explain proper names and obscure words in footnotes. Below the translation is a prose commentary with a heading summarizing the subject matter when possible, for those who wish to skip quickly through the book. The quatrains which I cannot decipher I leave to the ingenuity and patience of the reader.

I have omitted the Preface to the first edition and the Epistle to César, which is placed before the Seventh Century, because of length and obscurity.

December 1979

CENTURY I

76	Napoleon I
77	Battle of Trafalgar, 1805
78	
79	
80	
81	
82	Austria 1914–18
83	Italian Occupation of Greece, 1940
84	Murder of Duke de Berry, 1820
85	Fate of the de Guise family, 1568
86	Flight of Mary Queen of Scots, 1568
87	Earthquake, San Andreas fault, New York
88	Charles I and Parliament
89	Peninsular Wars, 1808
90	
91	America in Vietnam
92	Franco-Prussian war
93	Napoleon's Italian Campaign, 1795
94	Lepanto, 1571
95	
96	Cults, such as Moonies, etc.
97	Assassination of Henri III, 1589
98	Napoleon's Expedition to Egypt, 1798
99	
100	Comte de Chambord

1

Estant assis de nuict secret estude
Seul reposé sur la selle d'aerain;
Flambe exiguë sortant de solitude
Fait prosperer qui n'est à croire
    vain.

Sitting alone at night in secret study; it is placed on the brass tripod. A slight flame comes out of the emptiness and makes successful that which should not be believed in vain.

DIVINATION

Both this and the following quatrain describe Nostradamus' method of divination, they are not predictions. Nostradamus used the methods of the 4th Century neo-Platonist Iamblichus, a reprint of whose book *De Mysteriis Egyptorum* was published at Lyons in 1547 and almost certainly read by Nostradamus. It may well have been the source of his experiments with prophecy, for soon afterwards his Almanacs started to appear.

All the ingredients for magical practices are in this quatrain. It is night. Nostradamus is alone in his study reading the secret forbidden books which inspire his prophecies; the brass tripod is a method used by Iamblichus—on it was placed a bowl of water into which the seer gazed until the water became cloudy and pictures of the future were revealed. *Flambe exiguë* is the light of inspiration which seizes Nostradamus as he begins to prophesy.

2

La verge en main mise au milieu
    des BRANCHES[1]
De l'onde il moulle[2] & le limbe[3]
    & le pied:
Un peur & voix fremissant par
    les manches:
Splendeur divine. Le divin pres
    s'assied.

The wand in the hand is placed in the middle of the tripod's legs. With water he sprinkles both the hem of his garment and his foot. A voice, fear; he trembles in his robes. Divine splendour; the god sits nearby.

[1]*Branches*—Capitals in original = (*a*)The three limbs or branches of the tripod. (*b*) Indirect reference to the prophetess of Branchus.
[2]*moulle*—Modern french *mouille* = to moisten.
[3]*limbe*—Latin, *limbus* hem of a garment.

DIVINATION

Nostradamus continues to explain his method. He touches the middle of the tripod with his wand, and then moistens his robe and his feet with the water placed on it. This is the same method as was used to obtain inspiration by the Apollonian prophetess at the Oracle of Branchus in Classical times. Nostradamus is afraid of the power he evokes when it comes to him; he hears it, as well as sees it; it appears to speak to him and he writes down the prophecies. He is unafraid once the gift has possessed him. This dual aspect of his vision is most important when interpreting the Centuries.

3

Quand la licture du tourbillon versee,	When the litters are overturned by the whirlwind and
Et seront faces de leurs manteaux convers:	faces are covered by cloaks, the new republic will be trou-
La republique par gens nouveaux vexée,	bled by its people. At this time the reds and the whites will
Lors blancs & rouges jugeront à l'envers.	rule wrongly.

FRENCH REVOLUTION

The French Revolution of 1789, which Nostradamus calls the Common Advent, the coming of the ordinary men in the Preface, is here described. The aristocracy were always carried in litters, and this, their symbol, is overturned by the violent whirlwind of revolution. Could the line mentioning the heads covered by cloaks refer to the many exiles who fled from France, or possibly to the heads which fell from the guillotine and were hidden from sight? It is interesting that Nostradamus should here refer to France as a republic, and to one that was greatly troubled by its new rulers. The era of Danton, Murat and Robespierre during the terror springs vividly to mind. White was the colour of the Bourbon kings and red, of course, that of the revolutionaries. The last line 'à l'envers' may also imply that the law givers, i.e. the church and aristocracy, were chosen by the populace who were unsuited for this work.

4

Par l'univers sera faict un monarque,	In the world there will be made a king who will have little peace and a short life. At this time the ship of the Papacy will be lost, governed to its greatest detriment.
Qu'en paix & vie ne sera longuement,	
Lors se perdra la piscature[1] barque,	
Sera regie en plus grand detriment.	

NAPOLEON AND PIUS VII

Napoleon crowned himself king and Emperor of France on 18th May 1804 and abdicated in April 1814, ruling for the short time of ten years. Peace was certainly not a characteristic of his era. Pius VII (1800-23) first came to France to crown Napoleon as Emperor, but on his second visit he came as a prisoner. The French army, under General Miollis, captured Rome in 1809 and the Papal States were joined to the French Empire in 1810; the Pope was held prisoner by Napoleon and only released by the abdication at Fontainbleau on 23rd January 1814. The last line refers to the general religious anarchy that existed in France from the time of the dissolution of the Clergy in 1792.

5

Chassés seront pour faire long combat,	They will be driven away for a long drawn out fight. The countryside will be most grievously troubled. Town and country will have the greater struggle. Carcassonne and Narbonne will have their hearts tried.
Par le pays seront plus fort grevés:	
Bourg & Cité auront plus grand debat,	
Carcas[2] Narbonne auront coeur esprouvéz.	

HUGUENOT STRUGGLES IN PROVENCE, 1562–98

The whole of southern France was greatly afflicted by the religious wars which broke out between Huguenots and Catholics before the accession of Henri IV. Carcassonne declared

[1]*piscature*—Latin, = fishing, but a common synonym for the Papacy.
[2]Apocope of Carcassonne.

itself for the Catholic League but the Huguenots seized part of the town, and Narbonne also suffered a great deal of fighting. A general quatrain covering a wide period of over thirty years. Nostradamus was always greatly interested in the fate of France and those towns he knew and had lived in during his wanderings.

6

L'oeil de Ravenne sera destitué,
Quand à ses pieds les ailles failliront:
Les deux de Bresse auront constitué,
Turin, Derseil¹ que Gaulois fauleront.

The eye of Ravenna will be forsaken, when his wings will fail at his feet. The two of Bresse will have made a constitution for Turin and Vercelli, which the French will trample underfoot.

FRENCH OCCUPATION OF BRESSE, 1601, TURIN, 1640 etc. VERCELLI 1904 etc. CAPTURED FROM THE PAPAL STATES

Ravenna has been part of the Papal States since 1509, and the most likely interpretation of this quatrain concerns the fates of the states mentioned above, Bresse, Turin and Vercelli, which were all occupied by the French at some period. Bresse was ceded to France in 1601, Turin was taken by the French in 1640 and 1798–1814. Vercelli was also captured in 1704 and 1798–1814. All that is certain is that each of these places, except for Ravenna, suffered French occupation after the Centuries were written.

7

Tard arrivé l'execution faicte,²
Le vent contraire lettres aux chemin prinses:
Les conjurez xiiii d'une secte:
Par le Rousseau semez³ les entreprinses.

Arrived too late, the act has been done. The wind was against them, letters intercepted on their way. The conspirators were fourteen of a party. By Rousseau shall these enterprises be undertaken.

---

¹Read *Versail* = Vercelli, Piedmont, Italy.
²*faicte*—Normal spelling of the period for fait.
³Two alternatives. Either *semez*, to spread, which I accept, or *senez* = wise.

DREYFUS CASE, 1894–1906.
M. WALDECK ROUSSEAU, 1899

Alfred Dreyfus, a Jewish French soldier was condemned for treason for selling military secrets to the Germans in 1894, and publicly degraded and transported to a penal colony, l'Ile du Diable in 1895. In 1899 he was brought back to France for a public retrial but due to strong anti-semitic influences was again found guilty, but with extenuating circumstances. President Loubet pardoned him ten days later and the courts ordered further investigation of the case. The letters which convicted him were declared forgeries and Dreyfus innocent. The case troubled French society for some years to come. Nostradamus describes the proof of Dreyfus' innocence as arriving too late, for his sentence has already been passed and he is in the penal colony. *Vent contraire* is interpreted as political, i.e., anti-semitic, feeling running high against Dreyfus. The minister who was called upon to revise the Dreyfus case in 1899 was M. Waldeck Rousseau, whose name is given in the last line. He was violently anti-Dreyfus, finding him guilty a second time until the public pardon. The number of conspirators may well have been fourteen, but it is impossible to prove at this date.

8

Combien de fois prinse cité solaire	How often will you be captured, O city of the sun?
Seras changeant les loix barbares & vaines:	Changing laws that are barbaric and vain. Bad times approach you. No longer will you be enslaved. Great Hadrie will revive your veins.
Ton mal s'approche. Plus sera tributaire,	
La grand Hadrie[1] recourira des veines.	

HENRI IV. SIEGE OF PARIS, 1590

After his accession to the French throne Henri IV de Navarre had to besiege Paris for six months before he could enter the city in September 1590. It is called Solaire, city of the sun,

---

[1]*Hadrie*—Henry by anagram, one letter being altered according to Nostradamus' rules.

a suitable epithet if one thinks of Louis XVI, the Sun King, 1774–1793. The barbarous laws refer to the innovations of the Seize which was the first truly revolutionary faction to govern Paris. *'Ton mal s'approche';* the siege occurred less than thirty years after Nostradamus' death and he seems to feel the accession of a Huguenot king deeply. The last line is interesting in that throughout the siege from April to September Henri IV allowed food to be passed through the lines to the starving people of Paris. Perhaps this line is to be taken in its most literal form, or more metaphorically in that the new line of the Navarre family will revive the greatness of France and the French kings?

9

De l'Orient viendra la coeur Punique	From the Orient will come the African heart to trouble Hadrie and the heirs of Romulus. Accompanied by the Libyan fleet the temples of Malta and nearby islands shall be deserted.
Facher Hadrie & les hoirs[1] Romulides	
Accompagné de la classe[2] Libyque	
Temples Mellites[3] & proches isles vuides.	

1. HENRI IV AND THE DUC DE PARME.
2. THE SIEGE OF MALTA

This quatrain should be divided into two parts. Lines 1–2 continue from the last verse and refer again to Henri IV. The man who troubles him from the East is the Duke of Parma who compelled Henri to raise his siege of Paris in 1590 in order to meet the Spanish army advancing from Flanders. This annoyed the Pope (the heir of Romulus) who favoured the Navarre claim and was hostile to Spanish policy at this point.

Lines 3–4 most probably refer to the siege of Malta in 1565 and the Libyan fleet is then the Turkish navy which roamed the Mediterranean. It is unlikely to refer to Gadaffi.

[1] *hoirs* = heirs. The heirs of Romulus are of course the Italians.
[2] *classe*—Latin, *classis* = fleet.
[3] *Mellites* = adjective, Maltese.

10

Serpens¹ transmis dans la caige de fer,
Ou les enfans septaines² du Roy sont pris:
Les vieux & peres sortiront bas de l'enfer,
Ains mourir voir de fruict mort & cris.

A coffin is put into the vault of iron, where the seven children of the king are held. The ancestors and forebears will come forth from the depths of hell, lamenting to see thus dead the fruit of their line.

FATES OF VALOIS CHILDREN AND HENRI III's DEATH, 1610

This complicated quatrain refers to the fall of the House of Valois and in particular to the removal of the remains of the last Valois king, Henri III, in 1610 to the family sepulchre at Saint Denis. The theme of the seven Valois children of Catherine de' Medici, Queen of France, wife of Henri II, recurs several times in the quatrains. Nostradamus seems clearly aware that the line will die out although it is only fair to admit that Henri III was not the last to die, as Marguerite de Navarre lived until 1615. Line three is a poetic reference to the family ghosts who return to mourn the end of the Valois line.

11

Le mouvement de sens, coeur, pieds & mains,
Seront d'accord Naples, Lyon,³ Sicille:
Glaves, feux, eaux puis aux nobles Romains,
Plongez tuez mors par cerveau debile.

The motion of senses, heart, feet and hands will be in agreement between Naples, Lyon and Sicily. Swords, fire, floods, then the noble Romans drowned, killed or dead because of a weak brain.

¹*Serpens*—From *serpos*, Gk. = Shroud.
²*enfans septaines* = (*a*) François II, 1559–60. (*b*) Elisabeth 1545–68. (*c*) Claude 1547–75. (*d*) Charles IX 1560–74. (*e*) Henri III 1574–89. (*f*) Marguerite 1552–1615. (*g*) François, duc d'Alençon 1554–84.
³*Lyon*—Alternative reading = Leon.

All the places mentioned, if one accepts the reading Leon for Lyon, were part of the Spanish Hapsburg Empire. The weak mind may imply that some Pope would cause trouble between the Vatican and the Empire?

12

Dans peu dira faulce brute fragile,
De bas en haut eslue prompte-ment:
Puis un instant desloyale & labile,
Qui de Veronne aura gouverne-ment.

There will soon be talk of a treacherous man, who rules a short time, quickly raised from low to high estate. He will suddenly turn disloyal and volatile. This man will govern Verona.

From 1405–1562 Verona was governed by podestas, the office of a captain which was meant to change yearly. After that date it was ruled by a council of proveditors. The last podesta was Jacapo Sansebastiani 1539/62, but he was not a traitor.

13

Les exilez par ire, haine intestine,
Feront au Roy grand conjuration:
Secret mettront ennemis par la mine,
Et ses vieux siens contre aux sedition.

Through anger and internal hatreds, the exiles will hatch a great plot against the king. Secretly they will place enemies as a threat, and his own old (adherents) will find sedition against them.

CONSPIRACY OF AMBOISE, 1560 (?)

This is a generally worded quatrain concerning the Conspiracy of Amboise 1560. The coming to power of the Guise family in France, caused other parties, in particular the Montmorencys and the Bourbons, to conspire to kill the Duc de Guise and kidnap the King, Francis II. However the plot leaked out in advance and was suppressed.

14

De gent esclave[1] chansons, chants
& requestes,
Captifs par Princes & Seigneur[2]
aux prisons:
A l'avenir par idiots sans testes,[3]
Seront reçus par divines oraisons.

From the enslaved populace, songs, chants and demands, while Princes and Lords are held captive in prisons. These will in the future be received by headless idiots as divine prayers.

FRENCH REVOLUTION, 1789

Most commentators accept this quatrain as referring to the songs and demands of the populace while Louis XVI was imprisoned with his family in the Temple. The idiots who lose their heads are the early ringleaders of the terror who in their turn will follow the aristocracy to the guillotine, but who are regarded at first as inspired leaders of the Revolution.

15

Mars nous menace par la force
bellique,[4]
Septante fois fera le sang es-
pandre:
Auge[5] & ruine de l'Ecclesiastique,
Et plus ceux qui d'eux rien voud-
ront entendre.

Mars threatens us with the force of war and will cause blood to be spilt seventy times. The clergy will be both exalted and reviled moreover, by those who wish to learn nothing of them.

DIFFICULTIES FACING THE CHURCH

Commentators of the early 19th Century, such as Nicollaud, take lines 1–2 as referring to Napoleon (Mars) and the many wars of the Empire. The church was both humbled and exalted during this period. In 1792 the clergy were disbanded and religion almost vanished from France during the early days of the Directoire. However by 1804 Napoleon had recognized the Pope and the position of the clergy in order to legitimize his coronation. The troubles facing the Catholic Church in the future is a common theme through the Prophecies. Religious

[1]*esclave* = (*a*) enslaved, (*b*) Slav or Russian?
[2]Singular use of *Seigneur* may indicate King Louis XVI.
[3]*testes*—O.F. for *têtes* = heads.
[4]*bellique*—Latin, *bellicus* = warlike.
[5]*Auge*—Latin, *augere* = to increase.

practice is certainly declining in most western countries at the present time.

16

Faulx¹ à l'estang² joint vers le Sagitaire,³	A scythe joined with a pond in Sagittarius at its highest
En son hault AUGE⁴ de l'exaltation,	ascendant. Plague, famine, death from military hands;
Peste, famine, mort de main militaire,	the century approaches its renewal.
La siecle approche de renouvation.	

WAR TOWARDS END OF THIS CENTURY

When Saturn and Aquarius are in conjunction with Sagittarius in the ascendant, towards the end of a century, we should expect a great war, together with disease and famine. This description is general and it could fit our century as well as any other. Nostradamus refers in later centuries to the possibility of a third war towards the end of this century, dating it at any time from 1981 onwards. However, Nostradamus is not completely correct as Aquarius can not be in conjunction with Sagittarius. When Saturn is in Aquarius and Sagittarius is exalted it will either be in the signs of Cancer, Scorpio or Pisces. Saturn is never exalted in Sagittarius. When Saturn is in a water sign and Sagittarius is exalted towards the end of the century gives no clear dating. Saturn goes into a water sign every seven years. See I. 67. II. 41, 46, 62, 75. III. 34, 42. VI. 97. VIII. 59, 77. X. 4, 49, 72, 74, 75.

17

Par quarante ans l'Iris n'apparoistra,	For forty years the rainbow will not be seen. For forty
Par quarante ans tous les jours sera veu:	years it will be seen every day. The dry earth will grow more
La terre aride en siccité croistra,	parched and there will be
Et grans deluges quand sera aperceu.	great floods when it is seen.

¹*Faulx* = a scythe, the sign of Saturn.

²*l'estang* = a pond or water sign, i.e. Saturn in Scorpio, Pisces or Cancer.

³*Sagitaire* = Sagittarrius.

⁴*Auge*—Latin, *augere* = increase.

FLOODS AND DROUGHT

This must be left to the reader. There is no record of a forty-year drought followed by forty years of flooding. One of the general quatrains of gloom and doom.

18

Par la discorde negligence Gauloise,
Sera passaige à Mahommet ouvert:
De sang trempé la terre & mer Senoise,
Le port phocen[1] de voiles & nefs convert.

Because of French discord and negligence an opening shall be given to the Mohammedans. The land and sea of Siena will be soaked in blood, and the port of Marseilles covered with ships and sails.

SECOND WORLD WAR

This refers to the chaos in France during 1940 which allowed the Italian armies to march into North Africa without hindrance. The Italian blood spilt would refer to the battles in the desert; the harbour at Marseilles was constantly operative, although in German hands.

19

Lors que serpens viendront circuir[2] l'are,[3]
Le sang Troyen vexé par les Espaignes:
Par eux grand nombre en sera faicte tare.
Chef fruict,[4] caché aux mares[5] dans les saignes.[6]

When the snakes surround the altar, and the Trojan blood is troubled by the Spanish. Because of them, a great number will be lessened. The leader flees, hidden in the swampy marshes.

CATHERINE DE' MEDICI

Catherine de' Medici, Queen mother of France, changed her emblem after her husband's death to a serpent biting its

[1] *phocen* = Marseilles, founded by the people of Phocaea, the mother city in W. Asia Minor.
[2] *circuir*—Latin, circuire = to encircle.
[3] *are*—Latin, ara = altar.
[4] *fruict*—fuit = flee.
[5] *mares*—O.F. = swamp, marsh.
[6] *saignes*—O.F. = swamp, marsh.

tail curled round a star, not an altar. Trojan blood is the usual
Nostradamus description of Royal blood derived from the
medieval legend that the French Royal family were descended
from Francus, a mythical son of Priam. The French trouble
with Spain did not really occur until the interregnum 1589–94,
and the later war of the Spanish succession. Another suggestion is that the snakes refer to the Huguenots pressing hard
around the Catholic altar, but the reference to Trojan blood
links it to Catherine de' Medici and the French royal line. The
last line is unclear.

20

Tours, Orleans, Blois, Angiers,
   Reims, & Nantes,
Cités vexées par subit change-
   ment:
Par langues estranges seront ten-
   dues tentes,[1]
Fleuves, dards Rones, terre &
   mer tremblement.
	The cities of Tours, Orléans,
	Blois, Angiers, Reims and
	Nantes are troubled by sud-
	den change. Tents will be
	pitched by (people) of foreign
	tongues; rivers, darts at
	Rennes, shaking of land and
	sea.

OCCUPATION OF LOIRE TOWNS

All the cities, except for Reims, are situated on the Loire
and have suffered several foreign invasions, mainly the Prussian and Russian armies in 1815, the Prussians again in 1871
and 1940, and also the Americans in 1917–19 and 1944–5.
There is no record of an earthquake at Rennes since publication.

21

Profonde argille blanche nourrit
   rochier,
Qui d'un abisme istra[2] *lacti-*
   neuse:[3]
En vain troublez ne l'oseront
   toucher,
Ignorans estre au fond terre
   argilleuse.
	The rock holds in its depths
	white clay which will come out
	milk-white from a cleft.
	Needlessly troubled people
	will not dare touch it, una-
	ware that the foundation of
	the earth is of clay.

[1] *tentes* = (*a*) Tents pitched by invaders. (*b*) Latin, *tentare*, to attack.
These cities will be attacked by invaders. The meaning is substantially
the same.
[2] *istra*—O.F. = *aller* to go (ira).
[3] *lactineuse*—Latin, *lac* = milk. *lacticineum* = milk food.

No connection with local historical events can be found to explain this odd verse. I wonder whether the language has alchemistic undertones?

22

Ce que vivra & n'ayant ancien sens,	A thing existing without any senses will cause its own end
Viendra leser à mort son artifice:	to happen through artifice.
Austun, Chalan, Langres & les deux Sens,	At Autun, Chalan, Langres and the two Sens there will be
La gresle & glace fera grand malefice.	great damage from hail and ice.

RARE MEDICAL EVENT 1613

A very interesting solution to this quatrain occurs in Garancieres. He states that in 1613 a petrified embryo was removed by operation (artifice) from the womb of a woman called Colomba Chantry who lived at Sens. This was quite a rare event; examples can be found in medical textbooks, and a woman living in Italy two years ago was found to have been carrying a petrified embryo well into her sixties; an interesting medical sideline from Nostradamus the doctor. All the towns mentioned belong to the Duchy of Burgundy. The reference to the weather seems very general, the quatrain implying that it occurred around the same period, 1613. The second town of Sens is near Louhans.

23

Au mois troisiesme se levant le soleil	In the third month, at sunrise, the Boar and the Leopard meet on the battlefield.
Sanglier, Liepard au champ Mars pour combattre:	The fatigued Leopard looks
Liepard laissé, au ciel extend son oeil,	up to heaven and sees an eagle playing around the sun.
Un aigle autour du Soleil voit s'esbattre.	

BATTLE OF WATERLOO. 18th JUNE 1815.
NAPOLEON'S 100 DAYS

This is one of Nostradamus' most fascinating quatrains. The background to the battle of Waterloo was that Blücher, the Prussian Boar, had been beaten back at Ligny and the joining up of the British and Prussian forces had therefore not been able to take place when Wellington decided to make his stand at Waterloo. This was in June, just over three months after Napoleon's return from Elba in February 1815 (*au mois troisiesme*). It may also contain a reference to Napoleon's reign of 100 days which this battle brought to an end. Equally, dating from the March solstice, which Nostradamus would have done, we are given the month of June for the date of the battle. This is a typical example of Nostradamus' convoluted style where meaning after meaning appears to be contained in one phrase. The French troops battered the English Leopard all day from sunrise to evening while Wellington waited for his ally Blücher to turn the French flank. Wellington's position was facing south so he would have seen Napoleon's Imperial eagles flying against the sun. As the day drew to a close, the British were exhausted. A cloud of dust was seen. Napoleon thought it was Grouchy, but it was Blücher. The end had come. This is a vivid and poetic quatrain of a much higher standard than most. The Imperial Eagle is often used in the Centuries as a synonym for Napoleon himself. On this occasion it refers both to the standards and to the man. Napoleon used to call the English heraldic lion the Leopard of England.

24

A cité neufue pensif pour condemner,
L'oisel de proye au ciel se vient offrir:
Apres victoire à captifs pardonner,
Cremone & Mantoue grands maux aura souffert.

At the New City he is thoughtful to condemn; the bird of prey offers himself to the gods. After victory he pardons his captives. At Cremona and Mantua great hardships will be suffered.

NAPOLEON AT VILLA NOVA, AND THE SIEGE OF MANTUA, 1796–97

During Napoleon's Italian campaigns 1795–7, he arrived at Villa Nova uncertain how to proceed, having received no orders from the Directoire in France. In June 1796 Napoleon besieged Mantua which, despite terrific bombardments, held out until February 1797. Napoleon is reputed to have treated the prisoners generously on their defeat. Cremona is situated near Mantua and must have suffered from the French invasion. Mantua's peace, however, lasted a very short time. In

1799 it was again taken by the Austrians and, although restored to the French in 1801 (Lunéville) it became Austrian again from 1814 to 1866. Cremona and Mantua both suffered severe political persecution as did the whole of Lombardy between 1849–59 after the peace of Villafranca. Note again the use of the metaphor of the bird of prey, the eagle, for Napoleon.

25

Perdu trouvé, caché de si long siecle,	The lost thing is discovered hidden for many centuries.
Sera Pasteur demi Dieu honoré:	Pasteur will be celebrated almost as a god-like figure. This
Ains que la lune acheve son grand siecle,	is when the moon completes her great cycle, but by other
Par autres vents sera deshonoré.	rumours he shall be dishonoured.

LOUIS PASTEUR, 1822–95.
FOUNDING OF INSTITUTE, 1889

Another fascinating quatrain which contains not only the name of Pasteur but also a very specific dating although not apparent at first. Pasteur's discovery that germs polluted the atmosphere was one of the most important in medical history, and led to Lister's theory of sterilization. The Encyclopaedia Britannica says that Pasteur, the 'demi-Dieu', 'was now the acknowledged head of the greatest chemical movement of the time'. He founded his Institute Pasteur on 14th November 1889; the cycle of the moon ran from 1535 to 1889. The rumours that dishonoured him may mean the violent opposition to his methods which were roused among powerful members of the Academy, against the new practices of the Institute such as vaccines against hydrophobia etc.

26

Le grand du fouldre tumbe[1]   The great man will be struck
   d'heure diurne,   down in the day by a thun-
Mal & predict par porteur postu-   derbolt. An evil deed, fore-
   laire: told by the bearer of a peti-
Suivant presage tumbe[1] d'heure   tion. According to the
   nocturne,   prediction another falls at
Conflict Reims, Londres, Etr-   night time. Conflict at Reims,
   usque pestifere.   London, and pestilence in
                                       Tuscany.

KENNEDY ASSASSINATIONS

The first three lines here may apply to the assassinations
of the two Kennedy brothers. John F. Kennedy was shot down
(thunderbolt) in broad daylight at Dallas, Texas on 22nd November 1963 by the psychopath, Lee Harvey Oswald. The
other man linked with him who is killed at night, was his
brother Robert F. Kennedy who was shot down on 5th June
1968 in the early morning while celebrating his victory in the
presidential primary elections at an hotel. Line 2, the fact that
the assassination had been told by the bearer of a petition may
refer to the many death threats John F. Kennedy and his
brother received during their terms of office. The troubles in
France, England and Italy would refer to the world repercus-
sions to these assassinations. See VIII. 46, 77, IX. 36, X. 26.

27

Dessouz de chaine[2] Guien du ciel   Beneath the oak tree of Gi-
   frappé,   enne, struck by lightning, the
Non loing de là est caché le tresor: treasure is hidden not far
Qui par longs siecles avoit esté   from there. That which for
   grappé,   many centuries had been
Trouve mourra, l'oeil crevé de   gathered, when found, a man
   ressort: will die, his eye pierced by a
                                       spring.

There are several puzzling quatrains linking the finding of a
tomb, a man dead for many centuries, and a treasure, see

[1]tumbe—tombe = fall.
[2]chaine—O.F., chene, oak tree but could possibly mean chaine = a
chain of mountains.

quatrain IX. 7, but none of them make much sense. Guienne was an ancient province of South-west France, therefore this quatrain cannot refer to the opening of Nostradamus' tomb, which was done during the Revolution when his remains were transferred to the chapel of Notre Dame in the church of St. Laurent, as Salon is not in that province. *Guien* could stand for *gui*, meaning mistletoe, which alters the first line to 'beneath the mistletoe covered oak tree etc.'. However, this gets us no further in solving the quatrain or the riddle of the spring guarding the tomb. I wonder whether the treasures could be the many antiquarian treasures of southern France, most of which were not seriously excavated until the end of the 19th Century.

28

La tour de Boucq craindra fuste[1] barbare	Tobruk will fear the barbarian fleet for a time, then much
Un temps, long temps apres barque hesperique.[2]	later the Western fleet. Cattle, people, possessions, all will be
Bestail, gens, meubles tous deux feront grand tare[3]	quite lost. What a deadly combat in Taurus and Libra.
Taurus & Libra quelle mortelle picque?[4]	

TOBRUK. SECOND WORLD WAR, 1941

It is possible that Tour de Boucq was the nearest Nostradamus could get to the place name Tobruk. The first line refers to Tobruk's chequered history as a trading port between Greeks and Libyans until the Italians became interested in it for strategic reasons. Tobruk then suffered the British invasion of 1941. Hesperique is a difficult word to interpret in the Centuries. It can mean either Western or Spanish, but I feel it cannot here mean Spain, and therefore is more applicable to America. Although it was the British Army which was fighting the Italians at Tobruk in January 1941, the attack upon Pearl Harbour occurred in November of that year in the same

---

[1]*fuste* = a low draught galley with sails and oars.
[2]*hesperique*—Spanish, Western or American.
[3]*tare* = loss.
[4]?—printers' error for *!*, if necessary at all.

month as Tobruk was retrieved, and so Hesperique can refer to the American fleet. Rommel reached Tobruk on 8th April (Taurus) and besieged it until November 1941, when it was relieved by British reinforcements. Libra is October, so Nostradamus was a month out in his calculations. Through all of 1941 Saturn and Uranus were in Taurus and this always indicates deadly combat or war.

29

Quand la poisson terrestre &
    aquatique,
Par forte vague au gravier sera
    mis:
Sa forme estrange sauve & horri-
    fique,
Par mer aux mure bien tost les
    ennemis.

When the fish that travels over both land and sea is cast up on to the shore by a great wave, its shape foreign, smooth and frightful. From the sea the enemies soon reach the walls.

POLARIS OR SUBROC

This is a perfect description of a Polaris ballistic missile fired from a submerged submarine, causing an enormous upheaval of water. Alternatively it describes the American equivalent, SUBROC, which although fired under water flies through the air to its target.

30

La nef estrange par le tourment
    marin,
Abourdera pres de port incogneu:
Nonobstant signes de rameau
    palmerin,[1]
Apres mort pille bon avis tard
    venu.

Because of the storm at sea, the foreign ship will approach an unknown port. Notwithstanding the signs of the palm branches, afterwards there is death and pillage. Good advice comes too late.

A very general quatrain. The rameau palmerin means palm branches indicating peaceful intent which is later reversed. It appears that the ship suffers the damage rather than the port, which lures it in feigning peaceful intentions.

[1]palmerin—Latin, palmarius = of a palm tree.

31

Tant d'ans les guerres en Gaule dureront	The wars in France will last for so many years beyond the reign of the Castulon kings. An uncertain victory will crown three great ones, the Eagle, the Cock, the Moon, the Lion, the Sun in its house.
Outre la course du Castalon¹ monarque:	
Victoire incerte trois grands couronneront,	
Aigle, coq, lune, lion, soleil en marque.	

DOWNFALL OF THE SPANISH MONARCHY BEFORE THE SECOND WORLD WAR

There are many ingenious interpretations offered for this quatrain concerning the French Revolutionary struggles and the Spanish Empire after the death of Charles V. It seems to indicate a great war in France after the downfall of the Spanish monarchy. Although some Spanish monarchs resigned and others were deposed, the real downfall of the monarchy must be dated from the founding of the Spanish Republic in 1923. This brings us to the 1930–40s, the period of the Second World War in which France was totally involved in *guerres en Gaule*. The three great powers who won an uncertain victory are America (Eagle), France (Cock), and Britain (Lion). The final capitulation of the Japanese which ended the war was proffered on 12th August (in Leo the Sun sign). See I. 73, which refers to the restoration of Spanish monarchy which took place during the last decade. See III. 54, IX. 16.

32

Le grand empire sera tost translaté,²	The great Empire will soon be exchanged for a small place, which soon will begin to grow. A small place of tiny area in the middle of which he will come to lay down his sceptre.
En lieu petit, qui bien tost viendra croistre:	
Lieu bien infime d'exigue comté,	
Ou au milieu viendra poser son sceptre.	

NAPOLEON I. ELBA AND ST. HELENA

The great Empire of the Imperial Napoleon (note the use of the word empire, not kingdom) is soon changed into the

---

¹*Castalon* = ancient Iberian city, standing for Spain.

²*translaté*—Latin, *translatus* = transferred, exchanged.

tiny island of Elba. However, on Napoleon's escape and the victorious 100 Days his Empire begins, but only begins, to grow again. From here he is sent to an even smaller realm of no account, St. Helena, where he finally relinquishes all claims to power. This is one of the better quatrains, succinct and moving in its simplicity. See V. 62.

33

Pres d'un grand pont de plaine spatieuse,	Near a great bridge near a spacious plain the great lion with the Imperial forces will cause a falling outside the austere city. Through fear the gates will be unlocked for him.
Le grand lion par forces Cesarees:[1]	
Fera abbattre hors cité rigoureuse,	
Par effrai portes lui seront reserées.[2]	

The austere city of line 3 is probably Geneva, home of Calvinism. The plain may be Lombardy, and the Lion the commander of the Imperial forces. But if Nostradamus hoped for the fall of Geneva through the pressures of the Holy Roman Empire he was grievously wrong. The bridge is probably to be interpreted as a mountain pass. One must remember Nostradamus' strong pro-Catholic, anti-Huguenot feelings which seem to come out periodically in the prophecies.

34

L'oiseau de proie volant à la semestre,[3]	The bird of prey flying to the left, before battle is joined with the French, he makes preparations. Some will regard him as good, others bad or uncertain. The weaker party will regard him as a good omen.
Avant conflict faict aux François pareure:[4]	
L'un bon prendra l'un ambigue sinistre,	
La partie foible tiendra par bon augure.	

[1] *Caesareus*—Latin = imperial.
[2] *reserées*—Latin, *reseratus* = unlocked.
[3] *semestre*—Latin, *sinistre* = left.
[4] *pareure*—O.F. = preparation.

HITLER AND FRANCE. *c.* 1938/40

Nostradamus is describing one of the great warmongers of all time, Hitler, as a bird of prey, which name he also gives to Napoleon. The former seems more appropriate here however. The left would mean nothing to Nostradamus other than in a geographical sense, that is the Low Countries. Hitler invaded France through Holland and Belgium having made his preparations (*pareure*) well in advance. The third line refers to the corruption and uncertainty rife among French politicians in the early days of the war, culminating in the Pétainists who accept Hitler's authority and the Vichy cabinet (*partie faible*). See II. 24, III. 35, 53, 58, 61, IV. 40, 68, V. 94, IX. 90.

35

Le lion jeune le vieux surmontera,	The young lion will overcome the older one, in a field of combat in single fight: He will pierce his eyes in their golden cage; two wounds in one, then he dies a cruel death.
En champ bellique par singulier duelle:	
Dans caige d'or les yeux lui crevera,	
Deux classes une, puis mourir, mort cruelle.	

DEATH OF HENRI II, 10th JULY 1559

This quatrain was understood in France during Nostradamus' lifetime, and was one of the verses that caused Catherine de' Medici to send for Nostradamus to interpret it. The Italian prophet Luc Gauric had warned Henri II that both the beginning and the end of his reign would be marked by a duel. The first took place soon after his accession, so it seems strange that the king did not take more care in the tournaments held in honour of the double marriage of his sister Elisabeth to Philip II of Spain, and Marguerite his daughter to the Duke of Savoy in the summer of 1559. During the festivities, which lasted for three days, the king joined in the competitions in the lists at the rue St. Antoine. He was victorious for the first two days, but on the third rode against Montgomery, the captain of the Scottish Guard. Henri failed to unseat his opponent and insisted on refighting the bout. On the third try they splintered lances successfully, but Montgomery failed to pull up his lance in time, and the splintered shaft pierced the king's gilt helmet and entered his head just above the eye. Some reports say that he suffered a second wound in the throat.

Henri's end was cruel indeed, he lay in agony for ten days before death released him. Montgomery was seven years younger than Henri who was forty when he died. Henri sometimes used the lion as his emblem. The word *classes* is understood here to come from the Green *klasis* meaning a break, or fracture, rather than the Latin *classis*, a fleet. The English ambassador to the French Court at the time, Throgmorton, wrote to Queen Elizabeth I of England about this prediction and the effect it had upon the more credulous courtiers, long before it occurred.

36

Tard le monarque se viendra re-pentir *De n'avoir mis à mort son adver-saire:* *Mais viendra bien à plus hault consentir,* *Que tout son song par mort fera deffaire.*	Too late the king will repent that he did not put his adversary to death. But he will soon come to agree to far greater things which will cause all his line to die.

HENRI III. DEATH OF GUISE BROTHERS AT BLOIS 1588. LOUIS XVI?

This is a quatrain which seems to fit two historical events equally well. The first and most probable interpretation is that it refers to Henri III and his determination to quash the influence of the Guise family in French politics. The king caused both the Duke and his brother Louis to be murdered at Blois on 25th December 1588. However he did not kill the third brother, the Duc of Mayenne, the real ringleader, and was forced to further action to eliminate their power (*à plus hault consentir*). Other commentators prefer to interpret it as describing Louis XVI and his brother and adversary, the Duke of Orléans. Certainly Orléans intrigued against the king and was a sworn enemy of the Queen, Marie Antoinette. At one point he debated joining up with the revolutionaries. Here line 3 then refers to the constitutional monarchy that Louis was forced to accept and the later imprisonment of himself and his family, leading to their deaths on the guillotine. But Louis' brother did not die, *tout son sang*: he returned to France in 1814 as Louis XVIII so this is rather a less satisfactory interpretation.

37

Un peu devant que le soleil s'excuse,	Shortly before sun set, battle is engaged. A great nation is uncertain. Overcome, the sea port makes no answer, the bridge and the grave both in foreign places.
Conflict donné grand peuple dubiteux:	
Profliges, port marin ne faict response,	
Pont & sepulchre en duex estranges lieux.	

I cannot explain this quatrain but offer these possible clues to the ingenuity of the reader. *Pont* in line 4 often stands for Pontifex, Pope, in Nostradamus. If it is so in this case, one might connect the Pope who died away from Rome in a foreign grave, with Pius VI, who died at Valence in 1799, captured by the French. His death occurred in August so could the first line mean the summer? The French nation were still *dubiteux* in 1799; the Directoire had suffered defeats both in Italy and Germany and Napoleon's Egyptian campaign was by no means completed. I can only suggest a reference to French naval action in Egypt for line 3; it cannot refer to the British fleet which were scouring the seas for Napoleon's ships.

38

Le sol & l'aigle au victeur paroistront	The Sun and the Eagle will appear to the victor. An empty answer is assured to the defeated. Neither bugle nor shouts will stop the soldiers. Liberty and peace, if achieved in time through death.
Response vaine au vaincu l'on asseure:	
Par cor ne cris harnois n'arresteront,	
Vindicte paix par mors si acheve à l'heure.	

WATERLOO, 1815

This quatrain probably followed on I. 23 in the original. It continues the vivid description of Waterloo with Napoleon, the Imperial Eagle, coming out of the mist into the sun to attack the victor, Wellington. Both sides knew this was a fight to the finish, but for Napoleon it was the final stand after the frantic 100 Days. No reasonable terms awaited him if he lost (*response vaine*), nothing but life exile on St. Helena. Once the men joined in battle they could not be stopped. Napoleon's Grenadiers fought until the last man dropped, and refused to retreat. Freedom and peace can once again come to Europe, but only by means of the bloody slaughter of battle, and possibly also Napoleon's end, his political, if not actual, death.

39

De nuict dans lict le suspresme[1] *estrangle,*	At night the last one will be strangled in his bed because
Par trop avoir sejourné, blond esleu:	he became too involved with the blond heir elect. The Em-
Par trois l'empire subrogé[2] *exanche,*[3]	pire is enslaved and three men substituted. He is put to
A mort mettra carte, et pacquet ne leu.[4].	death with neither letter nor packet read.

DEATH OF LOUIS BOURBON CONDÉ, 1830

The last of the Condés, Louis, was found strangled one night in 1830, not however in his bed, but hanging in his bedroom. He was probably murdered for the support he gave to the cause of the Duke of Bordeaux, the Comte de Chambord, whom Nostradamus rightly describes as *esleu* as he was the grandson of Charles X and heir to the French throne. The three who usurped power can be interpreted either as the three regimes which followed Charles X, Louis Philippe, the Republic and then the Bonapartes, or it could refer more specifically to the three men who intrigued against the Condé family, Charles X, the Duke of Angoulême and the Duke of Bourgogne. Le Pelletier says that Condé was fair-haired and had written a will (*carte et pacquet*) in favour of the Duke of Bordeaux. This is said to have been replaced by an earlier will written in favour of the Duke of Aumale, son of Louis Philippe who became king in 1830.

[1]*supresme* = either great or last, both meanings possible here.
[2]*subrogé*—Latin, *subrogatus* = substitute.
[3]*exanche*—Latin, *exancilatus* = enslaved.
[4]*leu.*—O.F., lu = read.

40

La trombe[1] *fausse dissimulant folie,*	The false trumpet concealing madness will cause Byzantium to change its laws. From Egypt there will go forth a man who wants the edict withdrawn, changing money and standards.
Fera Biscance[2] *un changement de loix:*	
Istra d'Egypte qui veut que l'on deslie,	
Edict changeant monnaies & alois[3].	

PRESIDENT SADAT AND IRAN 1979

The false trumpet of this quatrain seems remarkably like a reference to Ayatollah Khomeini calling the faithful to prayer from top of a mosque. The false trumpet almost certainly refers to the 1979 She'it Muslim Revival which caused a Middle Eastern country, probably Iran, to change its laws. This has certainly happened and the country is now in a state of anarchy. President Sadat of Egypt has tried to intervene and defuse the situation, the "edict". The changing money and standards presumably refer to Iran's wealth gained from its oil and the general political situation and power it had gained in the Middle East.

41

Seige en cité est de nuict assaillie,	The city is besieged and assaulted by night; few have escaped; a battle not far from the sea. A woman faints with joy at the return of her son, poison in the folds of the hidden letters.
Peu eschapés non loin de mer conflict:	
Femme de joie,[4] *retours fils defaillie,*	
Poison & lettres cachees dans le plic.	

This quatrain has been given many explanations by commentators who either refer it to the French invasion of Italy in 1556–57 or even to Dunkirk, 1940, where the Third Republic becomes the woman, the prostitute, and the poison the constitution (*lettres*) of the Nazi doctrines. None of these appears at all convincing.

[1] *trombe*—Misprint, *trompe* = trumpet.
[2] *Bisance* = Byzantium.
[3] *alois* = alloy, standard (of metal).
[4] *Femme de joie*—either a woman (fainting) with joy, or a prostitute.

42

Le dix Kalende[1] *d'Avril de faict Gothique,*	The tenth day of the April Calends, calculated in Gothic
Resuscité encor par gens malins:	fashion is revived again by wicked people. The fire is put
Le feu estainct assemblé diabolique,	out and the diabolic gathering seek the bones of the de-
Cherchant les os du d'Amant & Pselin.	mon of Psellus.

INSTITUTION OF THE GREGORIAN CALENDAR SYSTEM, 1582. DIVINATION

It is believed that the last line should read '*cherchant les os du Demon et Psellus*', but that Nostradamus suppressed it for fear that the authorities might accuse him of magic practices. There is a description of a similar evocation of spirits in Michael Psellus' book *De Demonibus*. Nostradamus seems to have understood the change of the Calendar from the old style to the Gregorian system, which took place (after his death) in 1582. The tenth day of the Calends of April would be 10th April, as the Calend was the first day of the Roman month. When the Gregorian system was introduced ten days were removed, so possibly Nostradamus means 1st April, new style. Good Friday was regarded as the best day for magical evocations, and it is possible that Nostradamus is implying that this was the day on which he started using these methods to inspire the Prophecies. Psellus mentions the use of a bowl of water 'which seems to boil over and a faint voice murmurs words which contain the revelation of future events'. Nostradamus may therefore have begun writing the Prophecies on a Good Friday which fell on 10th April, old style.

43

Avant qu'advienne le changement d'Empire	Before the Empire changes a very wonderful event will take
Il adviendra un cas bien merveilleux:	place. The field moved, the pillar of porphyry put in place,
Un champ mué, le pillier de pophire[2]	changed on the gnarled rock.
Mis translaté sur le rocher noilleux.	

---

[1]*Kalende*—Calend = 1st day of Roman month.
[2]*pophire* = porphyry—a type of red or white crystallized feldspar.

Line 1 probably places this quatrain after 1789 because of the word 'Empire'. There is another reference to a pillar of porphyry in IX. 32, but I cannot interpret the meaning of the pillar.

44

En bref seront de retour sacri-fices,	In a short time sacrifices will be resumed, those opposed will be put (to death) like martyrs. There will no longer be monks, abbots or novices. Honey shall be far more expensive than wax.
Contrevenans seront mis à mar-tyre:	
Plus ne seront moines, abbez, ne novices,	
Le miel sera beaucoup plus cher que cire.	

THE CULT OF REASON, 10th NOVEMBER 1793. ABOLITION OF CLERGY

The French Revolutionary government abolished the worship of God in 1793. The sacrifices in line 1 mean a restoration of paganism. On 10th November the Cult of Reason was established and in 1794 this was followed by a Festival of the Supreme Being, 8th June. The Constitution of 1790 declared the dissolution of the Clergy (no more monks) and of ecclesiastical orders. Many who refused to embrace the new ideology were persecuted, and all priests who refused to accept the Civil Constitution of the Clergy were expelled. The last line is a generalization implying that lack of demand for beeswax for church candles makes its price less than that of the honey it holds, a new state of affairs in France.

45

Secteur de sectes grand peine au delateur,	A founder of sects, much trouble for the accuser: A beast in the theatre prepares the scene and the plot. The author ennobled by acts of older times; the world is confused by schismatic sects.
Beste en theatre, dresse le jeu scenique,	
Du faict antique ennobly l'inven-teur,	
Par sectes monde confus & schis-matique.	

This is probably a tirade against Calvinism, like I. 33.

46

Tout aupres d'Aux, de Lestoure & Mirande,	Very near Auch, Lectoure and Mirande a great fire will
Grand feu du ciel en trois nuicts tumbera:	fall from the sky for three nights. The cause will appear
Cause adviendra bien stupende & mirande,	both stupefying and marvellous, shortly afterwards there
Bien peu aupres la terre tremblera.	will be an earthquake.

All three towns mentioned are in the Departement of Gers in South-Western France. Perhaps Nostradamus is referring to a hail of meteorites, which make the earth tremble, or which are followed by a minor earthquake?

47

Du lac Leman[1] *les sermons fascheront,*	The speeches of Lake Leman will become angered, the days
Les Jours seront reduicts par les sepmaines:[2]	will drag out into weeks, then months, then years, then all
Puis mois, puis an, puis tous defailliront,	will fail. The authorities will condemn their useless pow-
Les magistrats damneront leurs loix vaines.	ers.

LEAGUE OF NATIONS, 1919–47

Geneva was important as the setting of the League of Nations whose first assembly was held there on 15th November 1920. The quatrain describes vividly the years of fruitless argument and failure until the final formal disbandment after the war in August 1947, although in fact it ceased to be effective after early 1940. See also V. 85.

[1]*Leman* = Lake Geneva.
[2]*sepmaines—semaines* = weeks.

48

Vingt ans du regne de la lune passez,	When twenty years of the Moon's reign have passed an-
Sept mil ans autre tiendra sa monarche:	other will take up his reign for seven thousand years. When
Quand le Soleil prendra ses jours lassez,	the exhausted Sun takes up his cycle then my prophecy
Lors accomplit & mine ma prophetie.	and threats will be accomplished.

DATE OF PUBLICATION AND COMPLETION OF PROPHECIES

According to Roussat the cycle of the Moon lasted from 1535–1889, which places the date of the first line as 1555, the publication date of the first part of the Centuries. Nostradamus seems to envisage another 7,000 years from that date to the cycle of the sun when all will be accomplished. According to astrologers we have now entered the reign of Aquarius. This quatrain is interesting in that it gives the date of publication and associates this with the completion of the Prophecies. It is as though Nostradamus believes the Centuries are written at the start of a new era lasting 7,000 years. It was a commonly held theory in the Middle Ages that the world would come to an end at the beginning of the seventh millennium. This information originated from the book of Enoch which was general reading during the first and second centuries but removed by the Church from the Canon in AD 300. Nostradamus also refers to 7,000 years in quatrain X. 74, but no commentator is able to agree on the date from which to start calculating, and this theory does not agree with the statements of some of the other prophecies.

49

Beaucoup avant telles menees,	Long before these happen-
Ceux d'Orient par la vertu lunaire:	ings the people of the East, influenced by the Moon, in
L'an mil sept cens feront grands emmenees,	the year 1700 will cause many to be carried away, and will
Subjugant presque le coing Aquilonaire.[1]	almost subdue the Northern area.

[1]Aquilonaire—Latin, aquilonaris = northern.

EVENTS AROUND 1700

The astrologer Roussat also believed the years 1700–2 would show the start of great upheavals, but this seems a prophecy where both he and Nostradamus are wrong. It could apply to various invasions in the North (*Aquilonaire*). In February 1700, August II invaded Livania. Peter the Great took Azov and Kouban from the Turks; Charles XII occupied Iceland and Peter the Great then declared war on Sweden, but none of these actions reduced the North sufficiently in the sense Nostradamus means it.

50

De l'aquatique triplicité¹ naistra.	From the three water signs
D'un qui fera le jeudi pour sa feste:	will be born a man who will celebrate Thursday as his holiday. His renown, praise, rule
Son bruit, loz,² regne, sa puissance coistra,	and power will grow on land
Par terre & mer aux Oriens tempeste.	and sea, bringing trouble to the East.

AYATOLLAH KHOMEINI AND THE THIRD ANTICHRIST

This describes a person with the three water signs of Pisces, Cancer and Scorpio dominant in his birth chart, presumably not a Christian, "jeudi pour sa feste", whose power becomes so great that he brings trouble to countries in the East, as the Ayatollah has done. It may refer to the Third Antichrist. It is also interesting to note that Kaiser Wilhelm II, 1959–1941, who started World War I had in his ascendent Cancer in midheaven, Pisces in his birth sign, with the moon in Scorpio. See II. 5, 62, 89, IV. 50, VI. 33, VIII. 77, X. 66, 72, 75.

51

Chef d'Aries, Jupiter & Saturne,	The head of Aries, Jupiter
Dieu eternel quelles mutations?³	and Saturn. Eternal God, what changes! Then the bad times
Puis par long siecle son maling⁴ temps retourne	will return again after a long century; what turmoil in
Gaule, & Italie quelles emotions?	France and Italy.

¹*aquatique triplicité* = the three water signs of the Zodiac.
²*loz*—Latin, *laus* = praise.
³?printers' error for *!*
⁴*maling*—*malin*, old spelling.

POSSIBLE WAR IN 1995

The conjuntion of Jupiter and Saturn in Aries took place on 13th December 1702 during the War of the Spanish Succession under Louis XIV. The great changes of line 2 are the French Revolution which will occur before the century mentioned in line 3 is completed. By 1802 France is embroiled in the Italian campaign and it was in January of that year that Napoleon was declared President of the Italian Republic. The next time this conjunction occurs will be 2nd September 1995.

52

Les deux malins de Scorpion conjoinct,	Two evil influences in conjunction in Scorpio. The great lord is murdered in his room. A newly appointed king persecutes the Church, the lower (parts of) Europe and in the North.
Le grand seifneur meutri dedans sa salle:	
Pesta á l'Eglise par le nouveau roy joinct	
L'Europe basse & Septentrionale.	

DEATH OF SULTAN SELIM III 1807/8, AND NAPOLEON'S CONQUESTS

The last time that these evil influences occurred were in 1867 when Mars and Saturn were in Scorpio and when the Emperor Maximillian was shot. In 1886 Prussia attacked Austria.

53

Las qu'on verra grand peuple tourmenté,	Alas, how we will see a great nation sorely troubled and the holy law in utter ruin. Christianity (governed) throughout by other laws, when a new source of gold and silver is discovered.
Par la loi saincte en totale ruine:	
Par auttres loix toute la Chrestienté,	
Quand d'or, d'argent trouve nouvelle mine.	

DISESTABLISHMENT OF CLERGY 1790.
CREATION OF ASSIGNATS 1789

This quatrain again tells of the disestablishment of the French Clergy, 14th July 1790, and of its subsequent persecution during the Revolution. The laws other than Christian that governed France were those of the Cult of Reason, see quatrain I. 44. The last line is interesting. In 1789 the National Assembly passed a decree on 19th December creating an issue of 400 million assignats. This currency was in fact based on the confiscated goods of the clergy which were used as security for the notes, and was certainly a new source of wealth on which the country could draw.

54

Deux revolts faicte du maling[1] *falcigere,*[2]	Two revolutions will be caused by the evil scythe bearer mak-
De regne & siecles faict permu- tation:	ing a change of reign and centuries. The mobile sign thus
Le mobil signe[3] *à son endroit si ingere,*[4]	moves into its house: equal in favour to both sides.
Aux deux egaux & d'inclination.	

TWO REVOLUTIONS AND WAR
STARTING IN AUSTRIA

The evil scythe bearer is Saturn, and the two great Revolutions occurring in different centuries due to his malign influence are of course the French Revolution at the end of the 18th Century and the Russian Revolution in the early 20th Century. The mobile sign is Libra, the Balance, which governs Austria according to the astrologers. Apparently the influence of Libra was not strong enough to tip the balance in favour of Austria (*aux deux egaux*) and so the malign influence of Saturn is able to cause war in that country following on the second revolution. Nostradamus is referring to the assassination of the Arch Duke Ferdinand at Sarajevo, 1914, and its consequence, the First World War. See I. 51.

[1] *maling*—O.F. spelling = malin.
[2] *falcigere*—Latin, *falcam gerens* = bearing a scythe; the scythe was a sign of Saturn.
[3] Libra = the balance.
[4] *ingere*—Latin, *ingerere (se)* = to enter, penetrate. The *si* may be a misprint for *se*.

55

Soubs l'opposite climat Babylo- nique, *Grand sera de sang effusion:* *Que terre & mer, air, ciel sera* *inique,* *Sectes, faim, regnes, pestes, con- fusion.*	In the land with a climate op- posite to Babylon there will be great shedding of blood. Heaven will seem unjust both on land and sea and in the air. Sects, famine, kingdoms, plagues, confusion.

POSSIBLE HOLY WAR IN THE 20TH CENTURY

The land opposite to that of the climate of Babylon is almost certainly Russia, a land of snow and ice. Babylon stands for the Middle East and the quatrain refers to a battle between these two. The Middle Eastern country could possibly be Iran. This quatrain is definitely dated as being in the 20th Century because of the reference to air travel in line three. In August 1980 the Arabs declared that a Holy War against Israel was a strong possibility.

56

Vous verrez tost & tard faire *grand change,* *Horreurs extremes, & vindica- tions:* *Que si la lune conduicte par son* *ange,* *Le ciel s'approche des inclina- tions.*	Sooner and later you will see great changes made, dreadful horrors and vengeances. For as the moon is thus led by its angel the heavens draw near to the Balance.

Another astrological quatrain promising disaster in Libra, either the country, Austria, or using the sign as a date. It may follow on from the last verse, 1. 54, 55.

57

Par grand discord la trombe¹ *tremblera* *Accord rompu dressant la teste au* *ciel:* *Bouche sanglante dans le sang* *nagera,* *Au sol la face ointe² de laict &* *miel.*	The trumpet shakes with great discord. An agreement bro- ken: lifting the face to heaven: the bloody mouth will swim with blood; the face anointed with milk and honey lies on the ground.

¹*trombe = trompe,* trumpet.
²*ointe*—Latin, *unctus* = anointed.

EXECUTION OF LOUIS XVI.
21st JANUARY 1793

In 1793 amidst the horrors and discords of the Revolution
Louis XVI accepted the constitution decreed by the National
Assembly, (*accord rompu*). As Louis went to his execution he is
recorded as having recited the Third Psalm—*exaltus caput meum*
(*dressant la tête*). When a victim is guillotined the blood rushes
out through the mouth of the corpse. Nostradamus is nothing
if not meticulous about detail. Louis is described as anointed
with milk and honey because he was actually so anointed as
part of the coronation service. See also VI. 89.

58

Tranché le ventre, naistra avec deux testes,
Et quatre bras: quelques ans entiers vivra:
Jour qui Alquiloie[1] celebrera ses festes,
Fossen, Turin, chef Ferrare suivra.

Through a slit in the belly a creature will be born with two heads and four arms: it will survive for some few years. The day that Alquiloie celebrates his festivals, Fossana, Turin and the ruler of Ferrara will follow.

NAPOLEON AND THE BOURBONS

This is an involved quatrain dealing with both Napoleon
and the Bourbon family. It is possible to interpret the first line
literally as a Caesarian section, but it is more likely to refer to
Louis XVI as the belly. *Tranche* is the same adjective that Nostradamus uses for the king's death elsewhere, from whom
come the two comparatively short ruling heirs, Louis XVIII
and Charles X (*duex testes*). The four arms are understood to
be the Dukes of Angoulême, Normandy, Berry and Bordeaux.
Alquiloie, the rule of the Eagle, connects them with Napoleon
by whom the family was deposed, and the ruler of Ferrare was
the Pope who 'followed' Napoleon back to France as a prisoner;
the rest of Italy Fossana and Turin followed metaphorically,
in that they were captured by the French. This is one of the
quatrains in which Nostradamus has reversed the time sequence.

[1]*Alquiloie* = (*a*) *Aquila lex*, the rule of the eagle. (*b*) *Aquilene*, one of
the great cities of the Roman Empire.

59

Les exilez deportez dans les isles,	The exiles deported to the is-
Au changement d'un plus cruel	lands at the advent of an even
monarque	more cruel king will be mur-
Seront meurtris:[1] *& mis deux les*	dered. Two will be burnt who
scintiles,[2]	were not sparing in their
Qui de parler ne seront estez	speech.
parques.[3]	

Nicollaud ascribes this to the events of the Coup d'Etat in 1857, when many members of French secret societies were deported to the Cayenne Islands. The new king was Napoleon III, who caused people who spoke against the regime (*ne seront estez parques de parler*) to be imprisoned and deported. All the lines fit, but I am not convinced by the interpretation. Some commentators, such as Roberts, ascribe it to the cremation of the Jews, but this is impossible if one reads the line (*mis deux les scintiles*); not even Nostradamus would reduce six million tragedies to two.

60

Un Empereur naistra pres d'Italie	An Emperor will be born near
Qui à l'Empire sera vendu bien	Italy, who will cost the Empire
cher:	very dearly. They will say,
Diront avec quels gens il se ralie,	when they see his allies, that
Qu'on trouvera moins prince que	he is less a prince than a
boucher.	butcher.

NAPOLEON I, 1769–1821

This is one of the famous quatrains predicting Napoleon, the Emperor born near Italy in Corsica. He cost France dearly in both manpower and strength. The third line may be a reference to the Creole origins of his first wife, Josephine, or to his own brothers whom he raised to positions of great honour, kings of Naples and Spain, Holland and Westphalia. The reference to butchery also covers the enormous number of men who died in the Napoleonic campaigns.

[1]*meutrir*—O.F. = to kill.
[2]*scintiles*—Latin, *scintilla* = sparks, flames.
[3]*parques*—Latin, *parcus* = sparing, economic.

61

La republique miserable infelice[1]	The wretched, unfortunate
Sera vastee[2] *de nouveau magis-*	republic will again be ruined
trat:	by a new authority. The great
Leur grand amas de l'exile male-	amount of ill will accumu-
fice,	lated in exile will make the
Fera Sueve[3] *ravir leur grand*	Swiss break their important
contract.	agreement.

SWISS BANK NEUTRALITY BROKEN

After Germany's downfall, after the Second World War, the Swiss Banks (Latin, Suevi, meaning Swiss) will have to break the code of neutrality operated by their banks since they were founded. They will be forced to open up their accounts to inspection. These accounts may well refer to German monies amassed during the war linking up with lines 1 and 2. Certainly, they are now being forced to reveal some of their secrets.

62

La grande parte las que feront les	Alas! what a great loss there
lettres,	will be to learning before the
Avant la cycle de Latona[4] *par-*	cycle of the Moon is com-
faict:	pleted. Fire, great floods, by
Feu grand deluge plus par ig-	more ignorant rulers; how
nares sceptres,	long the centuries until it is
Que de long siecle ne se verra	seen to be restored.
refaict.	

1889

Nostradamus visualizes scholarship as suffering a great loss before the end of the Moon's cycle (1889). This may be open to two interpretations. First, that a work of scholarship becomes lost before that date, and reappears after many calamities after a century or so (*de long siecle*); second, a more general meaning that Nostradamus regarded scholarship as becoming vulgarized by the changing of scholastic standards and its

---

[1]*infelice*—Latin, *infelix* = unhappy.
[2]*vastee*—Latin, *vastatus* = ruined devastated.
[3]*Sueve*—Suevi = German Swiss tribe.
[4]*Latona* = mythological mother of Apollo and Diana; the Moon.

availability to what he would have called the common people. Like all scholars of his time, Nostradamus regarded himself as one of an élite.

63

Les fleurs[1] *passés diminue le monde,*	Pestilences extinguished, the world becomes smaller, for a long time the lands will be inhabited peacefully. People will travel safely through the sky (over) land and seas: then wars will start up again.
Long temps la paix terres inhabitées:	
Seur marchera par ciel, serre, mer & onde:	
Puis de nouveau les guerres suscitées.	

AIR TRAVEL FOLLOWED BY WAR
20th CENTURY

Nostradamus envisages a century in which the world becomes smaller because people can travel peacefully over land, sea and through the air. This gives us the 20th Century again. "The extinguished pestilence" may refer to disease or war. We should remember the many medical discoveries of this century, anti-biotics, the pill, etc. and realize that these words may refer to both. But war breaks out again after a long interlude of peace. This may refer to the third great war of this century. See re. air travel, I. 55, 64. II. 29. III. 69.

64

De nuict soleil penseront avoir veu,	At night they will think they have seen the sun, when they see the half pig man: Noise, screams, battles seen fought in the skies. The brute beasts will be heard to speak.
Quand le pourceau demi-homme on verra:	
Bruict, chant, bataille, au ciel battre aperceu:	
Et bestes brutes à parler lon orra.	

AIR BATTLE. 20th CENTURY

This seemingly nonsensical quatrain is one of the most interesting. Nostradamus describes a vivid picture of a battle in the air. The sun, appearing at night, is the searchlight piercing the sky, or possibly bombs exploding. The pig-like man, which

[1]*fleurs*—read *fléaux* = plague, pestilence.

no commentator to date has ever deciphered, seems a clear picture in silhouette of the pilot in oxygen mask, helmet and goggles. The oxygen breathing apparatus would look just like a pig's snout to Nostradamus. The air battle is a remarkable enough description for the 16th Century, and the screams may be the sound of the dropping bombs as they whine to earth. The battle is watched by people on the ground (*aperceu*) and it is important to understand the wording of the last line. The pilots (*brutes bestes*) are heard talking to others; could this be a forecast of radio? This quatrain convinces me that Nostradamus' inspiration was certainly partly visual and he describes as best he can in his limited vocabulary the puzzling glimpses of a future he didn't always understand.

65

Enfant sans mains jamais veu si grand foudre,	A child without hands, never so great a thunderbolt seen,
L'enfant royal au feu d'oesteuf blessé:	the royal child wounded at a game of tennis. At the well
Au pui¹ brises² fulgures³ allant mouldre,	lightning strikes, joining together three trussed up in the
Trois souz les chaines⁴ par le milieu troussés.⁵	middle under the oaks.

A definite quatrain about a specific event and a deformed royal child which has not been realized to date.

66

Celui qui lors portera les nouvelles,	He who then carries the news, after a short while will (stop)
Apres un peu il viendra respirer	to breathe: Viviers, Tournon,
Viviers, Tournon, Montferrand & Pradelles,	Montferrand and Pradelles; hail and storms will make
Gresle & tempestes les fera soupirer.	them grieve.

¹*pui*—well, or possible O.F. *puy* = hill? It does not help to interpret the quatrain.
²*brises*—O.F., *briser* = to fracture, break.
³*fulgures*—Latin, *fulgur* = flash of lightning.
⁴*chaines*—Either oak tree or *chaine* = chain of hills.
⁵*troussés*—Some interpreters translate this as carry off.

67

La grande famine que je sens ap-
  procher,
Souvent tourner, puis estre uni-
  verselle:
Si grand & long qu'un viendra
  arracher,
Du bois racine & l'enfant de ma-
  melle.

The great famine which I
sense approaching will often
turn (in various areas) then
become world wide. It will be
so vast and long lasting that
(they) will grab roots from the
trees and children from the
breast.

WORLD FAMINE

The shortage of food throughout the world and particularly
in the underdeveloped countries seems clear to Nostradamus.
He describes local famines, however dreadful, whether those
of France, 1709, Ireland, 1846, Biafra, 1969, India, 1971, as
appearing small in comparison with the problem of world hunger which will develop and become universal. See I. 16, 67,
II. 75, III. 34, 42.

68

O quel horrible & malheureux
  tourment,
Trois innocens qu'on viendra à
  livrer:
Poison suspecte, mal garde tra-
  diment,[1]
Mis en horreur par bourreaux
  envirez.

O to what a dreadful and
wretched torment are three
innocent people going to be
delivered. Poison suggested,
badly guarded, betrayal. Delivered up to horror by drun-
ken executioners.

69

La grand montaigne ronde de
  sept stades,[2]
Apres paix, guerre, faim, innon-
  dation:
Roulera loin abismant grands
  contrades,[3]
Mesmes antiques, & grand fon-
  dation.

The great mountain, seven
stadia round, after peace, war,
famine, flooding. It will spread
far, drowning great coun-
tries, even antiquities and their
mighty foundations.

[1]*tradiment*—O.F. = treason, betrayal.

[2]*stade*—Latin, *stadium* = measure roughly a furlong in length, seven
stades would be just under a mile in circumference.

[3]*contrades*—Provençal, *contrada* = country.

This probably describes a flood in southern France which may reveal many Graeco-Roman archaeological treasures sited somewhere near a mountain. Sites such as Glanum near the mountains of Les Beaux, very near Salon, may be indicated.

70

Plui, faim, guerre en Perse non cessée,	Rain, famine and war will not cease in Persia; too great a
La foi trop grand trahira le monarque:	trust will betray the monarch. Those (actions) started in
Par la finie en Gaule commencee,	France will end there, a secret
Secret augure pour à un estre parque.	sign for one to be sparing.

1979 EXILE OF SHAH THROUGH AYATOLLAH KHOMEINI

This is an amazing quatrain by any standards. Politicians could not have conceived of it in 1978, yet alone 1568. The monarch, the Shah of Persia, now Iran, will lose his grip on his kingdom partly through rain, famine and war. But as Nostradamus states the war was started in France, in Paris, in fact, where the Ayatollah Khomeini remained plotting his downfall. The secret sign for one to be sparing is difficult to interpret but certainly the Ayatollah's régime is extremely Spartan in its concept. See III. 47, 95.

71

La tour marine trois fois prise & reprise,	The marine tower will be captured and retaken three times
Par Hespagnols, Barbares, Ligurins:[1]	by Spaniards, Barbarians and Ligurians. Marseilles and Aix,
Marseilles & Aix, Arles par ceux de Pise,	Arles, by men of Pisa, devastation, fire, sword, pillage at
Vast,[2] feu, fer, pillé Avignon des Thurins.	Avignon by the Turinese.

This is an irritating quatrain because it appears to be indecipherable despite all the proper names given. The main prob-

---

[1]*Ligurins* = people of Liguria in Italy.
[2]*vast*—Latin, *vastus* = laid waste.

lem is the identity of the marine tower, which could then be related to conflict between the French and the Italians. Could it refer to the Tour de Bouq I. 78.?

72

De tout Marseille des habitants changee,	The inhabitants of Marseilles completely changed, fleeing
Course & poursuitte jusqu'au pres de Lyon,	and pursued as far as Lyons. Narbonne, Toulouse angered
Narbon Tholoze par Bordeaux outragee,	by Bordeaux; the killed and captive are almost one mil-
Tuez captifs presque d'un million.	lion.

FRENCH CASUALTIES. SECOND
WORLD WAR

The enormous number of dead places this quatrain in modern times, possibly in the last war, for which the official casualty lists give a figure of 675,000 Frenchmen dead or wounded. This sum does not include the Allies who fought alongside the French, so Nostradamus' total may be nearer the mark. When the German army entered Paris, June 1940, the French Government fled to Bordeaux. Narbonne, Toulouse and Lyons were all cities under the puppet Vichy régime. Marseilles, under German occupation, certainly had its *habitants changees*.

73

France à cinq pars[1] par neglect assaille,[2]	France shall be accused of neglect by her five partners.
Tunis, Argel[3] esmuez par Persiens:	Tunis, Algiers stirred up by the Persians. Leon, Seville and
Leon, Seville, Barcelonne faille	Barcelona having failed, they
N'aura la classe[4] par les Venetiens.	will not have the fleet because of the Venetians.

[1]*pars*—Used throughout Nostradamus to mean partner, rather than part. *See* IX. 20.

[2]*assaillir*—Literally assault. France has only been attacked on five sides once in 1813/4 and then by the European allies.

[3]*Argel*—Anagram or misprint for Alger = Algiers.

[4]*classe*—Latin, *classis* = fleet.

TROUBLE IN MIDDLE EAST
FROM IRAN

France is accused of neglect by her partner. She has recently broken the Common Market rules concerning the import of lamb and has angered her partners in 1979/80. Nostradamus relates this to trouble in Africa stirred up by the Iranians (Persians). This is an interesting reference to Iran's relationship with USSR again, because in his day Iran was part of the Ottoman Empire, an area of which is now a part of Russia. So, by implication, the Soviets are involved in the Middle Eastern troubles whether they like it or not. Perhaps this is another reference to Iran being invaded from the North at winter time?

74

Apres sejourné vogueront en Epire	After a rest they will travel to
Le grand secours viendra vers Antioch:	Epirus, great help coming from around Antioch. The
Le noir¹ poil crespe tendra fort à l'Empire,	curly haired king will strive greatly for the Empire, the
Barbe d'aerain se roustira en broche.	brazen beard will be roasted on a spit.

Both Epirus and Antioch were part of the Turkish Empire until the 19th Century. As the footnote states, '*noir*' is continually used as an anagram of '*roi*', king, in the Centuries. This dark-haired king recurs in other quatrains as does the red-bearded man. There was a family of Algerian corsairs named Barbarossa, whose plunderings were contemporary to Nostradamus. Other commentators refer this to Philip II of Spain who had a blondish beard, but his enigmatic fate is incomprehensible.

75

Le tyran Sienne occupera Savone,	The tyrant of Siena will occupy Savona, having won the
Le fort gaigné tiendra classe marine:	fort he will restrain the marine fleet. Two armies under
Les deux armees par la marque d'Anconne,	the standard of Ancona: the leader will examine them in
Par effrayeur le chef s'en examine.	fear.

¹ *noir*—Anagram for *roi*. IX. 20 etc.

Siena was a free town and held out with French help against
the Florentine states until April 1555. Savona was a protectorate of the Genoese Republic, and Ancona was part of the
Papal States.

76

D'un nom farouche tel proferé sera,	This man will be called by a barbaric name that three sis-
Que les trois soeurs[1] auront fato[2] le nom:	ters will receive from destiny. He will speak then to a great
Puis grand peuple par langue & faict dira	people in words and deeds, more than any other will have
Plus que nul autre aura bruit & renom.	fame and renown.

NAPOLEON I

This verse is always interpreted as fitting Bonaparte, because of the derivation of his name from the Greek NEA-
POLLUON, which means destroyer or exterminator. The
name was still spelt in this way during his lifetime, as the
inscription of 1805 in the Place Vendôme shows, NEAPOLIO.
IMP AUG. Napoleon was barbaric in a more general sense,
being the younger son of a Corsican family whose language
and standards were not those of Parisian society. He was also
renowned for the great speeches made to his troops (*par langue
dira*) before battle.

77

Entre duex mers dressera promontoire,	A promontory stands be- tween two seas: A man who
Que plus mourra par le mords du cheval:	will die later by the bit of a horse; Neptune unfurls a black
Le sien Neptune pliera voille noire,	sail for his man; the fleet near Gibraltar and the Rocheval.
Par Calpre & classe aupres de Rocheval.	

[1]The three Fates. In classical mythology they spin the web of a
man's destiny.
[2]*fato*—Latin, *fatum* = fate, destiny.

BATTLE OF TRAFALGAR, 1805

The promontory separating the seas is Gibraltar between the Mediterranean and the Atlantic. The French and English fleets fought the battle of Trafalgar between Gibraltar and Cape Roche (Rocheval), Trafalgar itself being a point between two bays. The leader of the French fleet, Admiral Villeneuve, was reputedly strangled by one of Napoleon's Mamelukes with the bridle of a horse at an inn in Rennes in 1806, when he returned to France having been taken prisoner by the English. When Nelson was mortally wounded his ship raised a black sail on its return voyage to England. Rocheval may just be an anagram for *roche*, rock, which is the name given to mean Gibraltar.

78

D'un chef viellard naistra sens hebeté	To an old leader will be born an idiot heir, weak both in
Degenerant par savoir & par armes:	knowledge and in war. The leader of France is feared by
Le chef de France par sa soeur redouté,	his sister, battlefields divided, conceded to the soldiers.
Champs divisez, concedez aux gendarmes.	

This has been referred to Marshal Pétain, who took over the government of France from Reynaud in 1940, but the sister is unsatisfactory and the whole quatrain too general.

79

Bazaz, Lestore, Condon, Ausch, Agine,	Bazas, Lectoure, Condom, Auch and Agen are troubled
Esmens par loix querelle & monopole:	by laws, disputes and monopolies. Carcasonne, Bor-
Car[1] Bourd, Toulouze Bay[2] mettra en ruine.	deaux, Toulouse and Bayonne will be ruined when they
Renouveller voulant leur tauropole.[3]	wish to renew the massacre.

[1]*Car*—Either apocope or Carcassonne, or *car* = because.
[2]*Bay*—Bayonne, as above.
[3]*tauropole*—Latin, *Taurobolium* = sacrifice of a bull; metaphorically, massacre, slaughter.

All these towns are in the south-west of France. It may contain
a reference to a trading dispute and the granting of rights to
monopolies in the locality. The massacre or sacrifice is unclear.

80

De la sixieme claire splendeur ce-leste,	From the sixth bright celestial light it will come to thunder very strongly in Burgundy. Then a monster will be born of a very hideous beast: In March, April, May and June great wounding and worrying.
Viendra tonner si fort en la Bour-gongne:	
Puis naistra monstre de treshi-deuse beste,	
Mars, Avril, Mai, Juin grand charpin[1] & rongne.	

Saturn being the sixth planet, apparently these portents will
occur during the time governed by him. Some commentators
date it as spring 1918.

81

D'humain troupeau neuf seront mis à part,	Nine will be set apart from the human flock, separated from judgment and advice. Their fate is to be divided as they depart. K. Th. L. dead, banished and scattered.
De jugement & conseil separez:	
Leur sort sera divisé en depart,	
Kappa,[2] Thita,[3] Lamda,[4] mors bannis esgarez.	

This has been applied by at least one commentator to the death
of the three Soviet cosmonauts. It is very obscure.

82

Quand les colomnes de bois grande tremblee,	When the great wooden columns tremble in the south wind, covered with blood. Such a great assembly then pours forth that Vienna and the land of Austria will tremble.
D'Auster conduicte couverte de rubriche:	
Tant videra dehors grand assem-blee:	
Trembler Vienne & le Pays d'Austriche.	

[1]*charpin*—O.F., rags to dress wounds. Wounds.
[2]Letter of the Greek alphabet K.
[3]Letter of the Greek alphabet Th.
[4]Letter of the Greek alphabet L.

AUSTRIA, 1914–18

In the autumn of 1918, when the trees trembled in the wind, Austria was overturned and the new revolutionary (rubriche) rule replaced the autocratic order of the Hapsburgs. The great assembly of the world Powers, which troubles Austria is the Triple Entente. Austria's troubles first started in the south (Auster) in Turkey and the Balkan States.

83

La gent estrange divisera butins, *Saturne en Mars son regard furieux:* *Horrible estrange aux Tosquans & Latins,* *Grecs qui seront à frapper curieux.*	The alien nation will divide the spoils. Saturn in dreadful opposition in Mars. Dreadful and foreign to the Tuscans and Latins, Greeks who will wish to strike.

ITALIAN OCCUPATION OF GREECE, 4 DECEMBER 1940

The last two lines seem to refer to the Greek struggles with the Italian occupying forces of 1940. The booty taken by the Germans was proverbial; it is still reappearing in sale rooms throughout the world, *divisera butins.* Mars is the God of War, and Saturn indicates a bad aspect, which indeed it was for the Italians who allied themselves with the losing side.

84

Lune obscurcie aux profondes tenebres *Son frere passe de couleur ferrugine:*[1] *Le grand caché long temps soubs les tenebres,* *Tiedera*[2] *fer dans la plaie sanguine.*	The moon obscured in deep gloom, his brother becomes bright red in colour. The great one hidden for a long time in the shadows will hold the blade in the bloody wound.

[1]*ferrugine*—Latin, ferruginus = rusty, blood-coloured.
[2]*Tiedera*—Read, *tiendra.*

MURDER OF THE DUKE DE BERRY.
13th FEBRUARY 1820

The Count of Artois is the man obscured, he was in exile, whose brother Louis XVI died (*passe*) in blood on the guillotine. D'Artois remained in exile for a long time before his return as Charles X, with his family. His son, the Duke de Berry, was attacked and fatally stabbed at the Opera on the night of 13th February 1820. As he died, he clutched the hilt of the knife and is reputed to have said, 'I am murdered. I am holding the hilt of the dagger.' See C. III. 96, IV. 73.

85

Par la response de dame Roi troublé,	The king is troubled by the queen's reply. Ambassadors will fear for their lives. The greater of his brothers will doubly disguise his action, two of them will die through anger, hatred and envy.
Ambassadeurs mespriseront leur vie:	
Le grand ses freres contrefera doublé	
Par deux mourront ire, haine, ennui.	

MURDER OF THE DUKE DE GUISE
AND HIS BROTHER, 1588

Catherine de' Medici, the Queen Mother, was furious at her son Henri III's action in killing not only the Duke de Guise, but also his brother the Cardinal because of their political power. The *Ambassadeurs* are probably the Estates whom the king assembled to meet him at Blois and who remonstrated strongly about the murders. The greater brother who survives was the Duke de Mayenne who then led the Catholic League, and became Lieutenant-General of France, *contrefera doublé*.

86

La grande roine quand se verra vaincue,	When the great queen sees herself conquered, she will show an excess of masculine courage. Naked, on horseback, she will pass over the river pursued by the sword: she will have outraged her faith.
Fera excés de masculin courage:	
Sus cheval, fleuve passera toute nue,	
Suite par fer: à foi fera outrage.	

FLIGHT OF MARY QUEEN OF SCOTS, 1568

This is a very close description of the flight of Mary Queen of Scots, in May 1568, when having been defeated a second time by Murray she fled to England possessing nothing but the clothes she wore, *toute nue*. Mary crossed the river by ferry, but fled on horseback, and had outraged her faith, whether the Catholics, or the Scots, by her behaviour with Boswell. See X. 39, 55.

87

Ennosigee[1] feu du centre de terre.
Fera trembler au tour de cité neu-fue:
Deux grands rochiers long temps feront la guerre,
Puis Arethuse[2] rougira nouveau fleuve.

Earthshaking fire from the centre of the earth will cause tremors around the New City. Two great rocks will war for a long time, then Arethusa will redden a new river.

EARTHQUAKE, SAN ANDREAS FAULT, NEW YORK

There will be a huge earthquake, the tremors of which will spread even as far as New York according to Nostradamus. Could this be the San Andreas' Fault? The experts describe the reason for this earthquake zone as being two plates of rock in the earth crust rubbing against each other and shifting the earth's surface. 'The two great rocks will war for a long time.' Ingenious commentators interpret Arethusa as Ares, the God of War plus the USA to give a location for the earthquake. This could be a typical Nostradamus' pun on words. The new, reddened river is either one of blood or of debris from wrecked buildings, or possibly even the poisoned water of New York mentioned in X. 49.

[1]*Ennosigaeus*—Greek = earth-shaking, a name given to Neptune.
[2]*Arethusa* = a Greek nymph who in one legend changed into a stream.

88

Le divin mal surprendra le grand prince,	The divine wrath overtakes the great Prince, a short while
Un peu devant aura femme espousee.	before he will marry. Both supporters and credit will
Son appuy & credit à un coup viendra mince,	suddenly diminish. Counsel, he will die because of the
Conseil mourra pour la teste rasee.	shaven heads.

CHARLES I AND PARLIAMENT

Divine wrath overtook Charles I of England when he was sentenced by his own Court, but the trouble with Parliament broke out originally around the time of his marriage in 1625 to Henrietta Maria of France. On his actual wedding day, Charles directed that persecution of the Catholics should cease. Parliament refused this and demanded subsidies for the war against Spain. This led to his death, demanded by the Roundheads (*teste rasee*) in 1649. *See* IX. 49.

89

Tous ceux de Ilerde[1] seront dans la Moselle,	Those of Lerida will be in the Moselle, killing all those from
Mettant à mort tous ceux de Loire & Seine:	the Loire and Seine. The sea-side track will come near the
Le cours[2] marin viendra pres d'haute velle,	high valley, when the Spanish open every route.
Quand Espagnols ouvrira toute veine.	

PENINSULAR WARS, 1808–14

This seems to be a general quatrain about the Peninsular Wars when Wellington pushed up through Spain and Portugal across the Pyrenees to Bordeaux. James Laver suggests that *haute velle* is Nostradamus groping towards the name of Wellington.

[1]*Ilerde* = Lerida, city in Spain.
[2]*cours* = path, progress.

90

Bourdeaux, Poitiers au son de la campane,	Bordeaux and Poitiers at the sound of the bell will go with a great fleet as far as Langon. A great rage will surge up against the French, when an hideous monster is born near Orgon.
A grand classe ira jusques à l'Angon:	
Contre Gaulois sera leur tramontane,	
Quand monstre hideux naistra pres de Orgon.	

This specifies an invasion by the French, great resistance, and the birth of a monstrous child near Organ, probably like the two-headed one Nostradamus saw and described in another book. In *The Times*, 20th November 1971, a report was given of the birth of a two-headed boy, so that Nostradamus is not completely in the realms of fantasy and two headed animals are not uncommon. I saw a two-headed lamb in 1979.

91

Les dieux feront aux humains apparence,	The gods will make it appear to mankind that they are the authors of a great war. Before the sky was seen to be free of weapons and rockets: the greatest damage will be inflicted on the left.
Ce qu'il seront auteurs de grand conflict:	
Avant ciel veu serein espee & lance	
Que vers main guache sera plus grand affiict.	

AMERICA IN VIETNAM

Nostradamus here declares that we will not know which side starts this war, although in later quatrains he places the blame upon China and the East. After a peaceful interlude, i.e. after the Second World War, the sky will be seen full of weapons and rockets pointing like lances in the skies. 20th Century dating again! The country on the left hand side of the map of the world is declared to be the loser. This is America and Vietnam has been its only, but spectacular, defeat in this century to date. See II. 89. 91, IV. 95, VIII. 59.

92

Sous un la paix par tout sera clamee	Under one man peace will be proclaimed everywhere, but
Mais non long temps pillé & re-bellion:	not long after will be looting and rebellion. Because of a
Par refus ville, terre, & mer entamee,	refusal, town, land and sea will be broached. About a
Mors & captifs le tiers d'un million	third of a million dead or captured.

FRANCO-PRUSSIAN WAR

The universal peace described here is the French Empire, bearing in mind Napoleon's statement, '*L'Empire, c'est la paix*'. The Franco-Prussian war is depicted in the rest of the quatrain, starting with the King of Prussia's refusal to agree to the humiliating French demands. The Encyclopaedia Britannica gives the figures of dead and wounded in this war as 299,000 which is very close to Nostradamus' estimate of 333,000.

93

Terre Italique pres des monts tremblera,	The Italian lands near the mountains will tremble. The
Lyon & coq non trop confederez:	Cock and the Lion not strongly united. In place of fear they
En lieu de peur l'un l'autre s'aidera.	will help each other. Freedom
Seul Catulon¹ & Celtes moderez.	alone moderates the French.

NAPOLEON'S ITALIAN CAMPAIGN, 1795

The mountains are the Alps and this is Napoleon's Italian Campaign which started in 1795. After capturing Toulon he set out on the Italian wars and France (*Coq*), saw the start of the enmity which grew up between her and England (*Lion*). This is followed by a period of mutual alliance, after the accession of Louis XVIII, the French (*Celtes*) regaining their freedom from tyranny.

¹*Catulon* = Liberty.

94

Au port Selin le tyran mis à mort,
La liberté non pourtant recou-
  vree:
Le nouveau Mars par vindicte
  & remort
Dame par force de frayeur hon-
  noree.

The tyrant Selim will be put
to death at the harbour but
Liberty will not be regained,
however. A new war arises
from vengeance and remorse.
A lady is honoured through
force of terror.

LEPANTO, 1571

At the battle of Lepanto fought on 7th October 1571, Ali
Pasha, the Admiral of the Turkish fleet, was killed while on
board his ship. Selim II was not killed himself but his aggres-
sion in the Mediterranean was finally crushed by the defeat
at Lepanto. However, Liberty was not regained as had been
hoped by the crusade of Christian countries to put down Turkish influence—this continued for some centuries. See IX. 42.
The Pope formally ascribed the victory of Lepanto to the in-
tercession of Our Lady, line 4.

95

Devant moustier[1] trouvé enfant
  besson,[2]
De heroic sang de moine &
  vestutisque:[3]
Son bruit par secte langue &
  puissance son,
Qu'on dira fort esleue le vopisque.

In front of a monastery will
be found a twin infant from
the illustrious and ancient line
of a monk. His fame, renown
and power through sects and
speech is such that they will
say the living twin is de-
servedly chosen.

Apparently the twin son of a monk will grow to be an important
leader. Many commentators refer this to the Man in the Iron
Mask who was possibly the son of Queen Anne and Cardinal
Mazarin.

[1]*moustier*—Provençal = monastery.
[2]*besson*—Provençal = twin.
[3]*vestutisque*—Latin, *vestutus* = old.

96

Celui qu'aura la charge de destruire
Temples, & sectes, changez par fantasie:
Plus aux rochiers qu'aux vivans viendra nuire,
Par langue ornee d'oreilles ressasie.

A man will be charged with the destruction of temples and sects, altered by fantasy. He will harm the rocks rather than the living, ears filled with ornate speeches.

CULTS, SUCH AS MOONIES, ETC.

A man will come whose religious destiny is concerned with people rather than the buildings, temples, bricks and mortar of accepted religions. It is possible that the rock in line 3 is the Rock of Peter, the Vatican, in which case this revival would harm the Catholic church.

97

Ce que fer, flamme n'a sceu paracheuer,
La douce langue au conseil viendra faire:
Par repos, songe, le Roy fera resver,
Plus l'ennemy en feu, sang militaire.

That which neither weapon nor flame could accomplish will be achieved by a sweet speaking tongue in council. Sleeping, in a dream, the king will see the enemy not in war or of military blood.

ASSASSINATION OF HENRI III, 1589

Henri III was killed not while at war but in council. The monk, Jacques Clément came to the king at St. Cloud saying he had a secret letter, and leaning towards Henri, as though to speak confidentially, he stabbed him in the stomach. Henri died the next day. The fact that he had dreamed of his death is well authenticated; he told his courtiers three days before his death that he saw the royal regalia, his blue cloak, two crowns, sceptre, sword and spurs all trodden underfoot by monks and the populace. An example of double precognition; by Nostradamus and the victim himself. Is the *douce langue* in line 2 a play on words on the name Clément? It would be a typical Nostradamus double meaning, as the two words mean the same in French.

98

Le chef qu'aura conduit peuple infiny	The leader who will conduct great numbers of people far from their skies, to foreign customs and language. Five thousand will die in Crete and Thessaly, the leader fleeing in a sea going supply ship.
Loing de son ciel, de meurs & langue estrange:	
Cinq mil en Crete & Thessalie fini	
Le chef fuyant, sauvé en marine grange.[1]	

NAPOLEON'S EXPEDITION TO EGYPT, 1798

When Napoleon left Egypt, he successfully eluded the British Navy to land in France, leaving behind for the Turks an army reduced to around 5,000 men. The Turks ruled Thessaly and Crete at this time, and Napoleon did flee in a wooden ship. This fact prevents the prophecy applying to the British Expeditionary forces in Crete and Thessaly in 1940, when ships were made of metal and the figures were also much greater.

99

Le grand monarque que fera compagnie,	The great king will join with two kings, united in friendship. How the great household will sigh: around Narbon what pity for the children.
Avec deux rois unis par amité:	
O quel soupir fera la grand mesgnie,[2]	
Enfans Narbon à l'entour quel pitié.	

100

Longtemps au ciel sera veu gris oiseau,	For a long time a grey bird will be seen in the sky near Dôle and the lands of Tuscany. He holds a flowering branch in his beak, but he dies too soon and the war ends.
Aupres de Dole & de Touscane terre:	
Tenant au bec un verdoyant rameau,	
Mourra tost grand & finera la guerre.	

[1]*grange*—Fr. = literally, barn.
[2]*mesgnie*—O.F. = household, court.

COMTE DE CHAMBORD

The grey bird is both the dove of peace and the Comte de Chambord, son of the Duchess de Berry and last legitimate heir to the French throne. At his birth he was called the Dove of Peace, but unfortunately he was usurped by the Orléans family and exiled to Venice, near Dôle, and Modena, near Tuscany. He also married the daughter of the Duke of Tuscany in 1846. He died without regaining the French throne, but he and the Comte de Paris, Duke d'Orléans, the Pretender, were reconciled when the latter was also sent into exile by the new republic. The death of the Comte de Chambord saved the possibility of another war between republicans and monarchists.

CENTURY II

34
35   22nd December
36   Abbé Tourné
37
38   Russia and Allies, c. 1940
39   Europe in 1939 and Germany
40   Second World War
41   Third World War, 1986
42   Death of Robespierre, 1794
43   Triple Alliance, 1881
44   France, 1813–14
46   Third World War, 1986
47
48   16th December 1986
49
50   1568, Revolt Netherlands
51   1666, Great Fire of London
52   War with United Provinces, 1665–7
53   Great Plague of London, 1665
54
55   France, 1594
56
57   John F Kennedy?
58
59
60   Zimbabwe Rhodesia
61
62   World Leader. Possible Third AntiChrist
63   Battle of Ivry, 1550
64   Cevennes, c. 1685
65   December 7, 2044
66   Napoleon's 100 days
67   James II, William III, 1688–90
68   Continued
69   Continued
70   Napoleon, 1815
71
72
73
74
75
76   Talleyrand, 1754–1838
77

1

Vers Acquitaine par insuls Bri-tanniques	Towards Aquitaine, by British assaults, and by them also
De pars eux mesmes grands in-cursions	great incursions. Rains and frost make the terrain unsafe,
Pluies gelées feront terroirs iniques,	against Port Selin they will
Port Selin fortes fera invasions.	make mighty invasions.

THE DARDANELLES. FIRST WORLD WAR, 1915

An important quatrain. When France (Aquitaine) and Britain were deadlocked on the Western Front during 1915, Winston Churchill persuaded the Allies to open a new front against Turkey (Port Selin is Constantinople, and Turkey, by extension). It was planned to attack the Dardanelles in order to reach Constantinople. The dreadful weather suffered by troops during the First World War is referred to in line 3.

2

La teste bleu fera la tete blanche	The blue leader will inflict
Autant de mal que France a faict leur bien,	upon the white leader as much damage as France has done
Mort à l'anthene grand pendu sus la branche,	them good. Death from the great antenna hanging from
Quand prins des siens le Roy dira combien.	the branch, when the king will ask how many of his men have been captured.

DEPOSITION OF THE AYATOLLA? THE BLUE LEADER?

If the white leader can be interpreted as the Ayatollah, white being the colour of the dress both of himself and his followers, especially those who have put on the white shirt of the martyr, to indicate that they will fight to death in a Holy War, then the Ayatollah is predicted as being eventually overcome by a Blue Leader who will make the position of Iran even worse than it is at present. The good being done by the

French influence must be understood as an ironic interpretation referring to the Ayatollah plotting the Shah's overthrow while in Paris. What tempts me to date this quatrain in this century is its use of the word antenna. This implies a sensitive machine that receives sound and/or touch. Could it refer to a wireless set? The rest is obscure. See V. 27, VI. 80.

3

Pour la chaleur solaire sus la mer
De Negrepont les poissons demi cuits:
Les habitans les viendront entamer,[1]
Quand Rhod, & Gannes leur faudra le biscuit.

Because of heat like that of the sun upon the sea the fish around Negrepont will become half cooked. The local people will eat them when in Rhodes and Genoa there is a lack of food.

ATOMIC EXPLOSION?

To produce such heat on the sea surface implies a very strong explosion, possibly of atomic force, somewhere in the Aegean sea, as Negrepont is the Italian name for the Island of Ruboéa. The second implication that in Italy and other parts of Greece people are starving, indicates either conditions of famine or war. Nostradamus mentions this explosion again in V. 98, when he says its source comes from the sky.

1

Depuis Monach[2] *jusque aupres de Sicile*
Toute la plage demourra desolée:
Il n'y aura fauxbourg, cité ne ville,
Que par Barbares pillé soit & vollée.

From Monaco as far as Sicily all the coast will remain deserted. There will be no suburbs, cities nor towns which have not been pillaged and robbed by barbarians.

[1]*entamer*—Literally to cut up, therefore = to eat.
[2]*Monach*—Latin, *Monoceus* = Monaco.

This may be a continuation of the last quatrain, II. 3. extending the area of the disaster through Italy to France. Nostradamus would describe as barbarian either Arab, Negro, Russian or Chinese, but from later quatrains the latter is the most likely interpretation.

5

Qu'en dans poisson, fer & lettres enfermée,
Hors sortira qui puis fera la guerre:
Aura par mer sa classe[1] bien pramée,
Apparoissant pres de Latine terre.

When weapons and documents are enclosed in a fish, out of it will come a man who will then make war. His fleet will have travelled far across the sea to appear near the Italian shore.

THE THIRD WAR, 1986? AND ITS ORIGINATOR

The fish is interpreted as a submarine rather than a ship as a fish travels under water; this one carries weapons and important papers as well as the man who is responsible for starting a new war. He is described as actually coming out (*hors sortira*) of the fish as are the hostile soldiers in I. 29, where the submarine is also called a fish by Nostradamus. The fleet brought by this unnamed man has travelled a great distance to appear in either the Mediterranean or Adriatic sea. It is tempting to link him with the man Nostradamus calls the Third AntiChrist whom he believes will start a third war in this century. The date may actually be given to us, because the first line contains a second, astrological meaning, 'When Mars and Mercury are in conjunction in Pisces'. According to Norab the next time this occurs is 23rd March 1986, and Nostradamus dates the war as starting around 1985 in I.51, in 1983 in II. 41, and mentions it indirectly in I. 16, all of which are uncomfortably close and consistent. See VI. 33.

[1]*classe*—Latin, *classis* = fleet.

6

Aupres des portes & dedans deux cités
Seront deux fléaux & oncques n'apperceu un tel:
Faim, dedans peste, de fer hors gens boutés,
Crier secours au grand Dieu immortel.

Near the harbour and in two cities will be two scourges, the like of which have never been seen. Hunger, plague within, people thrown out by the sword will cry for help from the great immortal God.

THE BOMBINGS OF NAGASAKI
AND HIROSHIMA, 1945

Both Nagasaki and Hiroshima are on the sea and experienced the plague of radiation which had never been seen before on earth. Two bombs were dropped (*deux fléaux*) and the survivors would have looked very similar to victims of the plague in Nostradamus' day, which turned them black, and for this was known as '*le charbon*'. Radiation burns turn black too, and there was hunger among the miserable survivors who were thrown out of the cities by the sword of war. The last line speaks for itself.

7

Entre plusiers aux isles deportés, deportés,
L'un estre nay à deux dents en la gorge:
Mourrant de faim les arbres esbrotés,
Pour eux neuf Roy, nouvel edict leur forge.

Among many people deported to the islands will be a man born with two teeth in his mouth. They will die of hunger having stripped the trees. A new king will pass new laws for them.

The islands are either the French penal colonies such as the Ile du Diable in South America or those along the south coast of France which are used for detention of dangerous criminals. It is quite common for children to be born with some teeth already formed. The last line may predict the closing of the penal settlements; most of the tropical ones are no longer in use.

8

Temples sacrez prime facon Romaine	Temples consecrated in the early Roman fashion, they
Rejecteront les goffres¹ fondements	will reject the broken foundations; taking their early human laws, expelling almost all the cults of the saints.
Prenant leurs loix premieres & humaines,	
Chassant, non tout des saincts les cultements.	

FRINGE CULTS

A general quatrain predicting a return to the simpler religious precepts and practices, and a rejection of the elaborate cult of Saints in the Roman Catholic Church. Many of the cults seem to be flourishing at present, such as Scientology, the Moonies, or the dreadful Peoples' Temple of Jim Jones and his followers who committed mass suicide in Guyana in 1978 could be referred to in this quatrain. Certainly the Roman Catholic Church is diminishing in its influence.

9

Neuf ans le regne le maigre en paix tiendra,	For nine years the thin man will keep a peaceful rule, then
Puis il cherra² en soif si sanguinaire:	he will fall into so bloody a thirst that a great nation will
Pour lui grand peuple sans foi & loi mourra,	die for him without faith or law; killed by a much better
Tué par un beaucoup plus debonnaire.	natured man.

Three specific elements combine in this quatrain, which do not seem to have occurred as yet. A very thin ruler will, after a nine year peace, plunge his nation into a disastrous war. His death, in turn, will be caused by someone with right or good on his side. It has been suggested that this could be the Nazi party coming to power in the elections of 1930, and that Roosevelt is the good-natured opponent, but this gives a wrong time factor.

¹*Goffre*—Romance = deep, broken.
²*cherra*—O.F., *choir* = to fall.

10

Avant long temps le tout sera rangé,	Before long everything will be organized; we await a very
Nous esperons un siecle bien senestre	evil century. The state of the masked and the solitary ones
L'estat des masques & des seuls bien changé,	greatly changed, few will find that they wish to retain their
Peu trouverant qu'à son rang vueille estre.	rank.

FRENCH REVOLUTION, 1789

A general description of the French Revolution in which the state of two particular social orders was dangerous to maintain and became greatly changed. The first were the Court (*masques*), and the second the Clergy, who were abolished in 1790. Both classes suffered financial loss and many faced death because of their social rank or function throughout the early years of the Revolution.

11

Le prochain fils de l'aisnier parviendra,	The following son the elder will succeed, very greatly
Tant esleue jusque au regne des fors:[1]	raised to a kingdom of privilege. His bitter renown will be
Son apre gloire un chacun la craindra,	feared by all, but his children will be thrown out of the king-
Mais ses enfans du regne gettez[2] dehors.	dom.

NAPOLEON

The first line is extremely difficult because of the multitude of possible meanings of *prochain* and *aisnier*. *Prochain* may mean next, nearest, younger or favourite, and *aisnier* either elder or a falcon (*l'ainier*) giving a metaphor of a bird of prey similar to Napoleon, the eagle. If it does refer to Napoleon, he was the second son and he was elected to a kingdom and privilege, from being the son of a Corsican middle-class family he became Emperor. He was feared in Europe and his children were

[1] *fors*—O.F., Privileges.
[2] *gettez*—Alternative spelling of jettez = to throw.

deprived of kingship by Louis XVIII. However, Napoleon's nephew, Louis Napoleon, re-established himself in 1852 and ruled until the Third Republic of 1871.

12

Yeux clos, ouverts d'antique fantasie,
L'habit des seuls seront mis à
   neant:
Le grand monarque chastiera
   leur frenaisie,
Ravir des temples le tresor par
   devant.

Their eyes closed, open to the old fantasy, the habit of priests will be abolished. The great monarch will punish their frenzy, stealing the treasure in front of the temples.

SUPPRESSION OF THE CLERGY, c. 1790

Nostradamus seemed greatly worried by the fate of the Catholic Church and its priests during the French Revolution and there are many references to it. The eyes of the people were closed to Christianity and the Cult of Reason was established in 1793. In 1789 the wearing of ecclesiastical costume was suppressed. The monarch can be interpreted either as Louis XVI, who had already helped despoil the monasteries, or as Napoleon, who continued to do so with great vigour until the time of his Coronation when he needed the Pope and found it necessary to restore the Roman Catholic religion to France.

13

Le corps sans ame plus n'estre en
   sacrifice.
Jour de la mort mis en nativité:
L'esprit divin fera l'ame felice,
Voyant le verbe en son eternité.

The body without a soul no longer at the sacrifice. At the day of death it is brought to rebirth. The divine spirit will make the soul rejoice seeing the eternity of the word.

RELIGIOUS BELIEFS

This is an ambiguous statement of Nostradamus' religious beliefs. Once dead, he can no longer communicate with the spirits, whether he means the Mass or some magical rite by the word sacrifice is impossible to say. His soul will be reborn at his death into happiness. The word ('verbe') is either Christ as is used in the Christian Gospel, *the word was made flesh,* or may be a promise made to Nostradamus in his magic studies which he expects to be fulfilled eternally at his death. If there is any occult meaning in this quatrain it is very deliberately hidden. Nostradamus foretold his own death to his confessor, Frère Vidal, and to his pupil, Chavigny, but he may have been able to do this by a medical diagnosis. He died on 1st July 1566.

14

A Tours, Gien, gardé seront yeux penetrans,	At Tours and Gien watchful eyes will be guarded, they will
Descouvriront de loing la grand seraine:	spy far off the Serene Highness. She and her suite will
Elle & sa suitte au port seront entrans.	enter the harbour, combat joined, sovereign power.
Combat, poussez, puissance souveraine.	

REGENCY OF CATHERINE DE' MEDICI, 1559–89

Tours and Gien are both on the Loire. This probably refers in general terms to the regency of Catherine de' Medici and the wars of religion which troubled France from 1562–98. The Queen died in 1599 having seen her three sons predecease her, as predicted.

15

Un peu devant monarque trucidé[1]	A short while before a king is murdered, Castor and Pollux in the ship, a bearded star.
Castor, Pollux en nef, astre crinite[2]	Public treasure emptied on land and sea, Pisa, Asti, Terrara and Turin are forbidden lands.
L'erain[3] public par terre & mer vuidé,	
Pise, Ast, Ferrare, Turin, terre interdicte.	

The second line of this quatrain gives a form of dating in June as Castor and Pollux, the twins, standing for Gemini. The ship of Argo obviously stands for the Papacy, and the bearded star

[1]*trucidé*—Latin, *trucidare* = to slaughter.
[2]*crinite*—Latin, *crinitus* = bearded.
[3]*erain*—Latin, *eranus* = public fund.

is a comet. Linked with these is an assassinated king, a great war effort, money being raised on land and sea, and the Italian states being placed in interdict. Could this refer to the Mussolini régime? Otherwise it seems unlikely that this prophecy will ever be fulfilled.

16

Naples, Palerme, Sicille, Syra- cuses,	In Naples, Palermo, Sicily and Syracuse new tyrants, thun-
Nouveau tyrans, fulgures¹ feux celestes:	der and lightning in the skies. A force from London, Ghent,
Force de Londres, Gand, Brux- elles, & Suses,	Brussels and Susa: a great massacre, then triumph and
Grand hecatombe, triomphe faire festes.	festivities.

Naples, Palerme, Sicille, Syra-cuses,
Nouveau tyrans, fulgures¹ feux celestes:
Force de Londres, Gand, Brux-elles, & Suses,
Grand hecatombe, triomphe faire festes.

In Naples, Palermo, Sicily and Syracuse new tyrants, thunder and lightning in the skies. A force from London, Ghent, Brussels and Susa: a great massacre, then triumph and festivities.

ITALY'S PART IN SECOND WORLD WAR

The new tyrants in the Italian towns are the Mussolini régime of the Fascisti. The thunder and lightning become the sound of war in Italy. London goes out in force against them, allied to Brussels, and wins the war after great slaughter.

17

Le camp du temple de la vierge vestale,
Non esloingé d'Ethne & monte Pyrenées:
Le grand conduict est caché dans la male²
North³ getez fleuves & vignes mastinées.⁴

The field of the vestal virgin's temple is not far from Ethne and the Pyrenees. The great one led is hidden in a trunk. In the North, the rivers overflow and the vines destroyed.

Ethne is probably a greek anagram for Elne, *th* in Greek being one letter. Elne lies near the Pyrenees between the Tech and the Réart which flow into the Mediterranean. I cannot decipher this quatrain further.

¹*Fulgures*—Latin, *fulgur* = lightning.
²*male*— (a) *malle* = trunk, or possibly, (b) *mal* = evil.
³*North* = very rare use of English by Nostradamus.
⁴*mastiner*—O.F. = to bruise, destroy.

18

Nouvelle & pluie subite impe-
  tueuse,
Empechera subit deux excercites:
Pierre ciel, feux faire la mere
  pierreuse,
La mort de sept terre & marin
  subites.
	News; unexpected and heavy rain will suddenly prevent two armies. Stones and fire from the skies will make a sea of stones. The death of the seven suddenly by land and sea.

HENRI III 1587–9

The clue to this quatrain lies in the last line, the death of the seven, the Valois children of Catherine de' Medici. When Henri III left Paris in 1587 the city was invaded by 35,000 German and Swiss troops. The Duc de Guise rushed with his troops of the League to Montargis, but the decisive battle was prevented by a violent rainstorm. In the following year, 1589, Henri III, the last of the Valois kings was assassinated; his death was the direct result of his clash with the Leaguers and the assassinations of the two Guise brothers. The fall of stones is not as ridiculous as it sounds. An authenticated case occurred on 27 October 1973. Two men were fishing at Skaneathes Lake, New York, and were disturbed by stones falling into the water around them. The rain of pebbles followed them in their car and started again when they stopped to go and have a drink. Analysis by the Geology Department at Syracuse University identified the falls as belonging to local rock types. See III. 42, 51, VI. 11.

19

Nouveau venus lieu basti sans
  defence.
Occuper la place par lors inhab-
  itable:
Pres, maisons, champs, villes
  prendre à plaisance,
Faim, Peste, guerre arpen[1] *long*
  labourable.
	Newcomers will build a place without defences, occupying a place uninhabitable until then Meadows, houses, fields, towns will be taken with pleasure. Famine, plague, war, extensive arable land.

[1]*arpen*—O.F. = measure of land, just under 1 acre.

20

Freres & soeurs en divers lieux captifs,	Brothers and sisters captives in differing places will find
Se trouveront passer pres du monarque;	themselves passing before the monarch. His attentive off-
Les contempler ses rameaux[1] ententifs,	spring will look at them, displeased to see the signs on
Desplaisant voir menton, front, nez, les marques.	their chins, foreheads and noses.

HENRI II 1557

The commentator Jaubert applies this to an event which occurred soon after the original publication. In September 1557 some Huguenots were captured in Paris during a raid and Henri II went to see them, taking his children with him. The King is reputed to have been angry that the captives had been wounded and bruised. But it is so general that it may apply to other similar events. These 'signs' could imply some form of family likeness.

21

L'ambassadeur envoyé par biremes,	The ambassador sent by the biremes is repulsed half way
A mi-chemin d'incogneus repoulsez:	by an unknown man. Four triremes come reinforced with
De sel renfort viendront quatre triremes,	salt; he is bound with cords and chains to Negrepont.
Cordes & chaines en Negre pont troussez.	

Biremes are oared galleys with two bridges, and triremes larger ones with three. Salt in the Centuries often stands for taxation, because of the famous French salt tax, the "gabelle", or for wisdom in the Biblical sense. Negrepont is the Italian name for Euboea which belonged to the Turks until 1831, when it became part of Greece. The ambassadors trap is reinforced with money, "gabelle", bribery, to get to Greece, but is ineffectual.

---

[1]*rameaux*—Literally branches, therefore offspring.

22

Le camp Ascop[1] d'Europe par-
tira,
S'adjoignant proche de l'isle sub-
mergée:
D'Arton[2] classe[3] phalange pliera,
Nombril du monde plus grand
voix subrogée.[4]

The aimless army will depart
from Europe and join up
close to the submerged island.
The NATO fleet folds up its
standard, the navel of the
world takes over from a
greater voice.

1980 NATO FLEET OFF BRITAIN

Nostradamus writes of the submerged island again in IX.
31 where it is identified with Britain. The army is described
as aimless; could this mean that it, just like the NATO fleet,
had no warlike intent as they were both only on exercises?
This view is reinforced by the fact that the fleet folds up its
standards showing no signs of war. The navel of the world,
and its centre, may be understood as Italy, presumably the
centre of the direction of operations. But again, Nostradamus
implies that NATO will be taken over (*subrogée*) by a more
powerful agency. European countries do combine at the present time to hold naval and military exercises both in Europe
and in the English Channel under the auspices of NATO. See
also IX. 31.

23

Palais, oiseaux, par oiseau des-
chassé,
Bien tost apres le prince parvenu:
Combien que hors fleuve ennemi
repoulsé,
Dehors sausi trait d'oiseau sous-
tenu.

Birds at the palace, chased
out by a bird very soon after
the upstart prince. How many
of the enemy are repulsed
beyond the river, the upheld
bird seized from without by
a trick.

This is very vague. Probably the birds are courtiers or supporters of one prince where power is taken by an upstart who
is finally captured by a trick. Some interpret line 4 as 'captured
outside, a shaft held by a bird', i.e. by an arrow, probably a
play on words here that I can't decipher.

[1]*Ascop*—Greek, *askopos* = incredible, aimless.
[2]*Arton*—Either anagram for NATO or Greek, *artos* = bread.
[3]*classe*—Latin, *classis* = fleet.
[4]*subrogée*—Latin, *subrogatus* = substituted.

24

Bestes farouches de faim fleuves tranner,[1]	Beasts wild with hunger will cross the rivers, the greater
Plus part du champ encontre Hister sera.	part of the battlefield will be against Hitler. He will drag
En caige de fer le grand fera treisner,	the leader in a cage of iron, when the child of Germany
Quand rien enfant de Germain observera.	observes no law.

HITLER

One of Nostradamus' most remarkable series of quatrains, with the name Hitler given in an anagram of Hister. There can be little doubt that Hitler is implied; who else could be so well described by the last line, the German who observed no law? In 16th-Century handwriting the resemblance is even closer with the use of the long *s*, Hifter. Commentators before 1930 understood the Hister to be the river Danube, from its Latin name Ister. But Hitler recognized himself in these quatrains by the mid 1930s and Goebbels made great propaganda out of them in the pre-war party years. Evidence for this is found in many sources, chiefly Ellic Howe's book 'Nostradamus and the Nazis'. During the first year of the Second World War the development of the war was to a great extent dependent upon the rivers crossed by the Germans who came into Europe in a never-ending stream looting and pillaging (*farouches de faim*). See I. 34, II. 24, III. 35, 53, 58, 61, IV. 40, 68, V. 29, 94, VI. 7, 51, IX. 90.

25

La garde estrange trahira forteresse	The foreign guard will betray the fortress, the shadowy hope
Espoir & umbre de plus hault mariage:	of an important marriage. The guard deceived, the fort
Garde deçeue,[2] *fort prince dans la presse,*	taken in the crush. Loire, Saône, Rhône, Garonne out-
Loire, Son, Rosne. Gar à mort oultrage.	raged to death.

[1]*tranner*—Latin, *tranare* = to swim across.
[2]*deçeue* = deceived, or Latin, *decisus* = to cut down.

CAPITULATION OF METZ, 1870

The defender of a fortress who betrays his trust chasing the illusion of a higher post (*plus hault mariage*) may be Bazaine who in 1870 handed over the fortress of Metz and his troops to the Germans, and thus allowed them into the French interior during the Franco-Prussian War.

26

Pour la faveur que la cité fera,
Au grand qui tost prendra camp de bataille,
Puis le rang Pau Thesin versera
De sang, feux mors noyés de coup de taille.

Because of the fervour that a city will show towards a great man who later loses on the battlefield, the ranks will flee, rushing into the Po and the Tessin, blood, firing, dead men drowned and slashed.

27

Le divin verbe sera du ciel frappé,
Qui ne pourra proceder plus avant:
Du reserant[1], le secret estoupé[2]
Qu'on marchera par dessus & devant.

The divine voice will be struck by heaven and he will not be able to proceed further. The secret is hidden with the revelation so that people will walk over and ahead.

One of the several quatrains which indicate some secret locked up with the grave. Someone over whom one can walk (*par dessus & devant*) in French means to be buried at the foot of a wall, or chained in an underground cell. Some person will be struck down and not be able to reveal his information. He may be a theologian or religious man (*le divin verbe*), possibly imprisoned for his beliefs.

[1] *reserant*—Latin *resarare* = to unlock.
[2] *estoupé*—O.F. = to shut up.

28

Le penultiesme du surnom du prophete,	The last but one of the prophet's name, will take
Prendra Diane pour son jour & repos:	Monday for his day of rest. He will wander far in his
Loing vaguera par frenetique teste,	frenzy delivering a great nation from subjection.
Et delivrant un grand peuple d'impos.[1]	

A MUSLIM LEADER

The last but one of the prophet's name has two possible meanings. Either that of a muslim leader who shall be the last but one, or of a person whose name begins with the penultimate syllables of the prophet's name, Mahomet or Mohamed. If the first interpretation is correct we come again to the Ayatollah Khomeini who certainly delivered Persia from the tyranny of the Shah and did so in a state of revolutionary fervour or frenzy as it is described here by Nostradamus. The reference to Monday as a holy day is not clear. See II. 62.

29

L'Oriental sortira de son siege,	The man from the East will
Passer les monts Apennins voir la Gaule:	come out of his seat and will cross the Apennines to see
Transpercera le ciel les eaux & neige,	France. He will cross through the sky, the seas and the snows
Et un chascun frappera de sa gaule.	and he will strike everyone with his rod.

MAN FROM THE EAST

This is a curious verse. The word *sortira* for *ira* indicates that the Easterner does not usually leave his country; could this refer to the North Vietnamese talks in Paris? France (*la Gaule*) to which he comes, was one of the few countries to maintain diplomatic relations with China until its acceptance into the United Nations in October 1971. The third line seems to indicate air travel—he goes through the air to his destination. The last line is very ambiguous. The word *gaule* means a stick or rod, it could mean a weapon, it also means France

[1]*impos*—O.F., *impost* = taxation.

and might be an indirect reference to the name of de Gaulle, which would certainly date the quatrain. There is a curiously threatening quality in the last line, as though no one is expecting any harm to come from the visitor. This verse becomes even more complex when one accepts that USA and China have now established diplomatic relations and that China is undergoing a revolution towards a more moderate line of thinking since the removal of the Gang of Four. See also V. 54.

30

Un qui des dieux d'Annibal infernaux,	A man who revives the infernal Gods of Hannibal, the terror of mankind. Never more horror nor the papers tell of worse in the past, than will come to the Romans through Babel.
Fera renaistre, effrayeur des humains:	
Oncq' plus d'horreur ne plus dire journaulx,	
Qu'avint viendra par Babel aux Romains.	

MIDDLE EASTERN TROUBLES

The theme of trouble in the Middle East is continued. The infernal Gods of Hannibal imply North Africa. This might refer to Colonel Gadaffi, the P.L.O. or President Sadat of Egypt and the near Middle East, which could tie in with I. 70. The word for newspapers is interesting as there were none in Nostradamus' time. However, this line is a definite reading from the first edition of Benoist Rigaud, 1568. Pamphlets existed, of course, and the word may be used in this sense. Babel implies a confusion of languages and is also the Hebrew word for Babylon.

31

En Campanie le Cassilin¹ sera tant,	In Campanie the Cassilin (river) will be so great that one will see only fields covered in water. Before and after the long lasting rain nothing green will be seen except for the trees.
Qu'on ne verra que d'aux les champs coumers:	
Devant apres le pluie de long temps,	
Hors mis les arbres rien l'on verra de vert.	

¹*Cassalin* = a town on the Volturno river.

This general quatrain predicts a flood of the Volturno river, perhaps of the town of Capua itself, in that it was built on the ruins of the Roman town of Casilinum.

32

Laict, sang grenouilles escoudre[1] en Dalmatie,	Milk, blood, frogs will be prepared in Dalmatia: battle engaged, plague near Balennes.
Conflict donné, peste pres de Balennes,	A great cry will go up throughout Slavonia, then will a monster be born near Ravenna.
Cri sera grand par toute Esclavonie,	
Lors naistra monstre pres & dedans Ravenne.	

AUTHENTICATED SHOWERS OF MILK, BLOOD AND FROGS

This prophecy covers both sides of the Adriatic. Showers of milk, blood and frogs have all been authenticated in recent times. In 1954 at Sutton Park, Birmingham, England, people sheltering from the rain were bombarded by hundreds of little frogs bouncing off umbrellas and scaring everyone with their leaping around. It is an interesting fact that whenever these "frog falls" appear the fall is never one of fully grown frogs or of tadpoles. Another such case happened in Arkansas on January 2, 1973, when a group of men playing golf were deluged with "thousands of frogs about the size of nickels which came right down with the rain from the sky." Rains of blood are among one of the oldest prodigies known to man, yet people still regard them as a myth. In Brazil, on August 27, 1968, a shower of blood and scraps of meat fell for between 5–7 minutes over an area of one square kilometer between Cocpava and São José dos Campos. There have also been instances of coloured rain. Professor Brun of Geneva investigated a case of blood-rain in 1880 in Morocco and found the rocks and vegetation at Djebel-Sekra covered with dried red scales which were identified as remains of colonies of a minute organism called Protococcus Fluvialis. His explanation was that they had been deposited by a whirlwind but he could not explain away the extraordinary selection involved. The whole colony was composed entirely of young organisms. Dalmatia is on the Eastern Adriatic, Balennes was Trebula, Bal-

[1]*Escoudre*—Latin, *excudere* = to prepare.

liensis near Capua, Ravenna is in Central Italy. The former
province of Slavonia is now part of Northern Yugoslavia and
part of the Hungarian Empire. See III. 18, 19 V. 61.

33

Par le torrent qui descent de Veronne,	Through the torrent which pours down from Verona
Par lors qu'au Pau guidera son entrée:	there where the entry is guided to the Po, a great wreck, and
Un grand naufrage, & non moins en Garonne	not less so in Garonne when the people of Genoa will
Quand ceux de Gennes marcheront leur contree.	march against their country.

This is similar to the last quatrain describing three 16th-Cen-
tury states, France, Venice and Genoa. Verona is on the river
Adige, which enters the Adriatic parallel to the Po about ten
miles distant. The flood may be connected with II. 31.

34

L'ire insensee du combat furieux,	The senseless rage of a fu-
Fera à table par freres le fer luire:	rious struggle will cause the brothers to draw their weap-
Les despartir, blessé, curieux,	ons at table. A wounded man parts them strangely: the
Le fier duelle viendra en France nuire.	proud duel will bring harm to France.

The duel that affects France must occur between her princes
or statesmen. Several French kings, including Henri III and
Louis XIV have hated their brothers but none have actually
duelled together to my knowledge.

35

Dans deux logis de nuict le feu prendra,	Fire will take hold in two houses at night, several peo-
Plusieurs dedans estouffes & rostis:	ple inside suffocated or burnt. It will happen near two rivers
Pres de deux fleuves pour seul il aviendra:	for sure, once the Sun, Sag- ittarius and Capricorn are all
Sol, l'Arq & Caper tous seront amortis.	diminished.

22nd DECEMBER

This event could occur on 22nd December of any year, for this is the day that the Sun moves out of Sagittarius into Capricorn. It is difficult to distinguish a town on two rivers, there are so many. Commentators who lived *c.* 1600 all related it to a fire at Lyons in December 1582, and this town is situated at the mouth of two rivers.

36

Du grand Prophete les lettres seront prinses,
Entre les mains du tyran deviendront:
Frauder son Roy seront ses entreprinses,
Mais ses rapines bien tost le troubleront.

The letters of the great prophet will be intercepted and fall into the hands of the tyrant. His efforts will be to deceive his King, but soon his thefts will trouble him.

ABBÉ TORNÉ

The Abbé Torné, a great interpreter of Nostradamus, believed this verse referred to him. It may just as well be Nostradamus talking of some personal vendetta of his own, against his pupil, Chavigny, who published the remainder of the Prophecies after his death, and obviously hoped to acquire the same authority among his contemporaries as Nostradamus had achieved. Needless to say he did not succeed.

37

De ce grand nombre que lon envoyera,
Pour secourir dans le fort assiegez,
Peste & famine tous les devorera,
Hors mis septante qui seront profligez.[1]

Of the great number that are sent to relieve the besieged fort, disease and hunger will destroy them all except seventy who will be killed.

---

[1]*profligez*—Latin, *profligare* = to destroy, kill, ruin.

38

Des condamnez sera fait un grand nombre,
Quand les monarques seront con-cilie⁷:
Mais l'un deux viendra si mal-encombre¹
Que guere ensemble ne seront re-liez.

There will be a great number of condemned people when the monarchs are reconciled. But one of them will be so unfortunate that they will hardly be able to remain allied.

RUSSIA AND ALLIES?

This may be interpreted as a general quatrain about the alliance of Hitler and Stalin between the years 1939–41. Others apply it to the breakdown of the Yalta conference of 1945, and interpret line one as referring to the Nuremberg Trials and the misfortune as the commencement of the Cold War by Russia towards the western powers.

39

Un an devant le conflict Italique,
Germains, Gaulois, Hespaignols pour le fort:
Cherra l'escolle maison de re-publicque,
Ou, hors mis peu, seront suffoque mors.

A year before the war in Italy, Germans, French and Spanish will be for the strong one; the school house of the republic will fall, where, except for a few, they will suffocate to death.

EUROPEAN ATTITUDES TOWARDS GERMANY, *c.* 1939

This quatrain summarizes very succinctly the general situation in Europe during 1939, the year before Italy was involved in the Second World War, which she declared on June 10, 1940. Many of the Spanish were on the side of the Germans as was obvious in the Spanish Civil War and there was a definite pro-German element in France as was proved by the Vichy régime. The strong man was Hitler who had enormous support in Germany at this time. The school-house republic which falls and crushes so many of its people could be either France or Italy. It is difficult to understand the meaning of the adjective here. This quatrain seems to continue on to the following one with the claim that after these alliances between Ger-

¹*malencombre*—O.F., 13th Century, *malencontre* = misfortune.

many, Spain and France there will be world battles on land
and sea, which were part of the Second World War.

40

Un peu apres non point longue
 intervalle
Par mer & terre sera faict grand
 tumulte:
Beaucoup plus grande sera pugne[1]
 navalle,
Feux, animaux, qui plus feront
 d'insulte.[2]

Shortly afterwards, not a very
long interval, a great tumult
will be raised by land and sea.
The naval battles will be
greater than ever. Fires, creatures which will make more
trouble.

SECOND WORLD WAR

Should this quatrain be linked with II. 39 it becomes a
continuation of the description of the Second World War. The
importance of power at sea was obvious, submarines played
a great part in the war game, and are probably described as
the creatures of line 4, as in I. 29, II. 5 etc. *Feux* could be
translated as firing, making them creatures with weapons.

41

La grand estoille par sept jours
 brulera,
Nuée fera deux soleils apparoir:
Le gros mastin toute nuict hur-
 lera.
Quand grand pontife changera
 de terroir.

The great star will burn for
seven days and the cloud will
make the sun appear double.
The large mastiff will howl all
night when the great pontiff
changes his abode.

THIRD WORLD WAR, *c.* 1986?

There are several Popes who have changed their abode in
the past, notably Pius VI who died in Valence, and Pius VII,
who was forcibly detained by Napoleon before returning to

---

[1]*pugne*—Latin, *pugna* = battle.
[2]*insulte*—O. Provençal = insult. Tumult, upheaval.

Rome. However the reference to the two suns, plus the great
star, which is probably a comet, may bring the quatrain to 1986
when Halley's comet will reappear and when the next Pope
but one, predicted by Malachy, may well be in the Vatican,
whose motto is given as *de laboris solis,* the toil of the sun. This
all fits in with Nostradamus' description of a Third World War
towards the end of this century. The then Pope might well
have to leave the Vatican, or even Europe, if this should arise.
See I. 16, II. 46, 62, VIII. 59, 77, X. 49, 72, 74, 75.

42

Coq, chiens & chats de sang *seront repeus*	The cock, cats and dogs will be replete with blood when
Et de la playe du tyran trouvé *mort.*	the tyrant is found dead of a wound in the bed of another.
Au lict d'un autre jambes & bras *rompus,*	Both arms and legs broken, he who was not afraid dies a
Qui n'avait peur de mourir de *cruelle mort.*	cruel death.

DEATH OF ROBESPIERRE, 1794

The cock is the emblem of France, and the dogs and cats
the rabble who have had enough of the reign of Terror under
the Committee led by Robespierre. Between 12th–28th July,
1,285 victims died on the guillotine. Robespierre was a tyrant
but so were many others of his Committee. On 26th July 1794,
he said the Terror should be ended and the Committee of
Public Safety renewed. Robespierre was arrested but freed by
troops of the Commune who took him to the Hôtel de Ville
(strange bed). Then the National Guard captured Robespierre;
he was shot in the jaw (not arms and legs) and after a long
night of agony he was executed without further trial on 29th
July at the Place de la Revolution.

43

Durant l'estoille chevelue¹ apparente,	During the appearance of the bearded star, the three great princes will be made enemies. The shaky peace on earth will be struck from the skies, the Po, the winding Tiber, a serpent placed upon the shore.
Les trois grans princes seront faits enemis:	
Frappés du ciel paix terre tremulante,	
Pau, Timbre undans, serpent sus le bort mis.	

TRIPLE ALLIANCE, 1881

Pope Leo XIII is given the motto 'Lumen in Caelo' by the prophet Malachy, and on his coat of arms was a comet (*estoille chevelue*). He is also referred to as this in VI. 6 by Nostradamus. During Leo XIII's reign the Triple Alliance (three great princes) was formed in 1881 by Germany, Austria and Italy against France. The fact that peace was disturbed is probably a reference to the Triple Entente, which ultimately led to the First World War. The snake which constricted the French leaders was that of the Triple Alliance.

44

L'aigle pousée entour de pavillions,	The eagle driven back around the tents will be chased by other birds around him. Then the sound of cymbals, trumpets and bells will restore sense to the senseless woman.
Par autres oiseaux d'entour sera chassée:	
Quand bruit des cymbres, tubes & sonaillons,	
Rendront les sens de la dame insensée.	

FRANCE, c. 1813–14

The Eagle is, as always, Napoleon, here driven back from Moscow and surrounded by the other birds of prey, Russia, Austria and Prussia. The last two lines may hold two separate interpretations. First, they may refer to the martial music of the armies which brings France back to her senses, that is, restore to her King Louis XVIII, or they refer to Napoleon's second marriage to Marie Louise of Austria and the grief and madness of the discarded Josephine (*dame insensée*). It was a

¹*estoille chevelue* = comet.

common popular belief that Napoleon's luck deserted him
when he discarded Josephine Beauharnais.

45

Trop le ciel pleure l'Androgyn[1] *procrée,*	The heavens weep too much for the birth of Androgeus,
Pres de ciel sang humain respondu:	near the heavens human blood is spilt. It is too late for the
Par mort trop tard grand peuple recrée,	great nation to be revived. Because of the death, soon,
Tard & tost vient le secours attendu.	yet too late, comes the awaited help.

Androgyn implies an hermaphrodite who causes some form
of aerial warfare in the second line? The rest is very generalized.

46

Apres grand troche[2] *humaine plus grand s'appreste,*	After great misery for man-kind an even greater ap-proaches when the great cycle
Le grand moteur des Siecles renouvelle:	of the centuries is renewed. It will rain blood, milk, fa-
Pluie, sang, laict, famine, fer & peste,	mine, war and disease. In the sky will be seen a fire, drag-
Au ciel veu feu, courant longue estincelle.	ging a trail of sparks.

THIRD WORLD WAR, *c.* 1986?

The great catastrophe of war that Nostradamus predicts
here is linked with a comet appearing at the end of a century.
The most likely is Halley's comet, last seen in 1910 and due
to reappear in 1986, which is consistent with the other dates
given by Nostradamus. He is obviously not exactly clear when
this war will break out and dates between the late 70s and 1999
are given. Comets were important to 16th-Century philoso-
phers and had significance according to their place in the
zodiac. It does not seem to apply to the 1910 dating, because

[1]*Androgyn* = (*a*) hermaphrodite. (*b*) Androgeus, son of Minos of
Crete, killed by the young people of Athens because he won all the
prizes at the Pantheon.

[2]*troche*—from the Greek, *trukos* = misery.

Nostradamus specifies that a great war has already taken place before the comet appears. This is important to remember when linking up the date of a war starting in 1980 in IX. 73. I have already discussed rains of blood in II. 32. See I. 91, II. 41, 62, 91, IV. 97, VIII, 59, 77, X. 49, 72, 74, 75.

47

L'ennemi grand vieil dueil meurt de poison,	The enemy watches with grief the old man dead from poison; the kings are overcome by an immeasurable (number). It rains stones, hidden under the fleece; vainly articles are asserted by the dead man.
Les souverains par infiniz subjugez	
Pierres plouvoir, cachez soubz la foison,	
Par mort articles en vain sont alleguez.	

For showers of stones see quatrains II. 18, 32, etc.

48

La grand copie¹ qui passera les monts,	The great army will pass over the mountains when Saturn is in Sagittarius and Mars moving into Pisces. Poison hidden under the heads of salmon, their chief in war hung with a cord.
Saturne en l'Arq tournant du poisson Mars:	
Venins cachés soubz testes de saulmons,	
Leur chef pendu à fil de polemars.²	

16 DECEMBER, 1986
The square mentioned in line 2 is rare and has only occurred on the 17 July, 1751, and will next occur on 16 December, 1986. The mountains may be the Alps but the third line seems incomprehensible. A saumon in Provençal means a donkey head, but gets one no further.

¹*copie*—Latin, *copia* = forces.
²*polemars* = (a) Greek *polemarches*, he who leads in war. (b) Provençal *polomar*, twine or thick string.

49

Les conseilleurs du premier monopole,[1]	The advisers of the first con- spiracy, the victors won over on behalf of the Maltese: Rhodes and Byzantium open- ing their towns for them, the pursuers in flight will need land.
Les conquerants seduits par la Melite:	
Rodes, Bisance pour leurs expo- sant pole,[2]	
Terre faudra les poursuivans de suite.	

The connection between Istanbul (Byzantium), Rhodes, Malta and a conspiracy is obscure. It almost certainly refers to an incident during the Ottoman Empire.

50

Quand ceux d'Hainault, de Gand[3] *& de Bruxelles,*[4]	When the people of Hainault, Ghent and Brussels see siege laid before Langres: behind their flanks will be dreadful wars, the former wound being worse than their enemies.
Verront à Langres la siege devant mis:	
Derrier leurs flancs seront guerres cruelles	
La plaie antique sera pis qu'ennemis.	

REVOLT IN NETHERLANDS, 1568

Hainault, Flanders (Ghent) and Brabant (Brussels) were the richest provinces of the 16th-Century Netherlands. Nostradamus sees them as involved with a siege upon Langres, which was an important city on the frontier during the Hapsburg wars. The third line then indicates the uprising of the Netherlands in 1568, but it is unclear what is meant by the 'former wound'; possibly some form of internal dissension?

[1]*monopole*—Greek, *monopolum* = conspiracy.
[2]*pole*—Greek, *polis* = town.
[3]*Gand* = Ghent, chief city of Flanders.
[4]*Bruxelles* = Brussels, chief city of Brabant.

51

Le sang de juste à Londres sera faulte,	The blood of the just will be demanded of London burnt
Bruslés par fouldres de vingt trois les six:	by fire in three times twenty plus six. The ancient lady will
La dame antique cherra de place haute,	fall from her high position, and many of the same de-
Des mesme secte plusieurs seront occis.	nomination will be killed.

GREAT FIRE OF LONDON, 1666

The only fire in London occurring in a year '66 is the great one of 1666. This was one of Nostradamus' more interesting quatrains where he gets very close to giving an accurate dating that can be checked historically. The *'dame antique'* who falls is interpreted as the Cathedral of St. Paul's, which was destroyed, and the others of the same denomination, either the churches or their occupants. Many people did flee from their wooden homes hoping to escape the flames in the stone-built churches, but the heat was so intense that even these buildings did not escape. The blood of the just is understood to mean that the victims of the fire were undeserving of their fate. This quatrain is linked with II. 53, by the words *'sang de juste'* and *'dame antique'*. It was very common at this period to give dates without a 'C' meaning 1,000 years, and was assumed as a contemporary date from the rest of the inscription.

52

Dans plusieurs nuits la terre tremblera:	For several nights the earth will shake; in the spring two
Sur le printemps deux effors suite:	great efforts in succession.
Corinthe, Ephese aux deux mers nagera,	Corinth and Ephesus will swim in the two seas; war will be
Guerre s'esmeut par deux vaillans de luit.[1]	stirred up by two valiant in combat.

WAR WITH UNITED PROVINCES 1665–7?

England was engaged in a naval war with the United Provinces from 1665–7, and if one can accept that they are represented by Corinth and Ephesus, even though the link is quite

[1]*luit*—Romance = fight, combat.

obscure, then this, the preceding and following quatrains
become a trio covering the same period.

53

La grande peste de cité maritime,
Ne cessera que mort ne soit vengée
Du juste sang par pris damné
*   sans crime,*
De la grand dame par feincte
*   n'outraigée.*

The great plague in the maritime city will not stop until
death is avenged by the blood
of a just man taken and condemned for no crime; the
great lady is outraged by the
pretence.

PLAGUE OF LONDON, 1665

Nostradamus clearly shows in the second line that he believes the Great Plague and Fire of London to be the result
of the killing of Charles I; see also quatrain IX. 49, where it is
predicted in detail. The maritime city is a description often
used for London, and the plague broke out the year before
the great Fire. It is suggested that the lady who is outraged,
and was interpreted as St. Paul's Cathedral in II. 51, stands
for the Church because soon afterwards Protestantism became
re-established in England under William III, and Nostradamus
was a fervent Catholic. His views towards all Protestant forms
of religion are very hostile throughout his writings, probably
a reflection of the development of Calvinism during his own
lifetime. Again in this verse is the theme that the people suffering from the plague are those of *'juste sang'*, the people of
II. 51, who are described as being in London.

54

Par gent estrange, & Romains
*   loingtaine,*
Leur grand cité apres eaue fort
*   troublée:*
Fille sans trop different domaine,
Prins chef, ferreure[1] *n'avoir este*
*   riblée.*[2]

By a foreign people, far from
the Romans, their great city
will be greatly damaged by
water. A girl without a greatly
different estate taken by the
leader, the iron not having
been removed.

[1]*ferreure* = iron—This may read in variants as *serreure* = lock.
[2]*riblée*—O.F., *ribler* = to rob, pillage.

55

Dans le conflict le grand qui peu valloit,	In the conflict the great man who is of little worth will per-
A son dernier fera cas merveil-leux:	form an astonishing deed at his death. While Hadrie sees
Pendant qu'Hadrie verra ce qu'il falloit,	what is needed, during a ban-quet he stabs the proud.
Dans le banquet pongnale l'orgueilleux.	

FRANCE, 1594

By 1594 the revolutionary ideas of the Paris Seize (Peoples' Parliament) were becoming too strong for the League to cope with, and the Duc de Mayenne, claimant to the throne through the House of Guise, carried out a *coup d'état*. He invited all the leaders of the Seize to a banquet in order to lull their suspicions and had them all killed on the following night. Mayenne hoped that he would be able to hold Paris for the Catholic League but Henri IV (Hadrie) realizing the situation, saw that he had to become Catholic and thus unite France.

56

Que peste & glaive n'a sceu de-finer,[1]	One whom neither plague nor sword could kill will die
Mort dans le puis sommet du ciel frappé:	on the top of a hill, struck from the sky. The abbot will
L'abbé mourra quand verra ruiner,	die when he sees the ruin of the people in the shipwreck
Ceux du naufrage l'escueil vou-lant grapper.	trying to hold on to the reef.

57

Avant conflict le grand tombera,	Before the battle the great
Le grand à mort, mort, trop subite & plainte,	man will fall, the great one to death, death too sudden and
Nay imparfaict: la plus part na-gera,	lamented. Born imperfect, it will go the greater part of the
Aupres du fleuve de sang la terre tainte.	way; near the river of blood the ground is stained.

[1]*definer*—O.F. = die, finish, decide.

JOHN F. KENNEDY?

'*Mort, trop subite*' probably implies assassination and '*nay imparfaict*', a person born with a physical deformity. Senator Jack Kennedy was born with a congenital illness. Many of John F. Kennedy's critics agree that he had a great deal of charisma but wonder whether his political judgement would have been altogether sound had he lived to serve another term of the Presidency. "It will go the greater part of the way" may well refer to Kennedy's stand against Mr Kruschev's attempt to set up missile bases in Cuba. The Russian fleet did, after all, get the greater part of the way from Russia. It was after this confrontation that Kennedy was killed at Dallas '*trop subite et plainte*'. See IV. 14.

58

Sans pied ne main dend aiguë & forte,	Without either foot or hand, with strong and sharp teeth
Par globe¹ au fort de port & lainé nay:	through the crowd to the fortified harbour and the elder
Pres du portail desloyal transporte,	born. Near the gates, treacherous, he crosses over; the
Silene² luit, petit grand emmené.	moon shines but little, great pillage.

This quatrain cannot refer to Napoleon although most commentators generally do so. Napoleon was the second son of the family and this quatrain is quite specific in mentioning the eldest son. I cannot decipher it further.

59

Classe Gauloise par appuy de grande garde,	The French fleet with the support of the main guard of
Du grand Neptune, & ses tridens souldars:	great Neptune and his trident warriors: Provence scrounged
Rongée Provence pour soustenir grand bande,	to sustain this great band, moreover, fighting at Nar-
Plus Mars Narbon, par javelots & dards.	bonne with javelins and arrows.

¹*globe*—Latin, *globus* = a crowd, throng.
²*Silene*—Greek, *selene* = moon, but the spelling *selin* is more normal for Nostradamus, so this may be an anagram.

Neptune apparently refers to Turkey, the dominant power in
the Mediterranean during Nostradamus' lifetime. The trident
warriors are probably French allied troops. Toulon was used
as a base against the Hapsburgs during the 1540s but not later,
and there does not seem to have been any trouble in Narbonne
at this period. A retrogressive quatrain.

60

La foy Punicque en Orient rom-
pue
Grand Jud.[1] & Rosne, Loire &
Tag[2] changeront.
Quand du mulet la faim sera re-
pue,
Classe espargie,[3] sang & corps
nageront.

Faith with Africa broken in
the East, Great Jordan, Rhone,
Loire & Tagus will change.
When the hunger of the mule
is sated, the fleet is scattered
and bodies swim in blood.

ZIMBABWE RHODESIA

Could line one refer to the governmental talks between
Britain and the Africans in September to December 1979? At
the time of these troubles the great rivers of Jordan in Palestine, the Rhone and Loire in France, the Tagus in Spain and
Portugal will suffer political changes. This may mean the borders of the parent countries change, and is in some way allied
to a great naval disaster. These are extremely obscure except
for the interesting typing up of Jordan with Palestine, with
reference to recent talks between King Hussein of Jordan and
President Carter of USA regarding giving the Gaza Strip to
the PLO.

61

Euge,[4] Tamins,[5] Gironde & la
Rochele,
O sang Troyen Mort au port de
la flesche:
Derrier la fleuve au fort mise
l'eschele,
Points feu grand meutre sus la
bresche.

Bravo, men of the Thames,
Gironde and la Rochelle; O
Trojan blood killed by an arrow at the harbour. Beyond
the river the ladder put against
the port, flashes of fire, great
slaughter in the breach.

[1]*Jud*—Short for Jordan.
[2]*Tag*—Short for Tagus.
[3]*espargie*—O.F., *espargier* = to sprinkle.
[4]*Euge*—Latin = bravo!
[5]*Tamins*—Syncope of Tamisiens = people of the Thames?

The French Royal Family is referred to by Nostradamus as being of Trojan blood, see I. 19, but it did not exist by the time that Englishmen fought side by side with Frenchmen. There is no record of a prince of the blood being killed or wounded at a harbour.

62

Mabus puis tost alors mourra, viendra,	Mabus will then soon die and there will come a dreadful
De gens & bestes une horrible defaite:	destruction of people and animals. Suddenly vengeance will
Puis tout à coup la vengeance on verra,	be revealed, a hundred hands, thirst and hunger, when the
Cent, main, soif, faim, quand courra la comete.	comet will pass.

WORLD LEADER. POSSIBLE
THIRD ANTICHRIST

This is yet another reference to Halley's comet of 1986 which probably connects it with quatrains II. 41 and 46. This quatrain could be referring to a future war and the word Mabus could be an anagram of the leader's proper name. Nostradamus as a doctor would know that most diseases do not kill people as well as animals, yet in this verse he specifically says it will happen. It has been suggested that he is referring to atomic fallout which kills all living creatures dreadfully, 'horrible defaite'. See I. 16, II. 5, 28, 62, 89, IV. 50, VI. 33, IX. 51, 77, X. 72.

63

Gaulois, Ausone[1] bien peu subiugera,	The French will subdue Ausonia in a little while, Pau,
Pan, Marne & Seine fera Perme l'vrie:	Marne and Seine, Perme will make drunk. He who raises
Qui le grand mur contre eux dressera,	the great wall against them,
Du moindre au mur le grand perdra la vie.	the great one will lose his life from the least at the wall.

[1]Ausone—Ausonia, Southern Italy.

BATTLE OF IVRY, 1590

If line 2 reads *Parme l'vrie* there is a most interesting possibility. In 1590 the Duke of Parma was ordered to France from the Netherlands to help the Catholic Leaguers against Henri of Navarre. Parma was defeated by Henri at the Battle of Ivry, 1590. However he did not die until 1592 from wounds received at another battle.

64

Seicher de faim, de soif, gent Genevoise,
Espoir prochain viendra au defaillir:
Sur point tremblant sera loi Gebenoise.[1]
Classe au grand port ne se peut acuillir.

The people of Geneva will dry up with thirst and hunger, hope at hand will come to failure: the law of the Cevennes will be at breaking point, the fleet cannot be received at the great port.

CEVENNES, c. 1685

After the revocation of the Edict of Nantes 1685 by Louis XIV, the people of the Cevennes revolted, so deeply rooted was their Calvinist faith. Presumably the fleet would be bringing supplies across Lake Geneva.

65

Le parc enclin grande calamité.
Par l'Hesperie & Insubre fera:
Le feu en nef peste et captivité,
Mercure en l'Arc Saturne fenera.

In the feeble lists, great calamity through America and Lombardy. The fire in the ship, plague and captivity; Mercury in Sagittarius, Saturn warning.

The only comment that can be made about this conjunction is that the last happened in 1839. Saturn equals evil, and, by extension, war. Insubria is definitely either Milan or Lombardy but the dangers to it and America (Hesperie, I. 28) are not clear.

---

[1]*Gebenoise*—Cevennes mountain chain in Switzerland.

66

Par grans dangiers le captif eschapé,	The captive escaped great dangers, his fortune greatly
Peu de temps grand a fortune changée:	changed in a short time. The people are trapped in the pal-
Dans le palais le peuple est attrapé,	ace, by good omen, the besieged city.
Par bon augure la cité assiegée.	

NAPOLEON'S 100 DAYS, 1st MARCH–28th JUNE 1815

The captive who escapes great dangers and whose fortune changes so dramatically in a short time, is Napoleon after his escape from Elba on 1st March 1815. The line can also be read inversely with the meaning that the good fortune will very soon change back again, meaning the defeat at Waterloo on 18th June. The third line is interesting. On Napoleon's victorious return to Paris after his escape, the Parisian mob invaded the palace and court of King Louis XVIII and carried their hero, Napoleon, on their shoulders into the private chambers once occupied by the king, and reinstated him themselves physically. Apparently the crowd was so enormous that no one could get in or out for some hours. The final line is interpreted as meaning that Paris, the city besieged by the Allies, will find its monarch restored (*par bon augure*) as he was on 8th July 1815.

67

Le blond au nez forchu viendra commettre,	The blonde one will come into conflict with the hook-
Par le duelle & chassera dehors:	nosed one, in a duel and will
Les exiléz, dedans fera remettre,	drive him out. He will have
Aux lieux marins commettant les plus fors.	restored the exiles committing the strongest to the marine places.

JAMES II AND WILLIAM III, 1688–9

The blond man was understood even by contemporary pamphlets to stand for William of Orange, who was in fact also fair-haired. William's party drives out James II in 1688, but the Stuart party (*les exiléz*) decided to reinstate him and put all their efforts into a sea battle. James based himself in Ireland and was aided by the French fleet. In 1690 the Allies

were badly beaten at sea off Beachy Head but on the same day
William III won the Battle of the Boyne and James was forced
to flee to France, from which he never returned. The British
fleet did not finally subdue the French and assure her maritime
supremacy for another two years at Cap la Hague in 1692.

68

De l'aquilon¹ les effors seront grands.	In the North great efforts will be made, across the seas the way will be open. The rule on the island will be re-established, London fearful of the fleet when sighted.
Sus l'Occean sera la porte ouverte:	
Le regne en l'isle sera reintegrand,	
Tremblera Londres par voille descouverte.	

JAMES II, *continued*

This seems to continue the last quatrain, and is one of the
pairs that Nostradamus overlooked when he separated them
to make interpretation more difficult. The great efforts made
in the North are those of the invader, William III of Orange.
The British fleet was so sluggishly commanded at this time by
the Earl of Torrington that he lost several sea battles to the
French and Stuart fleets, particularly Beachy Head and Bantry
Bay, and it was only William's strength on land that kept him
the throne. There could be a second interpretation of line 2;
that the seas were open and undefended allowing William to
cross to England. The island, in the singular, indicates Ireland
where James II took refuge; Nostradamus usually refers to
the British Isles in the plural. James naturally re-established
Stuart rule there until displaced by the Battle of the Boyne,
1690. The last line again refers to the bad government of the
British fleet under Lord Torrington. After the defeat at Beachy Head he withdrew his remaining ships to London where
he was courtmartialled for lack of aggressiveness, but acquit-
ted. However, the British paid heavily for his reluctance to act
during the next two years. It may also refer to the occasion
in 1667 before William III came to England when his Dutch
fleet sailed up the Thames on a raiding party.

¹*aquilon*—Latin = North Wind, North.

69

Le Roy Gaulois par la Celtique dextre,	A Gallic king from the Celtic right hand (side) seeing the discord of the great monarch will flourish his sceptre over the three leopards against the king of the great Hierarchy.
Voyant discorde de la grand Monarchie	
Sus les trois pars fera florir son sceptre	
Contre la Cappe¹ de la grand Hierarchie.	

The clue for this quatrain is in line 3, the use of the word *pars*. In another book of his called 'the Horapollo' Nostradamus translates this word as leopards, and these are the three leopards of England, as Napoleon called the English heraldic lions. Thus we seem to continue yet again the theme of James II and William III. William is the Celtic king from Northern Gaul (i.e. Holland) (*dextre* is the northern side on a map) who seeing England in trouble under James II takes over the kingdom. Note that Nostradamus makes no mention of war. It was not a bloody invasion but one of invitation, William having many supporters in Britain. Cappe, as in other quatrains, is Nostradamus' version of Capet, the line of the French kings. As has been explained in the last two quatrains the French bitterly opposed William's establishment in England and allied themselves with the deposed James II and supplied him with troops and naval aid.

70

Le dard du ciel fera son estendue,	The dart from heaven will make its journey; Death while speaking; a great execution. The stone in the tree, the proud nation brought down; rumour of a human monster, purge and expiation.
Mors en parlant: grand execution:	
La pierre en l'arbre la fiere gent rendue,	
Bruit humain monstre purge expiation.	

¹*Cappe*—Nostradamus' version of Capet. One of the names of the French royal line until the last of the Bourbons. See also IX. 20 etc.

NAPOLEON, 1815

This is often interpreted as referring to Napoleon but it seems too general in its meaning for this to be satisfactory. The theory is that the scene is Waterloo 1815, and the dart from the sky is the vengeance of heaven. The next line refers to the carnage and slaughter, and the stone to an axe cutting down the Bonaparte dynasty. Then France surrenders, is expiated, and the monster, Napoleon, is removed to St. Helena. Very ingenious if one can accept it.

71

Les exilés en Sicile viendront,
Pour delivrer de faim la gent es-
trange:
Au point du jour les Celtes lui
faudront
La vie demeure à raison: Roi se
range.

The exiles will come to Sicily in order to deliver the foreign nation from hunger. At daybreak the Celts will fail them, life remains by reason; the king joins in alliance.

72

Armée Celtique en Italie vexé,
De toutes pars conflict & grande
peste:
Romains fuis, ô Gaule repoulsé,
Pres du Thesin,[1] *Rubicon pugne*[2]
incerte.

The French army will be troubled in Italy, on all sides conflict and great loss. Flee the Italians, O France repelled; near the Ticino the battle at the Rubicon is uncertain.

A difficult quatrain, because it sounds so specific and yet has not occurred since 1555. It is best used as an example of retroactive prophecy, that is, describing an event occurring during the prophet's lifetime or earlier and which has sunk into his subconscious. If this is so, the first 3 lines are a good description of the Battle of Pavia 1525, the third line describing the strategy of the Imperial forces. But even then the outcome of Pavia was a definite victory for the Italians, not an uncertain one.

[1]*Thesin*—River Ticino flows into the Po below Pavia.
[2]*pugne*—Latin, *pugna* = battle.

73

Au lac Fucin¹ de Benac² le ri-
vaige,
Prins du Leman³ au port de
l'Orguion.⁴
Nay de trois bras predict bellique
image
Par trois couronnes au grand
Endymion.⁵

The shore of Lake Garda to Lake Fucino, taken from Lake Geneva to the harbour of Orguion. Born with three arms it foretells a warlike image with three kingdoms for the great Endymion.

A large number of wild interpretations have been made for this quatrain including (Allen 1943) that Endymion is a metaphor for the USA! The three arms and crowns may well be the triple tiara of the Pope, linking it with the Vatican States, or a state containing three kingdoms probably set in Italy.

74

De Sens, D'Autun viendront jus-
ques au Rosne,
Pour passer outre vers les monts
Pyrenées:
La gent sortir de la Marque
d'Anconne,
Par terre & mer suivra à grans
trainées.

From Sens, from Autun they will come as far as the Rhône to cross over the Pyrenees. The people going out from the Marches of Ancona will follow in great trails over land and sea.

This quatrain is very muddled. Leoni (1961) has a clever interpretation in which he suggests that the Pyrenees are a mistake for the Alps. This would certainly help the geography, as Sens and Autun are in North Eastern France, but the Rhône is not on the way to the Pyrenees. If we interpret the mountains as the Alps the quatrain describes an invasion of Italy. The Marches of Ancona stretch from Rimini to north of Guilianova.

¹*Fucin*—Lake Fucino, drained in 1876, in Italy.
²*Benac*—Lake Garda, Italy.
³*Leman*—Lake Geneva, Switzerland.
⁴*Orguion*—? possibly Orgon in Southern France, or Orgiano in Lombardy, not deciphered.
⁵*Endymion*—Youth in Greek mythology loved by Selene the moon, and having the gift of eternal sleep.

75

La voix ouie de l'insolite oiseau,	The call of the unwanted bird
Sur le canon de respiral estage:[1]	being heard on the chimney
Si hault viendra du froment le	stack; bushels of wheat will
boisseau,	rise so high that man will de-
Que l'homme d'homme sera An-	vour his fellow man.
tropophage.[2]	

GENERAL FAMINE

The unwanted bird on the chimney stack is an owl or similar bird of ill omen bringing warning of famine and the high price of corn, but one is given no indication as to what famine will be so dreadful that men will become cannibals. Possibly refers to the World Famine of I. 16, 67, III. 34, 42.

76

Foudre en Bourgongne fera cas	Lightning in Burgundy will
portenteux,	reveal portentous events. A
Que par engin[3] *oncques ne pour-*	thing that could never have
roit faire,	been done by trickery. The
De leur senat sacriste fait boiteux	lame priest will reveal matters
Fera sçavoir aux ennemis l'affaire.	of the senate to the enemy.

TALLEYRAND, 1754–1838

Charles Maurice de Talleyrand-Périgord fits this quatrain remarkably well. The starting point lies in the third line, the lame priest. Talleyrand became lame at the age of nearly four years when a chest of drawers fell on his foot injuring it permanently. He was destined by his family for the Church and took orders in 1778 and was Bishop of Antin by 1789. By 1790 he was totally identified with the Revolutionaries, and was banned by the Pope in the following year. By 1807 however, he resigned his position as Grand Chamberlain in Napoleon's service because he disapproved of the Emperor's policies, and secretly advised the Emperor Alexander I of Russia not to pressure Austria as Napoleon wished. By 1814 he was contemplating absolute treachery. When Alexander I came to the Hôtel Talleyrand he was advised by Talleyrand that the res-

[1] The line literally means—on the pipe of the breathing floor.
[2] *Antropophage*—Greek, *anthro-phagos* = man-eating.
[3] *engin*—Latin, *ingenium* = genius, ruse, trickery.

toration of the Bourbons was the only solution for the future of France, and on 1st April in the same year he convened the Senate (line 3) who pronounced Napoleon to have forfeited his crown.

77

Par arcs feux poix & par feux repoussés,	Repulsed by bows, burning pitch and fires, cries and shouts will be heard in the middle of the night. They will get in through the broken defences; the traitors escape through the underground passages.
Cris hurlements sur la minuit ouis:	
Dedans sont mis par les ramparts cassez	
Par cunicules¹ les traditeurs² fuis.	

78

Le grand Neptune du profond de la mer,	Great Neptune from the depths of the sea, of mixed African race and French blood, the islands remain bloody because of the slow one; it will harm him more than the badly concealed secret.
De gent Punique³ & sang Gaulois meslé:	
Les isles à sang pour le tardif ramer,⁴	
Plus lui nuira que l'occult mal celé.	

Neptune was used by Nostradamus in II. 59 to refer to the Turkish Moslem fleet, which brings line 2 into the Franco-Turkish agreements of Nostradamus' day. The famous Barbary pirates, whose leader Barbarossa is also referred to in I. 74, are probably the Punic people, as their base was in Northern Africa. The last two lines may apply to an event of 1558 when, according to Jaubert, the Turkish fleet attacked Minorca (les isles), and took Chidadela, killing and enslaving the entire population of the town. He also states that the Turks were bribed to delay co-operating with the French fleet (tardif ramer) and thus demoralize them instead of coming to their aid in an Italian raid.

¹cunicules—Latin, cuniculus = rabbit, interpreted as burrow, passage, mine.

²traditeurs—Latin, traditor = traitor.

³Punique—adjective for Carthage in North Africa.

⁴ramer—Romance = to remain, stay.

79

La barbe crespe & noir par engin, *Subjugera la gent cruelle & fiere:* *Le grand CHIREN ostera du* *longin,*[1] *Tous les captifs par Seline*[2] *ban-* *iere.*	The man with the curly, black beard will subdue the cruel and proud nation through skill. The great CHIREN will take from afar all those captured by the Turkish banner.

LEPANTO, 1571?

This quatrain poses a problem. All commentators have interpreted CHIREN as an anagram for HENRIC, an alternative spelling for Henri. This verse is then ascribed to the Battle of Lepanto 1571 which freed over 1,500 Christian slaves from the Turkish fleet (line 4). But at the time of Lepanto, Charles X was on the French throne, and Henri III was not to follow until 1574. Perhaps Nostradamus is a few years out in his dates, or uses Henri as a symbol for France? At Lepanto the Christian powers formed the last crusade against the Turks (Seline, because of their crescent-shaped banners). Command was given to Don John of Austria who was dark and bearded. The third line may mean that France benefited from the final removal of Turkish naval power from the Mediterranean. The clue lies in a definitive interpretation of CHIREN. See IV. 34, VI. 27, 70.

80

Apres conflict du lesé l'eloquence, *Par peu de temps se trame faint* *repos:* *Point l'on n'admet les grands à* *delivrance,* *Des ennemis sont remis à propos.*	After the battle, the eloquence of the one left behind for a short time brings a short respite. None of the great will be allowed to go free, they are left to their enemies at the proper time.

---

[1]*longin*—Provençal, *longinc* = far off, distant.
[2]*Seline*—Greek, Selene = moon, crescent.

81

Par feu du ciel la cité presque aduste,	The city is almost burned down by fire from the sky, water again threatens Deucalion. Sardinia is vexed by the African fleet after Libra has left Leo.
L'urne¹ menace encor Ceuca-lion,²	
Vexée Sardaigne par la Punique fuste,³	
Apres que Libra lairra son Phaëton.	

This quatrain appears to be modern for the first line implies the destruction of a city from the air with fire, by bombing or something similar. This devastation is followed by flooding, as Deucalion was the Noah of Greek Mythology. Then follows an African raid on Sardinia or Italy, and line four gives us an astrological dating. Phaeton was the youth who drove the chariot of the sun, Leo, when struck down by Zeus. Libra usually stands for Austria in astrological geography.

82

Par faim la proye fera loup pri-sonnier,	Through hunger the prey will make the wolf prisoner, the attacker then in great distress; the elder having the younger in front; the great man cannot escape in the middle of the crowd.
L'assaillant lors en extreme de-tresse,	
Le nay⁴ ayant au devant le der-nier,	
Le grand n'eschappe au milieu de la presse.	

It is possible to invert the translation of the first line but unfortunately this does not make the quatrain any more specific.

---

¹*urne*—Metaphor for waters, flooding.
²*Ceucalion*—Misprint for Deucalion in other editions, see commentary above.
³*fuste* = a kind of low oared galley.
⁴Probably corruption of *l'aîné* = elder.

83

Le gros traffic d'un grand Lyon changé,	The great trade of great Lyons changed, the greater part
La plus part tourne en pristine[1] ruine.	turns into early ruin. A prey
Proie aux soldats par pille vendengé[2]	to the soldiers through a harvest of pillage. Fogs through
Par Jura mont & Sueve[3] bruine.	the mountains of Jura and Switzerland.

LYONS, 1795

Nicollaud gives as the basis for interpreting this quatrain the Memoirs of the Marquis de Beauregard who says that during October 1795, when troops of the Revolution were putting down an uprising at Lyons, 'we saw large crowds of peasants...who with great empty sacks rushed to Lyons to pillage the town'. This was after a two month long siege and many of the town's inhabitants had been massacred. The fog mentioned in the last line was not recorded.

84

Entre Campaigne, Sienne, Flora, Tustie,	Between Campania, Sienna, Florence and Tuscany, it will
Six mois neuf jours ne ploura une goutte:	not rain a drop for six months and nine days. A foreign lan-
L'estrange langue en terre Dalmatie,	guage will be spoken in Dalmatia, it will overrun the
Courira sus: vastant la terre toute.	country, devastating all the land.

When Nostradamus wrote, Dalmatia belonged to the Venetians, but it was surrounded by the Ottoman Empire. Perhaps he thought it would be taken by the Turks (*estrange langue*)? It was not captured, nor has so specific a drought been recorded along the west coast of Italy.

[1] *pristine*—Latin, *pristinus* = former, early, first.
[2] *vendengé*—O.F. = *vendage* = harvest.
[3] *Sueve* = Switzerland, from the Latin Suevi, the German Swiss.

85

Le vieux plain barbe soubs le statut severe,	Under the severe authority of the old man with the flowing
A Lyon faict dessus l'Aigle Celtique:	beard, at Lyons it is put above the Celtic Eagle. The small
Le petit grand trop autre persevere,	great one perseveres too far;
Bruit d'arme au ciel: mer rouge Ligustique.[1]	noise of weapons in the sky, the Ligurian sea is red.

NAPOLEON

The small great man of line 3 is applied possibly to Napoleon in II. 58 and the theme may be continued here. During the 100 Days Napoleon arrived at Lyons on 10th March; the Eagle is certainly the French eagle since it is described as Celtic, which further develops the possibility. It cannot be identified with the Hapsburg Imperial Eagle in this quatrain. But the stumbling block is line one; who is the severe bearded man who accepts Napoleon at Lyons? Marshall Ney was not bearded, and he went over to Napoleon at Auserre. I leave this to the ingenuity of the reader.

86

Naufrage à classe[2] *pres d'onde Hadriatique,*	The fleet is wrecked near the Adriatic sea, the earth trem-
La terre tremble esmeüe sus l'air en terre mis:	bles, pushed into the air and falls again. Egypt trembles;
Egypte tremble augment Mahometique,	Mahometan increase; the herald is sent to call out for sur-
L'Herault soi rendre à crier est commis.	render.

1799. NAPOLEON IN EGYPT

In 1799 during Napoleon's Expedition to Egypt the British and French fleets met on the Nile and the latter were roundly defeated by the British led by Sir Richard Abercromby. It is suggested that the second line may refer to the French army who had disembarked but were frightened when they heard

[1] *Ligustique*—Ligurian, North Eastern Mediterranean.
[2] *classe*—Latin, *classis* = fleet.

that the French Admiral's vessel had been blown up and the
pieces strewn along the beaches. From this defeat Napoleon
led his troops against the Turks at Acre, but during the siege
his men were struck with the plague and so finally Napoleon
decided to withdraw to Egypt, if he could not break down the
Turkish resistance. A herald was sent to demand the surrender
of Acre but this was refused and Napoleon was compelled to
raise the siege. Equally this could be a dual quatrain referring
to the two severe earthquakes that occurred in Iran in 1979.
The Mahometan increase would then apply to the rise of Islam
in that area and to the change of régime when the Shah was
deposed by the Ayatollah Khomeini.

87

Apres viendra des extremes con-
treés
Prince Germain, dessus le throsne
doré:
La servitude & eaux recontrées,
La dame serve, son temps plus
n'adore.

Afterwards there will come
from a distant country a German prince upon the golden
throne. Servitude met from
over the seas. The lady sub-
ordinated, in the time no
longer adored.

GEORGE I, 1714

This prediction probably applies to the accession of the
Hanoverian George I to the throne of England in 1714.
George came from Germany, a distant country, and was a
German Prince. Should the word germain be used with the
second meaning of cousin or relative, he was also a cousin of
the Queen Anne, but the use of the capital letter makes the
first interpretation the most likely. However, it may be one of
Nostradamus' famous double meanings. The English throne
was a great prize and so is described as golden. Servitude refers
to the fact that George was invited to accept the throne; it was
not won in battle, while the final line is probably a reference
to the Mother Church (Catholicism) which was no longer to
be the main religion once the Hanoverians came to the throne,
or a reference to Queen Anne.

88

Le circuit du grand faict ruineux,	The completion of the great
Le nom septiesme du cinquiesme sera:	disastrous action, the name of the seventh will be that of the
D'un tiers plus grand l'estrange belliqueux,	fifth. Of the third (name) a greater, foreign warmonger,
Mouton, Lutece,[1] Aix ne garantira.	Paris and Aix will not be kept in Aries.

THE CHILDREN OF CATHERINE DE VALOIS AND ACCESSION OF HENRI IV

An interesting and detailed quatrain which becomes very clear on study. The clue again is the seven children of Catherine de' Medici of whom the fifth will be the seventh and last king, Henri III (*tiers*), as his younger brother the Duke d'Alençon had died earlier, and his sister Marguerite had married the foreigner of the same name, Henri IV, who would become even greater through acts of war. Henri IV was considered a foreigner because he was Prince of Navarre, separate from France at this time. He had to besiege Paris before France capitulated and accepted his rule, and he started the siege in the sign of Aries (March, April) after the Battle of Ivry in February 1590. The first line probably refers to the massacre of St. Bartholomew which really sowed the seeds of final destruction for the Valois line (*circuit*) as it was partly because of this dreadful deed (*fact ruineux*) that Henri III was assassinated by the Jesuit Clément and left the throne free for Henri of Navarre.

89

Un jour seront demis les deux grands maistres,	One day the two great leaders will be friends; their great
Leur grand pouvoir se verra augmenté:	power will be seen to grow. The new land will be at the
La terre neufue sera en ses hauts estres,	height of its power, to the man of blood the number is
Au sanguinaire le nombre racompté.	reported.

[1]*Lutece*—Latin, *Lutetia* = Paris.

AMERICA, RUSSIA OR CHINA AND THE MAN OF BLOOD

To solve this quatrain one must first decide on the translation of the word *'demis'*; in the first line. Nearly all versions have the word *'d'amis'* (friends) which is how I have translated it here, because to understand *'demis'* as meaning halved would make nonsense of line two. The power of the leaders cannot be seen to increase if they are halved. The two great leaders sound as though they may be the great powers, and line 3 (the New Land) links them with America, as Nouvelle Lande was one of the contemporary names for America. This may well refer either to President Nixon's initial rapprochement with China or to President Carter's new rapport with Russia. If not, it may refer to the modern usage of the New World. When America is at the height of its power and is allied with another great power, then the man of blood, the third Antichrist of Nostradamus, will start assessing his position. See VIII. 77 where the war is described, III. 60 and IV. 50 where he seems to be placed somewhere in Asia. There are many other references to him.

90

Par vie & mort changé regne d'Ongrie,[1]	Through life and death the rule in Hungary will be
La loi sera plus aspre que service:	changed, the law will become
Leur grand cité d'hurlements plaincts & crie,	more bitter than servitude. Their great city calls out with
Castor & Pollux[2] *ennemis dans la lice.*	howls and laments, Castor and Pollux are enemies in the field.

REVOLUTION IN HUNGARY, 1956

The life and death change in Hungary certainly occurred during the Revolution of 1956 after Premier Nagy renounced the Warsaw Pact on 1st November of that year, and found Russian troops advancing into his country on 4th November.

[1]*Ongrie* = Hungary.

[2]*Castor & Pollux*—Identified with Gemini or the twins.

The strictness of the régime that followed, from which many thousands fled to the West, is well known. There was a general policy of severe repression and there were many executions. The great city of Budapest was occupied and badly damaged by the fighting during the Revolution. The last line means that the pro-Russian Hungarians were fighting against their brother Hungarians, as indeed happened. I do not think this is intended as an indirect form of dating.

91

Soleil levant un grand feu l'on verra,
Bruit & clarté vers Aquilon tendants:
Dedans le rond mort & cris l'on orra,
Par glaive, feu, faim, mort las attendants.

At sunrise a great fire will be seen, noise and light extending towards the North. Within the globe death and cries are heard, death awaiting them through weapons, fire and famine.

ATTACK ON USA OR RUSSIA?

This is a frightening quatrain if one applies it to the future. It seems to imply that a Northern Country, Russia or the USA will be bombed suddenly at sunrise, and this will be followed by a period of great devastation. In I. 92 Nostradamus states that America will suffer the greatest destruction. If we link this quatrain with I. 91, II. 5, 41 and 46, we are facing a very gloomy prospect.

92

Feu couleur d'or du ciel en terre veu,
Frappé du haut nay, faict cas merveilleux:
Grand meutre humain; prinse du grand nepveu,
Morts d'expectacles eschappé l'orgueilleux.

Fire the colour of gold from the sky seen on earth, struck by the high born one, a marvellous happening. Great slaughter of humanity; a nephew taken from the great one; the deaths of the spectators, the proud one escapes.

NAPOLEON III, 1870

The clue to this quatrain is the word nephew in line three. There are several references to Napoleon III as the nephew of Napoleon and this quatrain describes the German artillery; the second line an incident on 2nd August 1870 when a bullet hit the ground by the Prince Imperial's feet, an event much publicized by the newspapers. Napoleon III was captured during the general French capitulation of September 1870.

93

Bien pres du Timbre presse la Lybitine:[1]	Very near the Tiber hurries death a short while before a great flood. The captain of the ship taken and put into the bilges, the castle and palace burnt down.
Un peu devant grand inondation:	
Le chef du nef prins, mis à la sentine,[2]	
Chasteau, palais en conflagration.	

The word Tiber, in Rome, linked with the captain of a ship (the Bark of St. Peter) implies that the latter is a Pope who comes to a dreadful end before a flood. The castle and palace would be St Angelo and the Vatican.

94

GRAND Pau grand mal pour Gaulois recevra,	Great Po will receive great harm from a Frenchman, vain terror to the maritime Lion. An infinite number of people will cross the sea and a quarter of a million will not escape.
Vaine terreur au maritin Lyon:	
Peuple infini par la mer passera.	
Sans eschapper un quart d'un million.	

NAPOLEON IN ITALY AND EGYPT

As the first line says, Italy (the Po) suffered great harm from Napoleon who also terrified the maritime British lion, but vainly, because he did not manage to invade her. A great army did cross the seas to Egypt with Napoleon and certainly at least a quarter of a million men died during his campaigns.

[1]Lybitine—Latin, Libitina = Goddess of Death.
[2]sentine—Latin, sentina = (a) bilges, (b) dregs.

95

Les lieux peuplez seront inhabitables:	The populated lands will become uninhabitable, great
Pour champs avoir grand division:	disagreement in order to obtain lands. Kingdoms given to
Regnes livrez à prudents incapables,	men incapable of prudence. Then for the great brothers,
Lors les grands freres mort & dissention.	death and dissension.

THIRD WORLD WAR AND KENNEDY BROTHERS

The populated lands that become uninhabitable are probably those devastated as a result of the next war. Line 2 makes it clear that it is a territorial war. Kingdoms given to men incapable of prudence, could refer to any unstable political situation, but does seem at the present time to indicate the Middle East yet again. The line referring to the great brothers who suffered death and dissension contains two possible meanings. It can either refer to two great powers of the period, or possibly to the era of the Kennedy brothers. If Senator Edward Kennedy is elected President in 1984, Nostradamus has already given us a tentative dating for a war in 1981 in quatrain IX. 73. There is no other group of brothers known world-wide to link up with this period. See quatrains VIII. 46, 77, both of which refer to the three brothers and a war. Robert Kennedy was killed on June 5th 1968 by an Iranian, Shirhan Shirhan.

96

Flambeau ardent au ciel soir sera veu,	A burning torch will be seen in the sky at night near the
Pres de la fin & principe du Rosne:	end and source of the Rhône. Famine and weapon; help pro-
Famine, glaive: tard le secours pourveu,	vided too late, Persia will turn and invade Macedonia.
La Perse tourne envahir Macedoine.	

The last line of this quatrain, by far the most specific, seems to indicate that Nostradamus foresaw the Persians (never part of the Ottoman empire) inflicting a great defeat on the Turks (Macedonia) so as to open up the Balkans. The light in the sky

if the verse is to be accepted will be seen from the source of
the Rhône at the Furka Pass as far as the mouth of the river
west of Marseilles.

97

Romain Pontife garde de t'appro-
cher,
De la cité que deux fleuves ar-
rouse,
Ton sang viendras aupres de là
cracher,
Toi & les tiens quand fleurira la
rose.

Roman pontiff beware of approaching a city watered by
two rivers. You will spit blood
in that place, both you and
yours, when the roses bloom.

DEATH OF POPE PIUS VI AT VALENCE, 1799

The Pontiff in question is Pius VI who was imprisoned at
Valence by the French after they had taken Rome in 1799.
The two rivers are the Rhône and the Saône nearby at Lyons.
The Pope did die spitting blood, he suffered from an attack
of severe vomiting in the summer (when the roses bloom) and
died on 29th August 1799. His people referred to in the last
line were the thirty-two priests who were imprisoned with the
Pope. The word rose may have a typical Nostradamus double
meaning of red, and therefore revolutionary, as well as of
summertime. Both interpretations fit beautifully.

98

Celui de sang reperse[1] le visage,
De la victime proche sacrifiée,
Tonant[2] en Leo augure par pre-
sage,
Mis estra à mort lors pour la fi-
ancée.[3]

He whose face is spattered
with the blood of a newly sacrificed victim. Jupiter in Leo
forewarns through predic-
tion. He will be put to death
for the promise.

[1]*reperse*—Latin, *respergere* = to sprinkle, splash.
[2]*Tonant*—standing for Jupiter, Tonans, the Thunderer.
[3]*fiancée* = (*a*) marriage, bride. (*b*) Romance—promise or assurance.

99

Terroir¹ Romain qu'interpretoit augure,	Roman land that the augur interprets, will be greatly molested by the French nation. But the French will come to dread the time of the North wind having driven their fleet too far.
Par gent Gauloise par trop sera vexée:	
Mais nation Celtique craindra l'heure,	
Boreas,² classe³ trop loing l'avoir poussée.	

Terroir¹ Romain qu'interpretoit augure,
Par gent Gauloise par trop sera vexée:
Mais nation Celtique craindra l'heure,
Boreas,² classe³ trop loing l'avoir poussée.

Roman land that the augur interprets, will be greatly molested by the French nation. But the French will come to dread the time of the North wind having driven their fleet too far.

FAILURE OF NAPOLEON'S RUSSIAN CAMPAIGN, 1812

The Vatican States were taken into the French Empire in 1810, the French certainly molested Italy at this point. But soon afterwards, in 1812, Napoleon is suffering the defeat of his Russian campaign due to the cold weather (Boreas) and the folly of his general overcommitment. The fleet may refer to the earlier defeat at Trafalgar.

100

Dedans les isles si horrible tumulte,
Bien on n'orra qu'une bellique brigue
Tant grand sera des predateurs l'insulte,
Qu'on se viendra ranger à la grand ligue.

Within the islands will be so dreadful a tumult although one only hears the warlike party. So great will be the threat of the plunderers that they will come to join in the great alliance.

MALTA 1565

Malta 1565, when all the great powers of Christendom sent reinforcements and aid, the 'Grand Succorso', to La Vallette in order to save Europe. The great alliance is probably the supranational order of Malta plus the Christian powers.

---

¹ *terroir*—Latin, *terra* = land.
² *Boreas*—Latin = North wind.
³ *classe*—Latin, *classis* = fleet.

CENTURY III

1

Apres combat & bataille navale,
Le grand Neptune à son plus
haut befroi:
Rouge adversaire de peur vien-
dra pasle
Mettant le grand Ocean en effroi.

After the combat and naval
battle, great Neptune in his
highest belfry; the red adversary will become pale with
fear, putting the great ocean
into a state of terror.

RUSSIA AND NAVAL WAR

This quatrain may refer to the enormous sea power being
built up by Russia at the present time. 'Neptune in his highest
belfry', should be interpreted as a great sea battle. Strangely
enough, Nostradamus sees Russia, the red adversary, becoming pale with fear although it is it who commences the war and
creates terror on the high seas. He does not indicate on which
side the victory will lie. But see IV. 95.

2

Le divin verbe donrra¹ à la sub-
stance,
Comprins ciel, terre, or occult au
laict² mystique:
Corps, ame esprit ayant toute
puissance
Tant soubs ses pieds comme au
siege Celique.³

The divine word will give to
the substance (that which)
contains heaven and earth,
occult gold in the mystic deed.
Body, soul and spirit are all
powerful. Everything is beneath his feet, as at the seat
of heaven.

ALCHEMISTIC QUATRAIN

Although many commentators dismiss this verse I think it
is a rare and important description of Nostradamus' beliefs
and experiences. The divine word which takes on substance
is either Nostradamus literally calling forth the spirit who in-
spires him to prophecy, or an incantation which gives him
divine powers, 'the occult gold and the mystic deed'. He feels
his body to be possessed of great powers and possibly the last
line indicates that during his prophetic sessions he felt disem-
bodied, that his soul was outside his body looking down on
himself, at the foot of the heavenly seat, a psychic experience

¹*donrra*—Form of *donnera* = will give.
²*laict*—Misprint for *faict*, deed, found in other editions.
³*Celique*—O.F. = celestial, heavenly.

which is now accepted as fact. This is a common trance-like experience. Alternatively Nostradamus could mean that the spirit of inspiration came down to him and is as much present beneath his feet, and therefore under his control, as it is at its heavenly source.

3

Mars & Mercure & l'argent[1] joint ensemble,
Vers le midi extreme siccité:
Au fond d'Asie on dira terre tremble,
Corinthe, Ephese lors en perplexité.

Mars, Mercury and the Moon in conjunction, towards the south there will be a great drought. An earthquake will be reported from the depths of Asia, both Corinth and Ephesus then in a troubled state.

1977?

The astrological conjunction in line 3 could refer to 1977. It is obviously an astrological dating, but the great drought was in Britain not in the South, so this line is difficult to interpret. Alternatively, it may refer to India and the Far East. There were several earthquakes in both Turkey and Yugoslavia during this time and Greece, Corinth and Ephesus, were undergoing a revolution, the deposition of King Constantine and the substitution of the new Régime of the Colonels. This is the only quatrain which links these two towns together in the Prophecies. Quite an interesting quatrain. It is irritating that one can not be more specific.

4

Quand seront proches de defaut des lunaires,
De l'un à l'autre ne distant grandement,
Froid, siccité, danger vers les frontieres,
Mesme où l'oracle a prins commencement.

When the downfall of the crescent ones is close they will not be very distant from each other. Cold, drought, danger around the frontiers even where the oracle had its source.

[1] *argent*—synecdoche for the moon. An alchemistic term used because of its colour.

1980-81?

Joubert understands the first line as meaning a year when the solar and lunar eclipse come close together and arrives at the year 1556. He states that there was no rain from April to August followed by a very severe winter in 1556–7. The danger at the frontier was the Spanish invasion of Picardy. The last line must refer either to Salon where Nostradamus lived, or to St Rémy where he was born. At both towns there were local uprisings against the Huguenots by the peasantry, the Cabans, which continued well on into the 1560s. It is just possible that *lunaires* may mean 'people of the crescent', i.e. Mohammedans, and then the quatrain should be interpreted with regard to the contemporary struggles against the Ottoman Empire. Equally this may be a split quatrain and the first two lines may refer to the present time in the Middle East. The invasion of Afghanistan took place in the winter on the 'cold' frontiers of Iran.

5

Pres loing defaut de deux grands luminaires,	Then, after the eclipse of the two great stars which will occur between April & March. Oh, what a loss! but two great good influences will help on all sides by land and sea.
Qui surviendra entre l'Avril & Mars:	
O quel cherté mais deux grans debonnaires,	
Par terre & mer secourrant toutes pars.	

This quatrain probably continues on from III. 4, but is unclear as to what may happen between March and April. Perhaps the two good influences are those of planets and stars? Nostradamus may mean that the drought would have been even more severe except for their influence.

6

Dans temple clos le foudre y entrera,	Lightning will strike inside the closed temple and will harm the citizens inside their stronghold. Horses, cattle, men, the flood will reach the walls; through hunger and thirst beneath the weakest armed.
Les citadins dedans leur fort grevez	
Chevaux, boeufs hommes, l'onde mur touchera,	
Par faim, soif, soubs les plus faibles armez.	

CHATEAUNEUF 1819?

Lightning must have struck more than one church since 1555 when Nostradamus published this verse. There is however a famous occasion in 1819 at Châteauneuf when nine people were killed and eighty-two injured among those present. But this does not have any connection with a flood around this period, nor with people and cattle retiring to a fortified place on high ground to escape the waters. It is possible that the last two lines belong to another verse, and that this is one of the 'split' verses I mention in the Introduction.

7

Les fugitifs, feu du ciel sus les piques.
Conflict prochain des corbeaux s'esbatans,
De terre on crie aide secours celiques,
Quand pres des murs seront les combatants.

The fugitives, fire from heaven on to their weapons, the next conflict will be that of the crows. They call on earth for help and heavenly aid when the aggressors draw near the walls.

OCCUPIED FRANCE, 1940

The quatrain is usually understood as describing the Fall of France in 1940, when the French army and multitudes of refugees were driven back in confusion along the roads to Paris. The fire from the sky may mean the aerial attacks to which they were subjected, even the refugees were heavily bombed and strafed on the roads. The aggressors are the Germans about to enter Paris. The conflict of the crows probably refers to the habit of carnivorous birds devouring parts of dead bodies, the eyes in particular.

8

Les Cimbres joints avecques leurs voisins,
Depopuler viendront presque l'Espaigne:
Gens amassez, Guienne & Limosins,
Seront en ligue, & leur feront compaigne.

The Cimbrians, allied with their neighbours will come to ravage almost all of Spain. People gathered in Guienne & Limousin will be allied, and join their company.

SPANISH CIVIL WAR, 1936

The Cimbrians were a North German tribe who vanished as early as 100 BC becoming intermixed with the Teutones. This verse may refer to Germany and her neighbour Italy who supported the Fascist cause in Spain and Franco's armies, during the bloody Civil War of 1936–9. The last two lines may be a reference to the wide support for Hitler's policies that existed inside France at this period, or alternatively to the many Frenchmen who came to fight for the Insurgent armies in Spain, and to the fact that the Republican Spanish army after its defeat at Teruel in 1938 was actually driven into France for a time, followed by a mass exodus of Spanish refugees into France early in 1939. See III. 54, 68.

9

Bordeaux, Rouan, & la Rochelle joints,
Tiendront autour la grand mer Occeane,
Anglois, Bretons, & les Flamans conjoints,
Les chafferont jusque au pres de Rouane.

Bordeaux, Rouen & la Rochelle allied, will hold all around the open seas; The English, Bretons and Flemish allied will drive them as far as Roanne.

Although this quatrain gives detailed names and places it remains quite obscure. Bordeaux and La Rochelle are near each other, but Rouen is to the North. Roanne is on the upper Loire.

10

De sang & faim plus grand calamité,
Sept fois s'appreste à la marine plage:
Monech¹ de faim, lieu pris, captivité,
Le grand mené croc² en ferree caige.

With blood and famine even greater calamity; seven times it approaches the sea shore. Monaco, from hunger, captured, in captivity. The great golden one caught, in an iron cage.

¹*Monech*—Latin, *Moneceus* = Monaco.
²*croc*—(*a*) Latin, *croceus* = yellow. (*b*) O.F., *croquer* = to crunch. (*c*) Prov., *croc* = a hook.

HOUSE OF GRIMALDI, MONACO

Monaco was already a semi-independent state under the House of Grimaldi in Nostradamus' time. He refers to a series of disasters affecting the small state, none of which appear to have come true to date. The last line is particularly difficult to translate.

11

Les armes battre au ciel longue saison
L'arbre au milieu de la cité tombé:
Verbine,[1] rongne, glaive en face, Tison
Lors le monarque d'Hadrie succombé.

The weapons fight in the sky for a long period; the tree fell in the middle of the city. The sacred branch cut, a sword opposite Tison, then the King Hadrie falls.

ASSASSINATION OF HENRI IV, 1610

Hadrie is one of Nostradamus' anagrams for Henri IV, which seems at first sight to clash with line one, which suggests a modern battle in the air. But apparently when Henri was assassinated by Ravaillac on 14th May 1610 according to Guynaud there appeared in the *Mercure Français* of 1619 the story of a ghostly army marching in the skies at the time of the killing. It may have been a similar phenomenon to the Angels of Mons. Henri is the tree chopped down in the centre of the city of Paris, and he is also the last of the direct Valois family tree, as Louis XIII was the son of his second wife Marie de' Medici. He is described as sacred because he was anointed at his coronation; he was actually stabbed with a knife in the rue Ferronnierre, not far from the corner of which runs the Rue Tison. Nostradamus gives us another obscure but graphic proper name which helps sort out the whole quatrain.

---

[1]*verbine*—Latin, *verbene* = sacred branch.

12

Par la tumeur de Heb, Po, Tag, Timbre & Rome[1] *Et par l'estang Leman*[2] *& Aretin*[3] *Les deux grands chefs & citez de Garonne,* *Prins mors noyez. Partir humain butin.*	Because of the overflow of the Ebro, Po, Tagus, Tiber and Rhone and by the lakes of Geneva and Arezzo the two great and chief cities of the Garonne taken, dead, drowned. Human booty divided.

FLOOD

The flooding described in this quatrain is so vast that it covers Spain and Portugal (Ebro and Tagus), Italy (Po and Tiber) and France (Rhône). Lake Geneva is in Switzerland and Lake Trasimine is near Arezzo. The two chief cities of the Garonne are Bordeaux and Toulouse. There are other quatrains of this type predicting a vast general flood.

13

Par fouldre en l'arche[4] *or & argent fondu,* *De deux captifs l'un l'autre mangera:* *De la cité le plus grand estendu,* *Quand submergee la classe*[5] *nagera.*	Through lightning in the box gold and silver are melted, the two captives will devour each other. The greatest one of the city stretched when the fleet travels under water.

SUBMARINE FLEET

The first two lines are probably alchemistic and Nostradamus is referring to a chemical process that would fuse the two metals together. Line three is very obscure; the fourth line certainly indicates a fleet of submarines although it is difficult to know whether the metal of the first two lines is linked with the ships as a weapon, or a separate process. It has been suggested that this may be a reference to a generator for collecting cosmic rays.

[1]*Rome*—Misprint for Rhône, although it may be the city that is intended.
[2]*Leman*—Latin, *Lemannus* = Lake Geneva.
[3]*Arentin*—Latin, *Arentius* = now Arezzo.
[4]*arche*—Latin *arx* = box, ark.
[5]*classe*—Latin, *classis* = fleet.

14

Par le rameau¹ du vaillant per-
*   sonnage,*
De France infime, par le pere in-
*   felice:*
Honneurs, richesses, travail en
*   son vieil aage²*
Pour avoir creu le conseil d'homme
*   nice.³*

Through the offspring of a
valiant personage, of weakened France because of the
unhappy father; honours,
riches, labour in his old age,
because he believed the coun-
sel of an inexperienced man.

LOUIS XV AND FLEURY

Louis XV, son of the glorious Sun King, that valiant personage Louis XIV, caused the weakening of France. He came
to the throne aged five, and the Duke of Orléans exerted total
power during his Regency. France was in such a poor financial
state that it led to her bankruptcy under John Law in 1721.
The inexperienced man who brings trouble to the king, must
be Fleury, tutor and priest who did not come to power until
he was seventy-two in 1726. His policies helped the general
unrest leading to the attempted assassination of Louis XV by
Damiens in 1757.

15

Coeur, rigeur, gloire le regne
*   changera,*
De tous points contre ayant son
*   adversaire,*
Lors France enfance par mort
*   subjuguera,*
Un grand regent sera lors plus
*   contraire.*

The kingdom will change in
heart, vigour and glory. On
all sides having its adversary
opposed. Then through death
a child will rule over France,
the great Regent will then be
very contrary.

LOUIS XV

This quatrain continues with the subject of Louis XV. Again
we get a reference to the glory of the reign of Louis XIV (the
great kingdom will change in glory etc.) and a reference to the
Regent, Philippe, Duke of Orléans, who was the complete opposite both in public and private life, to his predecessor (*ad-*

¹*rameau*—literally branch.
²*aage*—O.F. spelling = age.
³*nice*—Romance = simple, inexperienced.

versaire). There has been no other male Regent of France since the publication of the Centuries. It is possible that in the words 'then through death a child will rule over France' there is a confirmation of popular opinion of the time which stated that both the Duke of Burgundy and the Duke of Bretagne, Louis XV's grandfather and father, had been poisoned by the Regent in order to obtain control over the throne.

16

Un prince Anglais Mars a son coeur de ciel,	An English prince, Mars has his heart in the heavens, will
Voudra poursuivre sa fortune prospere:	wish to follow his prospering fortune. In two duels, one will
Des deux duelles l'un percera le fiel,	pierce him in the gall bladder, hated by him, but well loved
Hai de lui, bien aimé de sa mere.	by his mother.

A quatrain which seems unfulfilled to date. There have been very few English princes, and even the Scottish ones do not satisfy this prediction. It seems unlikely that duels will take place in the future so this is probably a failure.

17

Mont Aventine brusler nuict sera veu,	Mount Aventine will be seen burning at night, the sky in
Le ciel obscur tout à un coup en Flandres:	Flanders will be suddenly obscured. When the King drives
Quand le monarque chassera son nepveu,	out his nephew their churchmen will commit scandals.
Leurs gens d' Eglise commettront les esclandres.	

Mount Aventine is one of the seven hills of Rome and therefore probably stands for the city itself. The sudden obscurity of the sky in Flanders may mean an eclipse of the sun, but I am unable to link it with a king driving out his nephew plus atrocities being committed in the Church. It sounds vaguely Napoleonic but Napoleon did not actually drive out his nephew, Napoleon III, however. He was driven out from Holland as a child when his father, King Louis, abdicated. The church scandals would relate to the Cult of Reason during the Revolutionary excesses. Presumably the first line may refer to Napoleon I's troops and their successful sack of Rome?

18

Apres la pluie laict assez lon-guette	After the rather long milky rain, several places in Reims will be touched by lightning. Oh what a bloody battle is approaching them, fathers and sons' Kings will not dare approach.
En plusieurs lieux de Reims le ciel touché:	
O quel conflict de sang pres d'eux s'appreste,	
Peres & fils Rois n'oseront approcher.	

The reference to a rain of milk is puzzling. It also occurs in the following quatrains, II. 32, III. 19. V. 62.

19

En Luques sant & laict viendra plouvoir,	In Lucca it will come to rain blood and milk, shortly before a change of governor. Great plague and war, famine and drought will be seen, far from where the prince and ruler dies.
Un peu devant changement de preteur:[1]	
Grand peste & guerre, faim & soif fera voir	
Loing où mourra leur Prince recteur.[2]	

Lucca was a duchy between Tuscany and Modena. It is impossible to try and identify the governor and the prince. Apart from the rain of milk we now also have a rain of blood, a favourite of Roman historians, but which can occur when red dust clouds meet rain clouds and the resultant drops fall red coloured. After the atomic bombs were dropped in 1945 the rain fell black, full of atomic dust. See II. 32, when showers of blood and fish fell over a town in Brazil in 1968. Also V. 62.

[1]*preteur*—Latin, *praetor* = governor.
[2]*recteur*—Latin = leader, governor, instructor, ruler.

20

Par les contrees du grand fleuve Bethique[1]	Through the lands of the great river Guadalquivir far
Loing d'Ibere[2] *au royaume de Grenade:*[3]	from Spain to the kingdom of Grenada; the cross spurned
Croix repoussees par gens Mahometiques,	by the Mohammedans, a man from Cordova will betray his
Un de Cordube trahira la contrade.[4]	country.

GONSALVO FERNANDEZ DE CORDOVA

Grenada, the last Moorish outpost of Iberia, North Eastern Spain, was conquered in 1492. It is south of the Guadalquivir river. The Jews in this area were allowed to remain after the conquest provided they accepted Christianity. In 1610, the remainder of the Jewish colony were accused of lack of sincerity in their religious practices and turned out of Spain by Philip II, despite the fact that a contract had been drawn up by Ferdinand and Isabella of Spain with Gonsalvo Fernandez de Cordova who helped negotiate the treaty. Here is another proper name produced by Nostradamus.

21

Au Crustamin[5] *par mer Hadriatique,*	Near the (river) Conca by the Adriatic sea will appear an
Apparoistra un horrible poisson:	horrible fish with human fea-
De face humaine & la fin[6] *aquatique,*	tures and an aquatic purpose,
Qui se prendra dehors de l'ameçon.	it will be caught without a hook.

Garencières (1672) says in his commentary that a mermaid-like creature, perhaps a manatee or dugong was seen near Rome in 1523 and by Rondeletius in 1531. But Edgar Leoni states in his commentary that the records of Cattolica, where the Conca flows into the Adriatic, shows no such event. Even

[1]*Bethique*—Latin, *Baetis* = Guadalquivir river.
[2]*Ibere*—Greek for Spaniards around river Ebro.
[3]*Grenade*—Southern Spain.
[4]*contrade*—Provençal = country.
[5]*Crustamin*—Latin, *Crustimius* flows into the Adriatic, now called river Conca.
[6]*fin*—Either means end or purpose.

Garencières seems to have been carried away by hearsay events in this case.

22

Six jours l'assaut devant cité donné:	Six days the assault is made in front of the city. It will be
Livree sera forte & aspre bataille:	freed in a strong and bitter fight. Three will hand it over,
Trois la rendront & à eux pardonné,	and to them pardon, to the
Le reste à feu & sang tranche traille.	rest fire and bloody slaughter and slashing.

Too general to be specifically identified.

23

Si France passes outre mer ligustique,[1]	If, France, you cross the Ligurian sea, you will find yourself besieged among islands
Tu te verras en isles & mers enclos:	and seas. Mahomet against
Mahommet contraire, plus mer Hadriatique,	you, more so the Adriatic, you will gnaw the bones of horses
Cheveux & d'Asnes tu rongeras les os.	and asses.

FRANCE, IRAN AND ADRIATIC

A general prediction which connects France with a leading Mohammedan country, probably Iran, and with war, danger starting in the Adriatic.

24

De l'entreprinse grande confusion,	From the expedition great confusion, immense loss of
Perte de gens, tresor innumerable:	men and treasure. You must never attempt to expand there
Tu n'y dois faire encore tension[2].	again. France, try to remember my prediction.
France à mon dire fais que sois recordable.[3]	

[1] *ligustique*—Latin, *ligusticus* = Ligurian.
[2] *tension*—Latin, *tensio* = extension.
[3] *recordable*—O.F. = memorable.

PERSONALIZED PREDICTION

This is one of the very few predictions that Nostradamus makes in the first person. It is clear he feels very strongly about the future of his country, France, and may well be the continuation of the warnings contained in the previous quatrain.

25

Qui au Royaume Navarrois par-
viendra,
Quand de Sicile & Naples seront
joints:
Bigore & Landres par Foix loron
tiendra,
D'un qui d'Espaigne sera par
trop conjoint.

He who attains the kingdom of Navarre when Sicily and Naples are allies; he will hold Bigorre and Landes through Foix and Oloron from one who will be too strongly allied with Spain.

HENRI IV

The man who inherits Navarre is Henri IV; Sicily and Naples were joined together sporadically for centuries but the title was only formalized three times, first by Philip of Spain when he was due to marry Mary Tudor in 1554, later by Joseph Buonaparte and Joachim Murat in the 19th Century. Henri became king of Navarre in 1562 and king of France in 1594. All the places mentioned in line 3 are in Navarre, and Bigorre has a double meaning as Bigorro was the rallying cry of the Huguenot armies, a typical Nostradamus 'pun'. The person too strongly allied with Spain from whom Henri IV keeps Navarre, is presumably his cousin Elizabeth, daughter of Henri II who married Philip of Spain in 1558. A rather generalized quatrain in many ways.

26

Des Rois & Princes dresseront
simulacres,
Augures, cruez eslueuz arus-
pices:[1]
Corne, victime dorée, & d'azur,
d'acre,
Interpretez seront les extipices.[2]

They will raise up idols of kings and princes, augurers and hollow priests elevated. A victim, its horns gilded with gold, azure, dazzling, the entrails will be interpreted.

[1]*aruspices* = auspices.
[2]*extispicus* = soothsayer, inspector of animal's entrails.

27

Prince libinique puissant en Occident,	The Libyan prince will be powerful in the West, the French will become so enamoured of Arabia; learned in letters he will condescend to translate the Arab Language into French.
François d'Arabe viendra tant enflammer,	
Scavans aux lettres sera condescendant,	
La langue Arabe en François translater.	

PRESIDENT GADAFFI AND LIBYA

This is another quatrain which made little sense when the book was first written but which now appears much clearer. It reiterates the connection that Nostradamus believed to exist between France and the Middle East and the Libyan reference is almost certainly one to President Gadaffi and his influence in the West, due to his involvement with Palestine and the oil problems of the West. The reference to a translation from Arabic to French is puzzling, as Algeria was French and has now become a country in its own right. The first French/Arabic dictionary appeared in 1505, but I can not think of any other work of literary merit that was translated under these conditions.

28

De ferre faible & pauvre parentele,[1]	One possessing few lands and of poor parentage through efforts and peace will attain to the empire. For a long time a young woman shall reign, never has a worse influence remained on the kingdom.
Par bout & paix parviendra dans l'empire:	
Long temps regner une jeune femelle,	
Qu'oncques en regne n'en survint un si pire.	

ENGLAND AND FRANCE, 1558

This is regarded by most commentators as a 'split' quatrain referring to two different people. The first two lines refer to Henri of Navarre whose court was renowned for its poverty and simplicity. Elizabeth and Henri only reigned contemporaneously between the years of 1594 and 1601, but Elizabeth's

---

[1] *parentele*—O.F. = parentage.

confirmation of Protestantism would rate the epithet 'worse influence' from the pro-Catholic Nostradamus. Elizabeth ruled for nearly half a century which was an extremely protracted reign for that period. However, the first two lines could perhaps refer to the lowly origin of Anne Boleyn, Elizabeth's mother, and the poverty to which she was subjected as a child. Alternatively, the two lines may refer to Elizabeth I of England, the virgin Queen, who would never admit that she was growing old and became a grotesque character in her old age. Nostradamus is extremely biased in describing her influence on the kingdom as a bad one. She did, however, reign for longer than any other English queen.

29

Les deux nepveux en divers lieux nourris:
Navale pugne,[1] terre peres tombez:
Viendront si haut esluuez enguerris,[2]
Venger l'injure ennemis succombez.

Two nephews will be brought up in different places, a naval battle, fathers fallen to the ground. They will be greatly elevated by making war, to avenge their injury, the enemies overcome.

The nephews mentioned here may be two of one of the many Popes, or alternatively the nephews of the then Constable of France, Anne de Montmorency, Coligny, Chatillon and d'Andelot; however there is nothing to show which of them were intended here.

30

Celui qu'en luitte & fer au faict bellique,
Aura porté plus grand que lui le prix:
De nuict au lict six lui feront la pique,
Nud sans harnois subit sera surprins.

He who in the struggle with a weapon in deed of war will have carried off the prize from one greater than he. At night six will bring harm to his bed, naked without his armour he will suddenly be surprised.

[1] *pugne*—Latin, *pugna* = battle.
[2] *enguerroier*—O.F. = to make war.

COUNT OF MONTGOMERY, 1574

The Count of Montgomery, Captain of Henri II's Scottish Guard, who unwittingly killed his king in a friendly joust, is the hero of this quatrain. Although Henri had pardoned him, Catherine demanded Montgomery's life, determined to avenge her husband. He fled to England as a Huguenot and came back to Normandy to lead the rebelling Protestants. After various successes, he was surrounded by the Marshal de Matignon at Domfront and compelled to yield. Under the terms of surrender his life was to be spared but Catherine secretly sent six men of the royal guard to arrest him. He was taken in his bedroom on 27th May 1574 and sent to the Conciergerie at Catherine's command. Note that Nostradamus does not mention his death, only the circumstances of his capture.

31

Aux champs de Mede, d'Arabe & d'Armenie,
Deux grans copies¹ trois fois s'assembleront:
Pres du rivage d'Araxes la mesgnie,²
Du grand Soliman en terre tomberont.

On the (battle)fields of Media, Arabia and Armenia, two great armies will assemble three times; near the border of Araxum the establishment of great Suliman will fall to the ground.

LEPANTO, 1571

A great deal has been written about this quatrain referring it to battles which had already occurred during Nostradamus' lifetime, in particular to the Battle of Araxes of 1514 or to the fighting with the Turks in Armenia and Media—but not Arabia—which continued until the general peace of 1555. It appears more probable that James Laver's interpretation is the correct one. The Battle of Lepanto, fought in 1571 in which Don John of Austria crushed Selim II, the son of Soliman (part of his establishment). Lepanto was fought off Cape Papa, then known as Cape Araxum, in the Mediterranean.

¹*copies*—Latin, *copiae* = forces.
²*mesgnie*—O.F. = household, establishment.

32

Le grand sepulchre du peuple Aquitanique,	The huge grave for the French people will approach from the direction of Italy. When war is near the German corner and in the lands of the Italian people.
S'approchera aupres de la Toscane:	
Quand Mars sera pres du coing Germanique,	
Et au terroir de la gent Mantuane.	

SECOND WORLD WAR AND MUSSOLINI

A general quatrain, but one which can best be applied to the Second World War because of Nostradamus' insistence on the involvement of Italy and Germany in a war that would kill many Frenchmen. Aquitaine stands for France, as do Tuscany and Mantua for Italy. It is possible that the lands of the Italian people refer to Mussolini, who joined with Germany in declaring war on the Allies in 1940. See III. 32, 68, IV. 68, VI. 31, 33.

33

En la cité où le loup entrera,	Into the city which the wolf will enter, the enemies will be very close by; A foreign army will devastate the great country, the friends will pass the walls and Alps.
Bien pres de là les ennemis seront:	
Copie estrange grand pays gastera,	
Aux murs & Alpes les amis passeront.	

A quatrain involving wars between Italy and France with a third friendly party, possibly crossing the Alps?

34

Quand le deffaut du Soleil lors sera.	Then when the eclipse of the sun will be in broad daylight the monster will be seen. It will be interpreted quite differently; they will not care about expense, none will have provided for it.
Sur le plain jour le monstre sera veu:	
Tout autrement on l'interpretera,	
Cherté n'a garde nul n'y aura pourveu.	

This quatrain is almost impossible to interpret because we are given no date for the eclipse of the sun, other than the coming of a monster which may be interpreted literally or metaphorically. The last line indicates an unexpected famine or drought for which no provision will have been made.

35

Du plus profond de l'Occident d'Europe	In the deepest part of Western Europe a child will be
De pauvres gens un jeune enfant naistra:	born of poor family, who by his speech will entice many
Qui par sa langue seduira grande troupe,	peoples. His reputation will grow even greater in the
Son bruit au regne d'Orient plus croistra.	Kingdom of the East.

HITLER OR NAPOLEON

This is an excellent example of the ambiguous quatrain, one that seems to apply equally satisfactorily to two distinct historical events, here separated in time by over a century. Is this an example of history repeating itself? It seems that throughout history certain situations have recurred which appear very similar when described only in general terms. Therefore we may take this quatrain as describing either Hitler or Napoleon. I prefer the former interpretation as Austria is better described as in deepest Europe, i.e. almost at the limits of the continent; Corsica is less apt in this context although it is near the borders of Africa; one must translate profond as lowest, if Corsica is preferred. Hitler came of lowly stock, as did Napoleon. Both were renowned for their personal magnetism and their famous speeches to their armies. Where Hitler is concerned we can see examples of this in the Nuremberg rallies on contemporary films. The crowd were completely in his hand. It is the last line which convinces me that the German leader is described here. The kingdom of the East, Japan, joined Hitler as an ally and his reputation there was obviously held in great esteem. As far as Napoleon was concerned the East means the Middle East, Egypt, and refers to the fact that Napoleon came to power on the Coup d'État on the 18th Brumaire 1798, on his return to France. See I. 34, II. 24, III. 35, 53, 58, 61, IV. 40, 68, V. 29, 94, VI. 7, 51, IX. 90.

36

Enseveli non mort apopletique,
Sera trouvé avoir les mains man-
*   gees:*
Quand la cité damnera l'heretique,
Qu'avoit leurs loix se leur sem-
*   bloit changees.*

Burned, apoplectic but not
dead, he will be found to have
gnawed his hands; when the
city will condemn the heretic
who, it seemed to them, had
changed their laws.

The word apoplectic obviously indicates a person in a state of
coma or stroke during which he is buried, believed dead. There
are several medical cases on record of this having occurred.
Presumably the hands of the wretched person are chewed by
rats before he returns to consciousness, or bleed as he strug-
gled to get out of the coffin. This event is meant to occur when
a city revolts against its leader, but this is unfortunately not
specific enough to identify it.

37

Avant l'assaut l'oraison[1] *pro-*
*   noncee,*
Milan prins d'aigle par em-
*   busches decevez:*
Muraille antique par canons
*   enfoncee,*
Par feu & sang à mercy peu
*   receus.*

Before the assault a speech is
proclaimed; Milan, deceived
by the ambush is captured by
the Eagle. The ancient walls
are breached by cannon; in
fire and blood few receive
quarter.

NAPOLEON DURING THE ITALIAN CAMPAIGN,
1796

Here again, Napoleon I is described as the Eagle, the rapacious bird of prey. He took Milan twice, first on 15th May
1796, and then on 2nd June 1800. However, the first attack
is referred to here, when Napoleon made that famous speech
to his troops before the battle which echoed around Europe.
'Soldiers, you are ill-fed and half-naked. The government owes
you much but can do nothing for you . . . Soldiers of Italy, are

[1]*oraison* = (*a*) Speech. (*b*) Prayer.

you wanting in courage?' This speech so rallied his men that the defending Austrians retired without trying to hold the city. The last two lines may refer to the following battle of Pavia whose inhabitants rose up against the French. The city walls were bombarded and breached and the city totally sacked.

38

La gent Gauloise & nation estrange,
Outre les monts, morts prins & profligez:
Au mois contraire & proche de vendage,[1]
Par les Seigneurs en accord redigez.[2]

The French people and a foreign nation beyond the mountains will be captured, killed and overcome. In a different month, near harvest time, by the Lords they will be put back into order.

1557

This is accepted by Jaubert as describing the peace declared between the Pope and the Spanish in September 1557, which could be either harvest time itself, or a month later, the grape harvest. In this peace the interests of the troops of the Duke de Guise belonging to the Pope, who were mainly French and Swiss, were completely ignored.

39

Les sept en trois mois en concorde,
Pour subjuguer des Alpes Apenines:
Mais la tempeste & Ligure couarde,
Les profligent en subites ruines.

The seven are in agreement for three months to subjugate the Apennines. But the storm and the cowardly Ligurian destroy them in sudden ruin.

1576 THE HOLY LEAGUE

This quatrain seems to refer to one of the leagues of 16th-Century Italy, probably the Holy League of 1576, and it implies that their agreement is upset by Genoa (Liguria).

[1]*vendage O.F.* = either harvest time, or the time of the vintage.
[2]Alternative translation. Drafted in agreement?

40

Le grand theatre se viendra re-dresser,	The great theatre will be raised up again, the dice thrown and the nets already cast. The great one who tolls the death knell will become too tired, destroyed by bows split a long time ago.
Les dez jettez & les rets ja tendus:	
Trop le premier en glaz viendra lasser,	
Par arcs prostrais[1] de long temps ja fendus.	

The second line referring to the dice and the nets is reminiscent of Ancient Rome but the quatrain remains completely obscure.

41

Bossu sera esleu par le conseil,	The hunchback will be elected by the counsel, a more hideous monster on earth was never seen. The deliberate shot will pierce his eye, the traitor whom the king received as loyal.
Plus hideux monstre en terre n'apperceu,	
Le coup[2] voulant[3] crevera l'oeil,	
Le traitre au Roi pour fidelle receu.	

DEATH OF LOUIS DE CONDÉ. 13th MARCH, 1569

This quatrain is one of Nostradamus' more notable successes and has been recognized by many commentators. Prince Louis de Condé was a hunchback and was proclaimed chief of the Huguenot Assembly in 1560. He was reconciled with the king several times (and made a public confession of his loyalty to Charles IX in 1560 and 1562) but continued to plot against him. He was eventually taken at the battle of Jarnac, 13th March 1569, and was deliberately shot by Montesquiou in the head, although a prisoner.

---

[1] *prostrais*—Latin, *prostratus* = destroyed, ruined.
[2] *coup* = (*a*) Blow. (*b*) Shot.
[3] *voulant* = deliberate. Variant, *volant* = flying.

42

L'enfant naistra à deux dents en la gorge,	The child will be born with two teeth in his mouth; stones
Pierres en Tuscie par pluie tomberont:	will fall like rain in Tuscany. A few years later there will be
Peu d'ans apres ne sera bled ni orge,	neither wheat nor barley, to satisfy those who will weaken
Pour saouler ceux qui de faim failliront.	from hunger.

FAMINE AND RAIN OF STONES

There is also a reference to famine and a person born with two teeth already formed in II. 7. Possibly it could refer to Louis XIV who reputedly was born with some of his teeth fully grown, as there were local famines during his reign? As to the falling stones, see the reference in II. 18, when two American fishermen were chased by showers of stones in October 1973, plus general references to famine and stone falls in the following: I. 16, 67, II. 18, 75. III. 34.

43

Gens d'alentour de Tarn Loth, & Garonne,	People from around the Tarn, Lot and Garonne, beware of
Gardez les monts Apennines passer:	crossing the Apennine mountains. Your tomb is near Rome
Vostre tombeau pres de Rome & d'Anconne,	and Ancona; the man with the dark, curly hair will set up
Le noir poil crespe fera trophee dresser.	a trophy.

There are two other references to the elusive *noir poil crespe* in I. 74, and II. 79, if one disregards the Aenobarbe quatrains. The Lot and Tarn are both tributaries of the Garonne, and Ancona is situated on the eastern coast of central Italy. In the two earlier quatrains the blackbeard applied very aptly to the Turks but they had no hold on central Italy which proved disastrous to the French.

44

Quand l'animal à l'homme domestique,	When the animal tamed by man begins to speak after
Apres grands peines & sauts viendra parler,	great efforts and difficulty, the lightning so harmful to
De fouldre à vierge[1] sera si male-fique,	the rod will be taken from the earth and suspended in the
De terre prinse & suspendue en l'air.	air.

WIRELESS COMMUNICATION AND ELECTRICITY

It is possible that Nostradamus is trying to describe wireless communication in this quatrain. He often used the word 'animal' to describe machines which have some of the qualities of life, i.e. that move or make a noise. Perhaps the tamed animal here is the discovery of the sound waves and the wireless as a form of communication. The lightning that is hostile to the rod, implies that the rod is either a radio mast sending out electric charges, or that it is being threatened by some electrical force, and the mast contains this force in the air. Some forms of electrical charges during storms go from the earth to the sky, although it is normally the other way round. One could alternatively interpret the last two lines as implying that the rod is a lightning conductor. Franklin discovered electricity by means of iron conducting rods in 1752, nearly two hundred years later.

45

Les cinq estranges entrez dedans le temple	The five foreigners having entered the temple; their
Leur sang viendra la terre pro-phaner:	blood will desecrate the land. The example made of the
Aux Tholousains sera bien dur exemple,	Toulousians will be very hard, made by the man who comes
D'un qui viendra les lois exter-miner.	to wipe out their laws.

BATTLE OF TOULOUSE, 1814

In this quatrain the five strangers are understood to be the five great powers who allied against Napoleonic France, Eng-

[1]*vierge*—O.F. spelling; *verge* = rod or wand.

land, Austria, Russia, Spain and Prussia. France is the land desecrated by their invasion. The battle of Toulouse fought by Wellington was very brutal and there were great casualties. The man who wipes out the laws is again the Allied Powers because they bring with them the end of Napoleon's reign.

46

Le ciel (de Plancus la cité) nous presage,	The heavens foretell, concerning the city of Lyons by
Par clers insignes & par estoilles fixes:	means of clear skies and fixed stars, that suddenly the time
Que de son change subit s'aproche l'aage,	of change approaches, neither for its good nor evil for-
Ne pour son bien ne pour ses malefices.	tune.

Plancus is Lyons, so called after its foundation by Lucius Munatuis Plancus in 43 BC. The quatrain is very general and similar to II. 83 in its prediction of a gloomy future.

47

Le vieux monarque dechassé de son regne	The old king chased out of his realm will go to seek help
Aux Orients son secours ira querre:	from the people of the East:
Pour peur des croix ployera son enseigne,	For fear of the crosses he will fold his banner; he will travel
En Mitylene ira par port & par terre.	to Mitylene by land and sea.

SHAH OF IRAN?

If the word 'crosses' refers to Christianity this quatrain may refer to the deposed Shah of Iran who eventually had to seek asylum in the West. He may well have approached Russia or China for help, people of the East, before fleeing to America and Panama. Mitylene is in Greece. There is a faint possibility that the crosses refer to the Swastika. Greece certainly was involved in World War II but was never occupied by the Germans. It seems unlikely that the fear of the 'crosses' refers to the present day political West. See I. 70.

48

Sept cens captifs estachez rudement,
Pour la moitié meurtrir, donné le sort:
Le proche espoir viendra si promptement,
Mais non si tost qu'une quinziesme mort.

Seven hundred captives roughly bound, the lots are drawn for half to be murdered; sudden hope will come so quickly, but not fast enough for about fifteen dead.

No definite information has come to light about this very general quatrain, despite the specific numbers of prisoners and dead involved.

49

Regne Gaulois tu seras bien changé,
En lieu estrange est translaté l'empire:
En autres moeurs & lois seras rangé,
Roan, & Chartres te feront bien du pire.

Kingdom of France you will be greatly changed, the Empire expands to foreign places. You will be set up with other laws and customs; Rouen and Chartres will do their worst towards you.

FRANCE AS AN EMPIRE AND ITS FUTURE

This is important because Nostradamus here calls France an Empire rather than a kingdom and clearly sees a change in the future from one form of rule to another. Rouen is in Normandy, Chartres in the Orléanais and it is implied that possible future trouble for France will come from these places. The last part of this prophecy may not yet be completed. Possibly this refers in a general way to the French attitude towards the Common Market and in particular to its agricultural policy.

50

La republique de la grand cité,
A grand rigeur ne voudra consentir:
Roi sortir hors par trompette cité.
L'eschelle au mur, la cité repentir.

The people's government of the great city will not consent to severe repression. The king, summoned by trumpets to leave the city, the ladder at the wall, the city will repent.

JOURNÉE DES BARRICADES. 12th MAY 1588

The Leaguers in France took Paris into their power after the Day of the Barricades when the people drove out the King, Henri III, and his followers. Henri retaliated by joining up with Henri of Navarre at St Cloud and resolved to besiege Paris. Before he could do this he was assassinated by Jacques Clément.

51

Paris conjure un grand meurtre commettre,	Paris conspires to commit a great murder. Blois will ensure that it is fully carried out.
Blois le fera sortir en plain effect:	The people of Orléans will want to replace their leader; Angers, Troyes and Langres will do them a disservice.
Ceux d'Orleans voudront leur chef remettre,	
Angiers, Troye, Langres leur feront un meffait.	

THE MURDERS OF THE DUKE DE GUISE AND HIS BROTHER, 1588

Henri III murdered the two brothers de Guise on 23rd December 1588. He planned the assassination in Paris and it was carried out at Blois whence the Duke de Guise had fled. He was killed by the king's bodyguard outside the royal apartment and the Cardinal, his brother, was killed the next day. At the same period the town of Orléans rose up against the governor, Balzac d'Entragues, and Charles de Lorraine, a prominent Leaguer and supporter of the Guise cause, took over. The last line is inaccurate; both Angers and Langres allied themselves with the League and Troyes remained neutral. See VI. 11.

52

En la campaigne sera si longue pluie,	In the countryside there will be rain for so long and such a great drought in Apulia; the cock will see the Eagle, its wing badly finished put into difficulties by the Lion.
Et en la Pouille si grand siccité:	
Coq verra l'Aigle, l'aesle mal accompli,	
Par Lyon mise sera en extremité.	

The Cock stands for France; it was the emblem both of the Gauls and of the French Revolutionaries. The Eagle may refer either to the Hapsburg Empire or to Napoleon. If the latter version is acceptable then the Lion stands for Britain who causes Napoleon's downfall. The rain and drought are not recorded but may possibly be metaphorical references to Napoleon's conquest of Italy.

53

Quand le plus grand emportera le pris,	When the greatest man carries off the prize of Nuremberg, of Ausberg and those of
De Nuremberg, d'Auspourg & ceux de Basle	Basle, Frankfurt retaken by
Par Agrippine¹ chef Frankfort repris:	the leader of Cologne: they will go through Flanders as
Traverseront par Flamant jusqu'en Gale.	far as France.

HITLER AND THE NUREMBERG RALLY
The only factor the places mentioned have in common is that they are all part of the Holy Roman Empire. Did Nostradamus think that after a new Emperor was elected France would be invaded from the North through Belgium? It is just possible that this quatrain connects with Hitler through the Nuremberg Rally. At that time he became the leader of Germany and did invade France from the North, but did not get any further than Flanders. See I. 34, II. 24, III. 35, 58, 61, IV. 40, 69, V. 29, 94, VI. 7, 51, IX. 90.

54

L'un des plus grands fuira aux Espaignes	One of the great men will flee to Spain which will bleed with
Qu'en longue playe apres viendra saigner:	a great wound thereafter. Troops will pass over the high
Passant copies par les hautes montaignes,	mountains devastating everything, then he will reign in
Devastant tout & puis en paix regner.	peace.

¹Agrippine—Latin, *Colonia Agrippina* = Cologne.

GENERAL FRANCO AND THE CIVIL WAR IN SPAIN, 1936–9

In 1936 General Franco was exiled from Spain to the Canary Islands as military governor. He then flew (*fuira*) to Morocco and back to Spain to start the rebellion that led to the Spanish Civil War. The wound from which Spain suffered so much was the war, with its appalling casualties, 611,000 men in all. The armies who crossed the Pyrenees, Spain's border, were the 50,000 Italians and 10,000 Germans who fought for Franco's Nationalist party, and the 20,000 Russian soldiers sent to support the Loyalist Republican army. It is ironic that after the Civil War Spain did, in a sense, remain in peace, in that she was neutral throughout the Second World War, and has remained so until this day. See the references to the general fate of Spain and the restoration of the monarchy. I. 31, IX. 16.

55

En l'an qu'un oeil en France regnera,	In the year that France has a one-eyed king the court will be in very great trouble. The great man from Blois will kill his friend, the kingdom put into difficulty and double doubt.
La court sera à un bien facheux trouble:	
Le grand de Blois son ami tuera,	
Le regne mis en mal & doubte double.	

THE DEATH OF HENRI II AND THE REIGN OF HENRI III, 1559–89

This famous quatrain was understood by Nostradamus' contemporaries. The one-eyed king was Henri II killed in the duel of 1559 (see I. 35) being wounded in the eye by Montgomery and dying after ten days of agony. The last two lines describe his son Henri III, who assassinates the de Guise brothers at Blois and the general civil unrest which followed this action. *Doubte double* probably refers to the two factions, the Leaguers and the Royalists.

56

Montauban, Nismes, Avignon & Besier,	Montauban, Nîmes, Avignon and Béziers, plague, lightning
Peste tonnere & gresle à fin de Mars:[1]	and hail at the end of March. Of the bridge at Paris, the wall
De Paris pont, Lyon mur, Montpellier,	at Lyons and Montpellier, since six hundred and seven
Depuis six cens & sept vingts trois pars.[2]	score three pairs.

The dating of this verse from the last line, see footnote, is extremely difficult. All the towns in the first line are in Southern France, but there does not seem to be much connection between the bridge of Paris and the walls of Lyons.

57

Sept fois changer verrez gent Britannique	Seven times you will see the British nation change, dyed
Taintz en sang en deux cents nonante an:	in blood for two hundred and ninety years. Not at all free
Franche non point par appuy Germanique,	through German support, Aries fears for the protecto-
Aries double son pole Bastarnien.	rate of Poland.

BRITISH HISTORY 1603–1995
FUTURE OF PRINCE CHARLES?

The great problem for this verse is to find the date from which to calculate the 290 years and the seven great changes which affect Britain. If the year 1603 is taken as the starting point, quite arbitrarily, the whole verse fits, including the last line which clearly links Poland (*Bastarnien*) with Britain in some manner connected with a war. Aries, the first sign of the Zodiac rules the East. Nostradamus indicates that there will be a critical state of affairs in Poland at the same time as Britain faces a great crisis connected with Germany. It also implies that the royal family on the throne at that time will be the last British dynasty of any note. This may mean that Prince Charles will

[1] Or in the wake of war.

[2] There are several possible readings for this. As above, which is 746 i.e. 1746 or 2301 (1555 plus 746) or 'six hundred and seven twenty three pairs' which gives 1653, or 2208 if added to 1555.

be the last King on the English throne. If an astrological dating is taken, the planet Pluto has a 265 year cycle which will next end in 1995, the new era of peace given by Nostradamus as a specific date in X. 72. Therefore, the seven year cycle should be presumed to start in 1730 approximately. See X. 100.

58

Aupres du Rhin des Montaignes Noriques,	Near the Rhine from the Norican mountains will be born
Naistra un grand de gens trop tard venu.	a great man of the people, come too late. He will defend
Qui defendra Saurome & Pannoniques,	Poland and Hungary and they will never know what became
Qu'on ne sçaura qu'il sera devenu.	of him.

HITLER

Hitler was born in Noricum, that is Austria, and he was the son of simple parents. He came too late in Nostradamus' view because his type of Empire was outdated. The third line must be read as describing Hitler's motives, his so-called 'defensive' attacks on Poland and Hungary to 'save' them from the Allies. The final line is interesting. Could Hitler possibly have escaped after all from the bunker at Berlin? Were the bodies found those of his mistress and himself? There has always been doubt about this question in many people's minds despite Hugh Trevor-Roper's very thorough research into the facts of Hitler's death at the end of the war. See I. 34. II. 24. III. 35, 58, 61. IV. 40, 69. V. 29, 94. VI. 7, 51. IX. 90.

59

Barbare empire par le tiers usurpé,	The barbarian empire is
La plus grand part de son sang mettra à mort:	usurped by a third, the greater part of its people will be put
Par mort senile par lui le quart frappé,	to death. The fourth man, senile, struck dead by his country,
Pour peur que le sang par le sang ne soit mort.	fears lest the line of his blood be dead.

THE FRENCH REVOLUTION. THE TIERS ÉTAT

The Third is usually accepted as meaning the Tiers État of the French Revolution 1789, although one wonders why Nos-

tradamus calls the Bourbons barbaric. There were also three
Committees of Public Safety during the Reign of Terror, those
of Danton, Robespierre and the Directoire. The fourth man
is Napoleon who took over from the Directoire in 1799 and
died a senile death, from old age, on Saint Helena. Napoleon
always feared that his line would not be continued and made
himself an hereditary monarch.

60

Par toute Asie grand proscription,	Throughout Asia there will be great proscription, also in Mysia, Lycia and Pamphilia. Blood will flow because of the absolution of a young dark man, filled with evil doing.
Mesme en Mysie, Lysie, & Pamphylie:	
Sang versera par absolution,	
D'un jeune noir[1] rempli de felonnie.	

MIDDLE EAST

The countries mentioned in line 2 are all to be found in
Asia Minor, the Middle East. 'The great proscription' could
describe military situation of many of these countries very
accurately. The influences of modern Iran, Iraq, Turkey,
Egypt, Israel, etc., have exercised a profound influence on
Western politics in recent eyars. The last two lines may refer
to the leader of students who imprisoned the Americans as
hostages in the Embassy in Iran. Alternatively, this bloodshed
and villainy may have yet to come. See footnotes.

61

La grande bande & secte crucigere,	The great following of the sect of the cross will arise in Mesopotamia. Light company of the nearby river who will regard such a law as inimical.
Se dressera en Mesopotamie:	
Du proche fleuve compagnie legiere	
Que telle loi tiendra pour ennemie.	

SECT OF THE CROSS

The solution to this quatrain obviously lies in the identification of the *secte crucigere*. Did Nostradamus mean the Cru-

[1]*noir* = (a) A young dark-haired man or a Negro. (b) The usual
Nostradamus anagram for *roi*, king.

sades or even the swastika, the *croix gammée*, as it was known in France. Mesopotamia is Iraq and the two rivers are the Tigris and the Euphrates. However some commentators insist that Mesopotamia stands for Paris between the rivers Seine et Marne and that this quatrain thus refers to the German occupation of France in 1940. See I. 34. II. 24. III. 53, 58. IV. 40, 68. IX. 90.

62

Proche del duero par mer Cyrene close,
Viendra percer les grands monts Pyrenées:
La main plus courte & sa percee[1] gloze,[2]
A Carcassonne conduira ses menées.

Near the Douro closed by the Cyrenian sea he will come to cross the great mountains of the Pyrenees. The shortest hand and his opening noted, he will take his followers to Carcassonne.

The river Douro rises in the mountains around Burgos in Spain and the Cyrenian sea is the Mediterranean. Apparently some leader will come across Spain into France. The third line is practically untranslatable, see footnote, and the fourth could carry the second meaning 'He will hatch his plots at Carcassonne'. Perhaps by the shortest hand means that this leader crossed the Carcassonne by the shortest route?

63

Romain pouvoir sera du tout abas,
Son grand voisin imiter les vestiges:
Occultes haines civiles & debats,
Retarderont aux bouffons leurs folies.

Roman power will be quite put down following the footsteps of its great neighbour. Secret hatreds and civil disputes will delay the crassness of these buffoons.

ITALY AND GERMANY 1937

This describes accurately the state of Italy under Mussolini and its relations with its great neighbour Hitlerian Germany after 1937, in whose footsteps Mussolini tried to follow. The

[1]*percee*—O.F., *perce* = stake pole, or opening.
[2]*gloze*—O. Provençal, *gloza* = commentary, notes.

name Mussolini literally means muslin maker—a craft regarded as the lowest of the low, and yet this man is dictator of Italy. The word 'buffoons' describes these two dictators horribly well with their histrionics and projects of Aryan purity and world domination. Hitler was certainly unbalanced and it is probable that Mussolini was also in his later years. See III. 68.

64

Le chef de Perse remplira grand Olchade,[1]	The Persian leader will fill up great Spain. A fleet of triremes against the Mohammedans from Parthia and Media, he will pillage the Cyclades: then a long wait in the great Ionian harbour.
Classe Trireme contre gent Mahometique:	
De Parthe, & Mede, & piller les Cyclades,	
Repos long temps aux grand port Ionique.	

IRANIAN LEADER

The connection between Spain and Iran, (Persia) is unclear at the present time. A trireme is a boat with three banks of oars. Parthia and Media are both parts of Iran. Presumably, they are connected with the invading leader who is also implied as being involved with trouble in Greece, the Cyclades. What is not clear is whether the fleet is destroyed by the Iranians before it retires to port or not. At the time of writing President Carter of the USA has just sent four aircraft carriers to keep an eye on events in that part of the world.

65

Quand le sepulcre du grand Romain trouvé,	When the tomb of the great Roman is found a Pope will be elected the next day; he will not be approved of by the Senate, his blood poisonous in the sacred chalice.
Le jour apres sera esleu Pontife:	
Du Senat gueres il ne sera prouvé,	
Empoisonné son sang au sacré scyphe.	

POPE JOHN PAUL I

There has been a lot of controversy over the recent death of Pope John Paul I. As is known, his reign lasted less than a

[1]Ochlade—Latin = race living in Southern Spain near Cartagena.

month. He was reputed to have been extremely unpopular in the Vatican, (Senate). I stated in the first edition of 1971 that line 4 might possibly indicate that a Pope would be poisoned. At the time of Pope John Paul I's death in 1979 a series of contradictory statements were issued by the Vatican to the newspapers concerning the time and manner of his death. He had dined the night before with some of his Cardinals. The church's refusal to allow an autopsy and the speed with which his body was cremated caused much amazement and speculation at the time. See also IV. 11. Line one suggests that the finding of the tomb, reputed to be that of St Peter, which happened a few years ago is not definitive, and that its authentication is still in dispute. See IX. 84.

66

Le grand Baillif d'Orléans mis à mort,	The great Bailiff of Orléans is condemned to death by one
Sera par un de sang vindicatif.	vindictive for blood. He will
De mort merite ne mourra, ne par sort,	not die a deserved death, nor one by jurors; they will keep
Des pieds & mains mal le faisoit captif.	him captive inefficiently (bound) by his hands and feet.

JERÔME GRESLOT, 1562–9

The Bailiff of Orléans was an hereditary post for the Greslot family since 1530, so Nostradamus clearly intended it for someone of the family. A certain Jerôme Greslot was put to death having opened the gates of the town in April 1562, but he was not condemned to death for this until 1569. Presumably this is what Nostradamus means by his being inefficiently guarded, a gap of seven years between action and execution?

67

Une nouvelle secte de Philosophes,	A new set of philosophers despising death, gold, honours
Mesprisant mort, or, honneurs & richesses:	and riches will not be limited by the mountains of Ger-
Des monts Germains ne seront limitrophes,	many, in their following will be crowds and support.
A les ensuivre auront appuy & presses.	

PROTESTANT SECTS

Nostradamus is probably referring to the sects of the Anabaptists which had been almost wiped out around 1536, and it seems as though he is expecting a revival of these or some similar Protestant sects from the direction of Germany, or could it be another reference to the endless spate of the so-called religious cults that have sprung up since the last war.

68

Peuple sans chef d'Espaigne &
    d'Italie,
Morts, profligez[1] dedans le Cher-
    ronesse:[2]
Leur dict[3] trahi par legiere folie,
Le sang nager par tout à la trav-
    erse.

Leaderless people from Spain and Italy dead and overcome in the Peninsula. Their dictator betrayed by stupid folly, blood will flow all about in the area.

SPAIN AND ITALY IN THE 20th CENTURY

This is an interesting quatrain in that Nostradamus gives us the two countries of Spain and Italy without their kings but with dictators, so this verse definitely describes the 20th Century. The dictator who is betrayed is Mussolini and a fascinating possibility is that by *à la traverse*, he was referring to Mussolini's being hanged. *La traverse* also means a cross roads, the usual place for a gibbet and is a typical Nostradamus play on words. For Franco see III. 8, 54. For Mussolini, see III. 32, 68, IV. 68, VI. 31, VIII. 31, 33.

69

Grand excercite conduict par
    jouvenceau,
Se viendra rendre aux mains des
    ennemis:
Mais le viellard nay au demi por-
    ceau,
Fera Chalon & Mascon estre
    amis.

The great army led by a young man, will come to give itself up into the enemy's hands. But the old man born to the half pig will make Châlon and Mâcon into friends.

---

[1]*profligez*—Latin, *profligatus* = overcome.
[2]*Cherronesse*—From the Greek word meaning peninsula.
[3]*dict*—Alternative, *duict* = leader, but meaning remains unaltered.

The half pig turns up also in I. 64 where Nostradamus describes a man wearing an oxygen mask. Probably here it is derived from the false etymology of Milan which according to legend derived its name from the finding of an animal half sheep, half pig at its foundation. Both Mâcon and Châlon are in Burgundy.

70

La grande Bretaigne comprinse l'Angleterre, *Viendra par eaux si haut à inonder* *La ligue neufue d'Ausone[1] fera guerre,* *Que contre eux ils se viendront bander.*	Great Britain, including England will be covered by very deep floods. The new league in Ausonne will make war so that they will ally against them.

GREAT BRITAIN 1604–7

A very interesting quatrain. England did not become Great Britain until the unification of the English and Scottish thrones under James I. He assumed the title of King of Great Britain on 24th October 1604. In January 1607 there were great floods recorded around Bristol and in Somerset, the country being covered for an area of approximately ten leagues, or thirty miles. The last two lines then refer to the renewal of the Holy League in 1606, Ausonia standing for Italy.

71

Ceux dans les isles de longtemps assiegez, *Prendront vigeur force contre ennemis:* *Ceux par dehors mors de faim profligez,* *En plus grand faim que jamais seront mis.*	Those besieged in the islands for a long time will take strong measures against their enemies. Those outside, overcome, will die of hunger, by such starvation as has never occurred before.

[1]*Ausonne* = Ausonia. Southern Italy, especially Naples but also used poetically for the whole country.

BLOCKADE OF BRITAIN 1939–45. CONCENTRATION CAMPS

The blockading of Britain by the German navy during the Second World War is vividly portrayed in this verse, as are the strong countermeasures taken, described in line 2, which opened the Atlantic routes for supplies. Britain apparently never had more than six weeks of food stocked in the country at one time, and all that was strictly rationed. The two final lines indicate that while the British islanders did not starve there was greater famine abroad, in Europe. The appalling concentration and labour camps of the Nazi régime describe a situation where starvation was a matter of policy and a convenient means of killing off many millions who did not go to the gas chambers.

72

Le bon vieillart tout vif enseveli,	The good old man is buried while still alive, near a great river through false suspicion. The newcomer is old, ennobled by wealth, having taken all the ransom gold on the way.
Pres de grand fleuve par fausse souspeçon:	
Le nouveau vieux de richesse ennobli.	
Prins à chemin tout l'or de la rançon.	

The theme of someone being buried alive is also found in III. 36, presumably to acquire the great wealth referred to. The identity of the usurper remains obscure.

73

Quand dans le regne parviendra le boiteux,	When the lame man comes into the kingdom, a bastard, close to him will compete with him. Both he and the kingdom will be greatly trimmed before he recovers, so that his action will be too late.
Competiteur aura proche bastard:	
Lui & le regne viendront si fort roigneux,	
Qu'ains qu'il guerisse son faict sera bien tard.	

THE DUKE OF BORDEAUX, 1820–71

This is an excellent quatrain full of interesting facts. The Duke of Bordeaux was the heir of Charles X of France. He became lame as the result of a riding accident in 1841. His close competitor was the Count of Paris, who was the illegal pretender to the throne. The trimming away of the kingdom refers to the Franco-Prussian war, so that by the time the Duke came to an agreement with the French they had declared the Third Republic and would not accept his terms, and he died in exile, as did the Count of Paris.

74

Naples, Florence, Favence &
Imole,
Seront en termes de telle fascherie:
Que pour complaire aux malheu-
reux de Nolle,
Plainct d'avoir faict à son chef
moquerie.

Naples, Florence, Faenza and Imola will be on terms of such disagreement that to comply with the wretches of Nola they complain that they had mocked its chief.

Nothing can be made of this quatrain. Faenza and Imola were in the Papal States; Florence, the capital of Tuscany, and Naples of the Two Sicilies. Nola is some eighteen miles East of Naples.

75

Pau, Verone, Vicence, Sarra-
gousse,
De glaives loings terroirs de sang
humides:
Peste si grande viendra à la
grand gousse,[1]
Proche secours, & bien loing les
remedes.

Pau, Verona, Vicenza, Saragossa, swords dripping with blood from distant lands. A very great plague will come with the great shell, relief near, but the remedies far away.

SEVESO JULY 1976

This is almost certainly a reference to the disastrous chemical explosion at Seveso, Italy, in July 1976, which caused many abortions and deformed foetuses among the local population over a wide area. The land is still regarded as contaminated.

[1]*gousse* Prov: = shell, scab, husk.

76

En Germanie naistront diverses sectes,	Various sects will arise in Germany which will come near to
S'approchant fort de l'heureux paganisme,	a happy paganism. The heart captive, the returns small, they
Le coeur captif & petites receptes,	will return to pay the true tithe.
Feront retour à payer le vrai disme.	

PROTESTANT SECTS, 16th CENTURY

This is another of Nostradamus's obsessions, the many Lutheran, Anabaptist and Calvinist sects that were springing up in Northern Europe throughout the 16th Century. He seems to imply in the last line that they will return to the true faith, Catholicism, which hardly seems likely at the present.

77

Le tiers climat sous Aries comprins,	The third climate included under Aries, in the year 1727
L'an mil sept cens vingt & sept en Octobre:	in October the king of Persia, captured by those of Egypt:
Le Roy de Perse par ceux d'Egypte prins:	battle, death, loss: great shame to the cross.
Conflit, mort, perte: à la croix grand opprobre.	

OCTOBER 1727. PERSIA

Here is a quatrain with not only the year, but the actual month and place! Nostradamus must have overlooked it when he went through the quatrains to make them more difficult to interpret. It is quite correct. In October 1727 a peace was concluded between the Turks and the Persians. Egypt belonged to the Ottoman Empire and stands for the Turks. The loss to Christianity is explained by the fact that the Shah Ashraf, in return for the recognition of his dynasty, gave the lands of Emvan, Tauris and Hamadan to the Turks and recognized the Sultan as legitimate successor to the Caliph. The Ottoman power continued in strength until this century, and no more Crusades were ever raised by the Christians.

78

Le chef d'Escosse avec six d'Alemaigne,
Par gens de mer Orienteaux captif:
Traverseront le Calpre & Espaigne,
Present en Perse au nouveau Roy craintif.

The leader from Scotland with six Germans will be captured by Eastern seamen. They will pass Gibraltar and Spain, presented in Persia to the new dreadful king.

79

L'ordre fatal sempiternal par chaisne,
Viendra tourner par ordre consequent:
Du port Phocen[1] sera rompu la chaisne,
La cite prinse, l'ennemi quant & quant.

The fatal and eternal order of the cycle will turn in due order. The chains of Marseilles will be broken, the city taken and the enemy at the same time.

The first two lines are astrological and extremely obscure making it impossible to date the downfall of Marseilles.

80

Du regne Anglois l'indigne dechassé,
Le conseiller par ire mis à feu:
Ses adherans iront si bas tracer,
Que le bastard sera demi receu.

The unworthy man is chased out of the English kingdom. The counsellor through anger will be burnt. His followers will stoop to such depths that the pretender will almost be received.

CHARLES I, 1600–49

Charles lost his kingdom mainly due to his own behaviour and irresponsibility towards Parliament. Of his counsellors Stafford was beheaded and Archbishop Laud burnt for treachery, the former in 1641, and the latter in 1645. His followers who stooped so low were the Scots who sold the king back to

[1]Phocen = Marseilles, after the Phocenses who founded the city.

Parliament in 1646. The Pretender, or bastard, who is almost received in the kingdom is Oliver Cromwell, a man who has no true right to rule and who becomes Lord Protector, not king. See VIII. 37, IX. 11, 49.

81

Le grand crier sans honte auda-cieux,	The great speechmaker, shameless and bold will be
Sera esleu gouverneur de l'armee:	elected governor of the army.
La hardiesse de son contentieux,	The boldness of his conten-
Le pont rompu cité de peur pas-mee.	tion, the broken bridge, the city faint from fear.

PONTEFRACT AND CROMWELL

The key to this quatrain lies in the broken bridge. If one can accept this as Pontefract from the Latin *pons*, a bridge, *fractus*, broken, then we have a description of this town which held out for Charles I and suffered two severe sieges during the Civil War. The speechmaker who takes over the army is Cromwell, for whom Nostradamus has little liking, as is apparent in other quatrains.

82

Friens, Antibor, villes autour de Nice,	Fréjus, Antibes, the towns around Nice will be greatly
Seront vastees fort par mer & par terre:	devastated by land and sea; the locusts, by land and sea,
Les saturelles terre & mer vent propice,	the wind being favourable, captured, dead, trussed up,
Prins, morts, troussez, pillés, sans loi de guerre.	plundered without law of war.

INVASION OF FRANCE?

An invasion of the coast of Southern France by air is probably implied by this quatrain. As we have seen, Nostradamus describes all his machines as types of animals, and locusts, if read literally, could not cause the death and destruction of the final line.

83

Les longs cheveux de la Gaule Celtique,	The long-haired people of Celtic Gaul, joined by foreign nations will capture the people of Acquitaine in order that they should succumb to their plans.
Accompaignez d'estranges nations:	
Mettront captif la gent Aquitanique,	
Pour succomber à internitions.	

LOUIS XVIII 1755-1824

Louis XVIII of France was known contemporarily as *le Chevelu*—the long-haired one, his long hair being a great contrast to the short cropped hair of the Revolutionaries and Bonapartists. The foreign nations who help him are the Allied Armies who defeat Napoleon. The last two lines are unclear. In IX. 6 Aquitaine means England or an English Colony.

84

La grand cité sera bien desolee,	The great city will soon be quite deserted, not a single one of the inhabitants will remain. Wall, sex, temple and virgin violated, people will die from plague and cannon shot.
Des habitans un seul n'y demoura:	
Mur, sexe, temple & vierge violee,	
Par fer, feu, peste, canon peuple mourra.	

SACK OF ROME UNDER PIUS VI, 1775–1799

If the word is *sexe* an abbreviation of Sextus, which it could well be, this verse then applies to the Sack of Rome by Napoleonic troops. Some commentators think the city is Paris.

85

La cité prinse par tromperie & fraude,	The city is taken by trickery and deceit, captured by means of a handsome young man. An assault is made by Raubine near LAUDE, he and all of them dead, for having deceived so well.
Par le moyen d'un beau jeune attrappé:	
Assaut donné Raubine pres de LAUDE,	
Lui & tous morts pour avoir bien trompé.	

---

[1]*Internitions*—Read intentions in all other texts.

The interpretation of this stanza is connected with the river Robine, a tributary of the Aude, and presumably the city which is taken lies upon either of these. The word, LAUDE, comes from the Latin meaning praise but this does not clarify the context.

86

Un chef d'Ausonne aux Espaignes ira,	A leader from Italy will go to Spain by sea and he will make a stop at Marseilles. He will linger a long time before dying, after his death great wonders will be seen.
Par mer fera arrest dedans Marseille:	
Avant sa mort un long temps languira,	
Apres sa mort on verra grand merveille.	

This implies that a ruler from a Southern Italian state, or of the two Sicilies in particular, because that was the home of the Ausones in ancient times, will die a lingering death at Marseilles. This does not seem to have occurred.

87

Classe Gauloise n'approches de Corsegue,	French fleet, do not approach Corsica; even less Sardinia, you will regret it. You will all die, the help from the cape in vain, captive, swimming in blood, you will not believe me.
Moins de Sardaigne tu t'en repentiras:	
Trestout mourrez frustrez de l'aide grogne,	
Sang nagera, captif ne me croiras.	

SINKING OF PART OF FRENCH FLEET, 1655

In 1655 part of the French fleet, under the command of the Chevalier de la Ferrière, was sunk in the Gulf of Lyons while sailing past the islands of Sardinia and Corsica. Many were lost because they were unable to reach the nearby Cap de Porceau. This is an interesting double meaning. Grogne can mean a cape, or the snout of a pig. Nostradamus uses it to describe two things with extreme economy of words.

88

De Barcellonne par mer si grand armee,	From Barcelona such a great army by sea, all Marseilles will
Tout Marseille de frayeur trem-blera:	tremble with terror. The islands seized, help cut off by
Isles saisies de mer aide fermee,	sea, your traitor will swim on
Ton traditeur en terre nagera.	land.

MARSEILLES, 17th FEBRUARY 1596

On this day in 1596, Philip II of Spain sent a fleet to Marseilles under the command of Charles Doria to divide French interests between the Leaguers and the king. It occupied the islands of Château d'If and Ratonneau and thus prevented help coming into Marseilles by sea. A certain Charles de Casau tried to betray Marseilles to the Spanish but was found out and assassinated by Pierre Libertat; he was killed by the sword and literally drowned in his own blood.

89

En ce temps là sera frustrée Cypres,	At that time Cyprus will be deprived of its help from those
De son secours de ceux de mer Egee:	of the Aegean sea. Old men slaughtered, but by cannons
Vieux trucidez, mais par mesles[1] & lyphres[2]	and supplications, the king is won over, the queen more
Seduict leur Roy, Royne plus out-ragee.	outraged.

ENOSIS, CYPRUS AND KING CONSTANTINE

This quatrain may describe Cyprus during the Troubles of the 1950s, when union with Greece was the great political problem. The quatrain clearly shows that Cyprus will not attain complete union with Greece, that the King (Constantine?) will be misled, and the Queen, probably Frederika, greatly upset by their enforced exile. 'Old men slaughtered' may well refer to the assassination attempts on Archbishop Makarios and his eventual death.

[1]*mesles*—Probably variant O.F., *masle* = cannon ball.
[2]*lyphres*—Possibly Greek, *lypros* = a supplication.

90

Le grand Satyre & Tigre d'Hyr-canie,	The great Satyr and Tiger of Hyrcania; gift presented to the people of the Ocean: the leader of a fleet will come forth from Carmania and land at the Phocea of Tyre.
Don presenté à ceux de l'Occean:	
Un chef de classe istra de Car-manie,	
Qui prendra terre au Tyrren Phocean.	

The key to this quatrain is in the last line. Phocea is Marseilles but it is not situated on the Tyrrhenian sea so Nostradamus is probably intending another seaport associated with the early Phoenician colonists of Tyre. Carmania and Hyrcania were both provinces of Persia but the expedition would have to cross by land as well as sea, as there was no Suez canal at this period. An uncertain quatrain.

91

L'arbre qu'estoit par long temps mort seché,	The tree which had been dead and withered for a long time will flourish again in one night. The old king will be sickly. The prince with a damaged foot, fear of his enemies will make him hoist sail.
Dans une nuict viendra à rev-erdir:	
Cron¹ Roy malade, Prince peid estaché,²	
Criant d'ennemis fera voile bon-dir.	

BIRTH OF THE DUKE DE BORDEAUX 1820, HIS EXILE & DEATH, 1838

The tree which sprouts again miraculously overnight is the line of the Bourbons, when the Duchesse de Berry gave birth to a son, the Duc de Bordeaux on 29th September 1820 seven months after her husband was assassinated. He was a sickly child and injured his foot in a fall from his horse in Austria which resulted in a permanent limp. He went into exile in 1830 with his grandfather Charles X and despite long negotiations with Republican France, did not succeed in regaining the throne.

¹*Cron*—From the Latin, *Cronus* = Saturn, an old man, in this case his grandfather.

²*estaché*—O.F. = stump, club foot.

92

Le monde proche du dernier pe- *riode,* *Saturne encor tard sera de retour:* *Translat empire devers nation* *Brodde,* *L'oeil arraché à Narbon par Au-* *tour.*	The world is near its final pe- riod, Saturn will again be late on his return. The empire will shift towards the Brodde na- tion; An eye at Narbonne plucked out by a goshawk.

TROUBLES IN AFRICA IN 1980s

This is an astrological quatrain dealing probably with the future of the African nations, as *Brodde* in old French means either black or dark brown. It also contains the meaning of decadent. Nostradamus speaks several times of an *'Empire translaté'* when referring to Napoleon. Here he implies that more power will be given to African nations as is happening at the present, before the final cycle of the world occurs. It might also mean that French power shifts towards Africa—which it did until France left Algeria. In which case we are now approaching this final period. There is a possibility that the word, empire, could refer to the infamous reigns of either Idi Amin of Uganda or the Emperor Ange Patasse Bokassa of the late Central Africa Republic, both of whom have lately been deposed. It is possible that the Rhodesian troubles are referred to here. Saturn in its planetary aspect always denotes trouble and conflict.

93

Dans Avignon tout le chef de *l'empire* *Fera arrest pour Paris desolé:* *Tricast¹ tiendra l'Annibalique ire,* *Lyon par change sera mal con-* *solé'.*	In Avignon, the leader of all the Empire will make a stop because Paris is deserted. Tri- cast will contain the African anger, the Lion will be poorly consoled by the change.

The quatrain hints at a great enemy of France, possibly also of Rome, in that Avignon belonged to the Vatican until 1791. The British lion will dislike this enemy in Africa—there is a temptation to link this quatrain with the British campaigns in Africa during the Second World War.

¹*Tricast—Tricasses* = city of Troyes.

94

*De cinq cens ans plus compte l'on
   tiendra
Celui qu'estoit l'adornement de
   son temps:
Puis à un coup grand clarté
   donra,
Que par ce siecle les rendra tres
   contens.*

For five hundred years more
they will take notice of him
who was the ornament of his
age. Then suddenly a great
revelation will be made which
will make people of that (same)
century well pleased.

This has been used by almost every interpreter of Nostradamus' quatrains to date as a guarantee of the inspired nature
of their works. No further comment is needed. The commentator has not yet appeared.

95

*La loy Moricque on verra defail-
   lir,
Apres un autre beaucoup plus
   seductive:
Boristhenes[1] premier viendra
   faillir,
Par dons & langue une plus at-
   tractive.*

The Moorish law will be seen
to fail, followed by another
that is more pleasing. The
Dnieper will be the first to
give way through gifts and
tongues to another more ap-
pealing.

FAILURE OF ISLAM AND RUSSIA

In this quatrain Nostradamus predicts the final fall of Moorish Islamic law which will be followed by a better influence.
The Dnieper is a river in Russia and presumably stands for
that country. As in IV. 95 Nostradamus indicates that Russia
will ally itself to another country, probably the USA.

96

*Chef de Fossan aura gorge cou-
   pee,
Par le ducteur du limier & leu-
   rier:
Le faict patré par ceux de mont
   Tarpee,
Saturne en Leo 13 de Fevrier.*

The leader from Fossano will
have his throat cut by the man
who exercised the blood-
hounds and greyhounds. The
deed will be committed by
those of the Tarpean rock,
when Saturn is in Leo on 13th
February.

[1] *Boristhenes*—Latin = the river Dnieper in the U.S.S.R.

13th FEBRUARY 1820

To trace the leader from Fossano is difficult. If he is the
Duke de Berry then he is called this because his maternal
grandfather was King of Fossano in Sardinia. The rest of the
quatrain fits very accurately. The assassin was Louvel, who
worked in the royal stables. He was a Republican, hence the
reference to the Tarpean rock from which Republican Rome
threw her criminals. Saturn rules Aquarius, so when it is in the
opposite sign of Leo it should be understood as maleficent.
The Duke de Berry was stabbed on 13th February 1820, as
Nostradamus stated, when leaving the Opéra. See I. 84.

97

Nouvelle loi terre neufve occuper,
Vers la Syrie, Judee & Palestine:
Le grand empire barbare corruer,
Avant que Phoebus son siecle de-
termine.

A new law will occupy a new
land around Syria, Judea and
Palestine. The great barbarian Empire will crumble before the century of the sun is
finished.

THE CREATION OF ISRAEL AND FINAL DEFEAT OF UAR. 20th CENTURY

The first two lines speak for themselves and describe the
creation of the state of Israel. By barbarian Nostradamus
means Arabic or Muslim and implies here that Israel will eventually triumph over her Arab enemies before the end of the
20th Century—the century of the sun. Considering the remarkable change in Egyptian and American attitudes towards
Israel during the past two years this prediction seems extremely impressive. See III. 95.

98

Deux royals freres si fort guer-
roierent,
Qu'entre eux sera la guerre si
mortelle:
Qu'un chacun places fortes oc-
cuperont,
De regne & vie sera leur grand
querelle.

Two royal brothers will fight
so fiercely and the feud between them will be so deadly
that both will live in fortified
places. Their great quarrel
will concern their lives and
the kingdom.

This is a fairly straightforward prophecy which suits the king of France, Henri III, and the Duc d'Alençon most closely (1574–84), but also fits Louis XIII and his brother the Duke of Orléans around the period 1632. A very good example of history, and prophecy, repeating itself!

99

Aux champs herbeux d'Alein et du Varneigne,	In the green fields of Alleins and Vernegues of the Luberon mountains near Durance, the fighting on both sides will be so bitter for the armies that Mesopotamia shall cease to be found in France.
Du mont Lebron proche de la Durance,	
Camps de deux parts conflict sera si aigre	
Mespotamie defaillira en la France.	

It is from the last line of this quatrain that commentators refer to Mesopotamia throughout the Centuries as referring to Paris. Both places in line one are villages near Salon, Nostradamus' home; the Luberon mountains are near the river Durance.

100

Entre Gaulois le dernier honnoré,	The man least honoured among the French will be victorious over his enemy. Strength and lands he explored in action, when suddenly the envious one dies from the shot.
D'homme ennemi sera victorieux:	
Force & terroir en moment exploré	
D'un coup de traict quand mourra l'envieux.	

GENERAL DE GAULLE?

This quatrain is normally applied to de Gaulle and the man who is assassinated is then identified as Admiral Darlan, who was killed on 24th December 1942. *Le traict* is the normal word for the shot of an arrow, but here may mean gunshot.

CENTURY IV

1

Cela du reste de sang non es-
   pandu,
Venise quiert secours estre donné.
Apres avoir bien long temps at-
   tendu,
Cité livrée au premier cornet
   sonné.

The remaining blood will not
be spilt, Venice seeks for help
to be given. Having waited
for a very long time the city
is handed over at the first
trumpet blast.

1560–1571
This probably describes the Turkish attack on Cyprus
(1560–73). Venice received very little help and Famagusta, the
capital of Cyprus, fell to the Turks after a prolonged siege in
1571.

2

Par mort la France prendra voy-
   age à faire,
Classe par mer, marcher monts
   Pyrenées,
Espaigne en trouble, marcher
   gent militaire:
Des plus grand Dames en France
   emmenées.

Because of a death France will
undertake a journey, the fleet
at sea, marching over the Pyrenean mountains. Spain will
be troubled, an army will
march, some of the greatest
ladies brought into France.

WAR OF SPANISH SUCCESSION 1701–1713
This is a successful quatrain. Philip V, grandson of Louis
XIV inherited the Spanish throne from Charles II in 1700.
This was not popular with Austria, England, Holland, Prussia
and Savoy, who formed a coalition to support the pretensions
of the Archduke Charles. The French fleet took to the sea,
and her army crossed the Pyrenees. The war in Spain lasted
for twelve years and it was all due to two Spanish princesses
who married into the French line, the wives of Louis XII and
Louis XIV respectively. See IV. 5.

3

D'Arras & Bourges[1], de Brodes grans enseignes, *Un plus grand nombre de Gascons batre à pied,* *Ceux long du Rosne saigneront les Espaignes:* *Proche du mont où Sagonte s'assied.*	From Arras and Bourges great banners from the Dark Ones, a greater number of Gascons fight on foot. Those along the Rhône will make the Spanish bleed. Near the mountain seat of Sagunto.

Brodes usually means dark-haired people, possibly the Spanish Moors in this context. If Bourges is understood as Bruges then line one describes another Hapsburg invasion from the North, probably that which resulted in the Battle of St Quentin, in 1557. The last two lines suggest that the French invaded Spain, which they did not do for another fifty years or so. The importance of Sagunto is unclear. See IV. 8, VIII. 34.

4

L'impotent prince faché, plaincts & querelles, *De rapts & pillé, par coqz & par Libiques:* *Grand est par terre par mer infinies voilles* *Seule Italie sera chassant Celtiques.*	The powerless prince is angered, complaints & quarrels, rape and pillage, by the cock and by the Libyans. It is great on land, at sea innumerable sails; Italy alone will be driving out the Celts.

DUKE COSIMO 1555

The cock is the French symbol and the Libyans are the Algerian corsairs who allied with them. The Prince is therefore probably a Hapsburg, possibly Duke Cosimo, who was in charge of the defence of Elba and the surrounding lands. These territories were ravished in 1555. The last line is confusing suggesting that the French will be defeated by the Italians but successful everywhere else. Exactly the reverse occurred. The French held their own in Italy but were defeated in the North. This prediction was fulfilled during Nostradamus' lifetime.

[1]*Bourges* = possibly Bruges.

5

Croix paix, soubz un accompli divin verbe, *L'Espaigne & Gaule seront unis ensemble:* *Grand clade¹ proche, & combat tresacerbe,* *Coeur si hardi ne sera qui ne tremble.*	Cross, peace under one the divine word achieved. Spain and Gaul will be united. A great disaster is close, the fighting very ferocious, no heart so brave as will not tremble.

WAR OF SPANISH SUCCESSION, 1701–1713

Spain and France were united for the short time that Louis XIV's grandson inherited the Spanish throne. Perhaps the revocation of the Edict of Nantes is hinted at in line one? Peace achieved under the divine word could be the Papal Bull, Unigenitus, which was issued in 1713, the year the war ended. The great disaster following upon the union of the countries is the War of the Spanish Succession of IV. 2, and the final line is self-explanatory, just used to fill up the quatrain.

6

D'habits nouveaux apres faicte la treuve,² *Malice tramme & machination:* *Premier mourra qui en fera la preuve,* *Couleur venise insidiation.³*	After the truce is made, new clothes will be put on, malice, conspiracy and plotting. He who will prove it is the first to die, the colour of Venetian treachery.

This is a very obscure quatrain. Perhaps the 'new clothes' imply a new order of things? There is a shade of yellow-brown paint which is known as venetian red. Perhaps this is meant rather than the city itself and is adopted to indicate the new régime? Equally the line could be politically orientated.

¹*clades*—Latin = disaster.
²*treuve*—O.F., *treve* = truce.
³*insidiation*—O.F. = snare, trap.

7

Le mineur filz du grand & hai Prince,	The younger son of a great and hated prince, will be
De lepre aura à vingt ans grande tache,	greatly marked by leprosy by the time he is twenty. His
De deuil sa mere mourra bien triste & mince,	mother will die of grief, very sad and thin, and he will die
Et il mourra là où tombe cher lache.	when the cowardly flesh falls (from his bones).

It seems impossible to identify the hated prince. There is no known record to date of a younger, or youngest son of a royal family dying of leprosy. Since Nostradamus was a doctor it is unlikely he would have used this word to indicate any other disease.

8

La grand cité d'assaut prompt & repentin,	The great city will be surprised at night by a sudden
Surprins de nuict, gardes interrompus:	and quick assault. The guards interrupted; the watch and
Les excubies & vielles sainct Quintin,	guards of St Quentin slaughtered, the guards and the
Trucidés gardes & les pourtails rompus.	gates broken down.

ST QUENTIN, 1557

There was a Battle of St Quentin in 1557 but the city was taken not in the way Nostradamus describes it, but by a seventeen-day siege. But at least the prediction of the town's capture is correct. See IV. 3. Yet another quatrain that was fulfilled during Nostradamus' lifetime.

9

Le chef du camp au milieu de la presse,	The leader of the army in the middle of the crowd is
D'un coup de fleche sera blessé aux cuisses,	wounded in the thighs with an arrow. When Geneva in
Lors que Geneve en larmes & detresse,	trouble and distress is betrayed by Lausanne and the
Sera trahi par Lozan & Souisses.	Swiss.

Presumably another anti-Calvinist tirade by Nostradamus. He seems to foresee that Lausanne and Switzerland generally return to the Roman Catholic faith with only Geneva led by the wounded leader, holding out. The identity of the leader of the army is unclear. A completely mistaken verse. There is a possible astrological meaning here in that Sagittarius governs the arrow.

10

Le jeune prince accusé faulsement,	The young Prince, falsely accused, will put the camp into quarrels and trouble. The leader is murdered for his support to appease the crown: then he cures the king's evil.
Mettra en trouble le camp & en querelles:	
Meutri le chef pour le soustenement,	
Sceptre appaiser: puis guerir escrouelles.	

This describes trouble between a Prince and his supporters which eventually ends in loss of his life. A new King comes to the throne, line 4, because French and English kings were reputed to cure scrofula by their touch, particularly on the day of their coronation.

11

Celui qu'aura gouvert de la grand cappe,[1]	He who will have government of the great cloak will be led to execute in certain cases. The twelve red ones will come to spoil the cover, under murder, murder will be perpetrated.
Sera induict a quelques cas patrer[2]	
Les douze rouges viendront fouiller la nappe.	
Soubz meutre, meutre se viendra perpetrer.	

POPE JOHN PAUL I, 1979
In the earlier edition of this book I said that this was detailed quatrain but one that had not yet materialized. A Pope would be condemned by his Cardinals. I also wrote that they would connive in a Pope's murder. The scandal surrounding the

[1]cappe = (a) Cloak. (b) Cape, standing for Pope and Vatican.
[2]patrer—Latin, patrare = to perform, execute.

death of Pope John Paul I and the discrepancies among the reports from the Vatican are now notorious. For details, see III. 65.

12

Le camp plus grand de route mis en fuite,
Guaires plus outre ne sera pour-chassé:
Ost recampé, & legion reduicte,
Puis hors ses Gaules du tout sera chassé.

The greatest army on the march put to flight will scarcely be pursued further. The army reassembled and the legion reduced, they will then be driven out of France completely.

This is a very general quatrain and the German invasions of France in the last two wars fit it most accurately. However, there is nothing sufficiently explicit to go on.

13

De plus grand perte nouvelles raportées,
Le raport fait le camp s'estonnera:
Bandes unies encontre revoltées,
Double phalange grand aban-donnera.

News of the great loss is brought; the report will astonish the camp. Bands unite against those revolting, the double phalanx will forsake the great one.

DUKE OF PARMA, 1580

This verse is normally applied to the 1580s when a rumour spread through the Duke of Parma's army of so great a defeat that they were quite demoralized and allowed the Dutch to capture Antwerp for a time. A phalanx was 800 men, so 1,600 men are understood to have revolted.

14

La mort subite du premier per-sonnage.
Aura changé & mis un autre au regne:
Tost, tard venu à si haut & bas aage,
Que terre & mer faudra que on le craigne.

The sudden death of the leading personnage will have changed and put another to rule. Soon, but too late come to high position, of young age, by land and sea it will be necessary to fear him.

J. F. KENNEDY

A general prophecy about a young leader who comes to power too late to alter the status quo of the country. It has been suggested that it may refer to J. F. Kennedy, succeeding the aged General Eisenhower, whose policies still could not lessen world tension. During the Cuba incident Kennedy's power was to be feared on land and sea. He was followed by the aged President Nixon and then by the younger President Ford. The words *mort subite* are also applied to the Kennedy brothers, and almost certainly to Edward Kennedy in II. 57. See I. 26, VIII. 77 and IX. 36.

15

D'où pensera faire venir famine, *De là viendra le rassasiement:* *L'oeil de la mer par avare canine* *Pour de l'un l'autre donra huile,* *froment.*	From the place where he will think to bring famine, from there will come the relief. The eye of the sea, like a covetous dog; the one will give oil and wheat to the other.

GREAT BRITAIN 1939–45. SUBMARINES

This verse describes Britain's predicament during the Second World War very accurately. The German blockade tried to starve her out, see also III. 71, but instead, she received large quantities of American aid. 'The eye of the sea, like a covetous dog' is understood as meaning the periscope of the German U-boats, which certainly hunted down the British convoys in packs.

16

La cité franche de liberté fait
    serve,
Des profligés & resveurs faict
    asile:
Le Roy changé à eux non si pro-
    terve[1]
De cent seront devenus plus de
    mille.
	The free city of liberty is enslaved, it becomes the refuge of profligates and dreamers. The king changes and is not so ferocious towards them. From one hundred they will become more than a thousand.

[1]*proterve*—Latin, *protervus* = violent.

Europe had many free cities when Nostradamus wrote. He may here be referring to Orange, which gave its name to the Dutch royal line, and did not belong to France until 1713. During Nostradamus' time it belonged to William the Silent, and line 2 may be intended as meaning that it had become a haven for Protestants, which it was.

17

Changer à Beaune, Nuy, Chalons & Dijon,	Changes at Beaune, Nuits, Chalon & Dijon, the Duke
Le duc voulant amander¹ la Barrée²	wishes to improve the Carmelites. Walking near the
Marchant pres fleuve, poisson, bec de plongeon,	river, a fish, a diving (bird's) beak, towards the tail; the
Vers la queue; porte sera serrée.	gate will be locked.

The first two lines may refer to St Theresa who reformed the order of Carmelite nuns in Spain in 1562. But nothing can be made of the following lines.

18

Des plus lettrés dessus les faits celestes	Some of the most learned men in the heavenly arts will
Seront par princes ignorans reprouvés:	be reprimanded by ignorant Princes; punished by an Edict,
Punis d'Edit, chassez comme scelestes,	driven out as scoundrels and put to death wherever they
Et mis à mort là où seront trouvés.	are found.

INQUISITION

Shades of the Inquisition linger over this verse, for in fact astrologers were never as grossly persecuted after Nostradamus' death as they were during the century before. However if he was also thinking of the witch hunts which bedevilled Europe they did not die out until somewhat later. Nostradamus was summoned to appear before the Inquisition at Toulouse and had to disappear for a while for his own safety.

¹*amander*—O.F. = to improve, to better.
²*Barrée*—This was the name for the Carmelite monks and nuns, from the O.F., *barré* = motley.

19

Devant Rouen d'Insubres mis le siege,	The Insubrians lay siege in front of Rouen, the passages
Par terre & mer enfermés les passages:	closed by land and sea. By Hainaut & Flanders, by Ghent
D'Haynault, & Flandres, de Gand & ceux de Liege,	and those of Liege, through cloaked gifts they will ravage
Par dons laenées[1] raviront les rivages.	the shores.

Rouen was first captured by the Duke of Parma who was helping de Guise faction against Henri of Navarre in 1592 but without much of a siege. Since Milan was part of his dominions there could have been Italians (Insubres) among his troops. Since then Rouen has never been captured by Italy, the Germans captured it in 1870 and 1940 and the Americans in 1944. All the other towns mentioned are in the Netherlands and Flanders. Although reasonably clear, this prophecy has not been fulfilled.

20

Paix uberté[2] long temps lieu louera;	Peace and plenty for a long time the place will praise: the
Par tout son regne desert la fleur de lis:	fleur de lis deserted throughout the kingdom. Bodies dead
Corps morts d'eau, terre là lon apportera,	by water, they will be brought to land there, waiting in vain
Sperants vain heur d'estre là ensevelis.	for the opportunity of being buried.

The fleur de lis was the emblem of many other families besides the French kings so this is not much help. The obvious time that it disappears throughout the kingdom is during the Revolution and the Empire. The last two lines would then be generalities about war and death.

[1]*laenées*—Latin, *laena* = cloak, mantle.
[2]*uberté*—Latin, *ubertas* = abundance.

21

Le changement sera fort difficile,
Cité, province au change gain
    fera:
Coeur haut, prudent mis, chassé
    lui habile,
Mer, terre, peuple son estat chan-
    gera.

The change will be very difficult. Both city and province
will gain by it. A prudent man
highly placed, will be chased
out by the cunning one. By
land and sea people will
change their estate.

FRANCE, 1940–4. DE GAULLE

The first two lines of this quatrain may refer to the fall of
France and Marshal Pétain's 'centralized decentralization'. The
prudent man is de Gaulle, who is chased out to England and
the last line refers to the general state of the country and the
war.

22

La grand copie[1] *qui sera des-*
    chassée,
Dans un moment fera besoing au
    Roi,
La foi promise de loing sera
    faulsée
Nud se verra en piteux desarroi.

The great army which will be
driven out at one moment will
be needed by the King. The
faith promised from afar will
be broken, he will see himself
with nothing, in pitiful disorder.

This is a general type of quatrain that may have occurred
several times. A king quarrels with an ally, and having dismissed its forces suddenly finds he needs them again. But
because one of them breaks a promise the king is left powerless.

[1]*copie*—Latin, *copia* — army, troops.

23

La legion dans la marine classe,
Calcine,[1] *Magnes*[2] *soulphre, &*
poix bruslera:
Le long repos de l'asseuree place,
Port Selyn,[3] *Hercle*[4] *feu les con-*
sumera.

The legion in the marine fleet
will burn, lime, magnesia, sulphur and pitch. The long rest
in a safe place; Port Selin,
Monaco will be consumed by
fire.

GREEK FIRE

This is a very strange quatrain. The second line appears to
be giving a recipe for Greek fire, the famous 'secret weapon'
of the Greeks and Byzantines. Nostradamus is quite correct
because after much research, Lieut.-Colonel H. Hime said that
it was the presence of quicklime which distinguished Greek
fire from all other known incendiaries of the period. The
mixture gave rise to heat on contact with water and thus took
fire spontaneously when wetted, and was used with great success in sea battles. But again, Port Selin, if I am correct in
identifying it with Genoa, and Monaco, have not been attacked
since Nostradamus' day. But the port of Toulon was used by
Barbarossa when he helped the French against the Emperor
during the 1540s.

24

Oui soubs terre saincte dame voix
fainte,
Humaine flamme pour divine
voix luire:
Fera les seuls de leur sang terre
tainte,
Et les saincts temples pour les im-
purs destruire.

The faint voice of a woman
is heard under the holy
ground. Human flame shines
for the divine voice. It will
cause the earth to be stained
with the blood of celibates
and destroy the holy temples
for the wicked.

PERSECUTION OF CLERGY

An impossible quatrain because of the many variants of the
first line. To which word does *saincte* belong? *Dame* is also given

[1]*Calcine*—Latin, *calcina* = lime.

[2]*Magnes*—Latin for loadstone or magnet. Also an abbreviation of
Magnesie, used loosely to describe Greek fire.

[3]*Port Selyn*—Genoa was a crescent-shaped republic and Selene
means crescent in Greek.

[4]*Hercle*—Latin, *Herculeis Monacei* = another name for Monaco.

as *d'ame*, of the soul, and *fainte* as *sainte*. The general idea seems to be the persecution of the church, perhaps personified in the Holy Lady of the first line, and its most probable fulfilment was the abolition and persecution of the clergy during the French Revolution.

25

Corps sublimes sans fin à l'oeil visibles:	The heavenly bodies endlessly visible to the eye come
Obnubiler viendront par ces raisons:	to cloud (the intellect) for these reasons. The body, to-
Corps, front comprins, sens chief & invisibles.	gether with the forehead, senses and head all invisible,
Diminuant les sacrees oraisons.	as the sacred prayers diminish.

OCCULT QUATRAIN

Some commentators regard this as referring to the invention of the telescope (1610) bringing new worlds and ideas which will be hostile to religion. But I think that Nostradamus is here describing the sensation of 'bodilessness' which he experiences when in a predictive trance, when his mind and intellect are used by the heavenly beings for their own purposes. The prayers of the last line are the invocations to the spirits made by Nostradamus. As they finish, he is possessed. See also I. 1 and 2, and III. 2.

26

Lou grand eyssame se levera d'abelhos,	The great swarm of bees will arise but no one will know
Que non sauran don te siegen venguddos:	whence they have come, the ambush by night, the sentinel
De nuech l'embousque, lou gach dessous las treilhos	under the vines, a city handed over by five tongues not na-
Cuitad trahido per cinq lengos non nudos.	ked.

NAPOLEON
THE COUP D'ETAT OF EIGHTEENTH BRUMAIRE
(9th NOVEMBER 1779)

This is one of the few quatrains written entirely in Provençal. It describes Napoleon's *coup d'état* of 1799 very accurately. The swarm of bees is Napoleon's emblem—they can still be seen on the embroideries at Malmaison and Fontainebleau. The five men (literally babblers), who handed over Paris were the members of the Directory who were bribed (*non nudos*) to give way to Napoleon's Consulate; they were also wearing official clothes as members of the Directory, as opposed to their everyday apparel. The coup was planned the night before it took place. Most commentators take *las treilhos* to be an anagram for the Tuileries into which Napoleon moved once he saw his action was successful. The exact French equivalent is *treilles*, but it is close enough and the quatrain fits very well in all other respects.

27

Salon, Mansol, Tarascon de SEX. l'arc,
Où est debout encor la piramide:
Viendront livrer le Prince Dannemarc,
Rachat honni au temple d'Artemide.

Salon, Mansol, Tarascon, the arch of SEX: where the pyramid is still standing. They will come to deliver the Prince of Denmark, a shameful ransom to the temple of Artemis.

PRINCESS ANNE AND MARK PHILIPS?

The complicated first line stands for St Rémy where Nostradamus was born, where there are two great historical monuments, a mausoleum with the inscription *SEX. L.M. JUILEI C.F. PARENTIBUS SUIS* and next to it a triumphal arch. *Mansol* is a misprint for Mausole, a priory just outside St Rémy. The problem lies in connecting them with Dannemarc. The word may well be one of Nostradamus' better concealed anagrams which I cannot decipher. Many people have suggested to me that this refers to Princess Anne and Mark Philips. It seems somewhat incredible but see VI. 41.

28

Lors que Venus du Sol sera couvert,
Soubs l'esplendeur sera forme occulte:
Mercure au feu les aura descouvert,
Par bruit bellique sera mis à l'insulte.

When Venus will be covered by the sun, under the splendour will be a hidden form. Mercury will have exposed them to the fire, by a rumour of war will be affronted.

OCCULT

This, and the following quatrains IV. 29, 30, 31, and 33 are all occult quatrains and probably describe Nostradamus' attempts to discover the elusive philosopher's stone which transmutes all other metals into gold, here described as the sun.

29

Le Sol caché eclipse par Mercure, *Ne sera mis que pour le ciel second:* *De Vulcan Hermes sera faicte pasture,* *Sol sera veu pur, rutilant & blond.*	The hidden Sun eclipsed by Mercury will be placed only second in the heavens. Hermes will be made the food of Vulcan, the Sun will be seen pure, shining and golden.

OCCULT

See IV. 28. Vulcan here stands for fire.

30

Plus onze fois Luna Sol ne voudra, *Tous augmenté & baissez de degré:* *Et si bas mis que peu or on coudra,* *Qu'apres faim, peste, descouvert le secret.*	More than eleven times the Moon will not want the Sun, both raised and lessened in degree. Put so low that one will sew little gold: after famine and plague the secret will be discovered.

OCCULT

See IV. 28. The Moon here probably means silver.

31

La Lune au plain de nuict sur le haut mont, *Le nouveau sophe d'un seul cerveau l'a veu:* *Par ses disciples estre immortel semond,* *Yeux au midi, en seins mains, corps au feu.*	The Moon, in the middle of the night over the high mountain, the young wise man alone with his brain has seen it. Invited by his disciples to become immortal, his eyes to the south, his hands on his breast, his body in the fire.

OCCULT

In this quatrain it is suggested that the young sage who finally makes this great discovery either experiences great ecstasy or, alternatively, comes to a violent end, racked by mental torment.

32

Es lieux & temps chair au poisson donra lieu,
La loi commune sera faicte au contraire:
Vieux tiendra fort puis osté du millieu,
Le Pánta chiona philòn mis fort arriere.

In those times and places that meat gives way to fish the common law will be made in opposition. The old (order) will hold strong, then removed from the scene, then all things common among friends put far behind.

DECLINE OF COMMUNISM

Pánta chiona philòn is the Greek for all things held in common among friends, that is, Communism in its strictest sense. Nostradamus has already described this in the USSR in quatrain III. 95, and seems definite that its appeal will fade and there will be strong attempts to revive the old order. One wonders whether this is associated with the theory that America and the USSR will ally together against the East, probably due to the reign of Islam, or less likely that of China. See II. 37, IV. 95, V. 78, VI. 21, 80.

33

Jupiter joinct plus Venus qu'à la Lune,
Apparoissant de plenitude blanche:
Venus cachée souz la blancheur Neptune
De Mars frappée par la gravée branche.

Jupiter joined more to Venus than to the Moon appearing in a white fullness. Venus hidden under the whiteness of Neptune struck by Mars by the engraved wand.

OCCULT

The translation of the last line is difficult. I take *gravée* to mean engraved, because *branche* is used by Nostradamus to

refer to the ceremonial wand and tripod used in his predictions
therefore that the wand is engraved with hieroglyphics. The
rest is very obscure.

34

Le grand mené captif d'estrange terre,	The great man led captive from a foreign land, chained in gold, offered to King CHYREN. He who in Ausonia, Milan, will lose the war and all his army put to fire and sword.
D'or enchainé au Roy CHYREN offert:	
Qui dans Ausone, Milan perdra la guerre,	
Et tout son ost mis à feu & à fer.	

DR HENRY KISSINGER?

  CHYREN is an almost definite anagram for the Old French
spelling of Henri, *HENRYC*, but the great problem lies in
deciding which Henri these verses refer to. Many commentators favour Henri IV, others of the 19th Century in particular, a new king of France yet to come. It has been suggested
that Henryc should stand for Henry Kissinger or Henry K, as
he is always known in the States, but since these quatrains are
not completely favourable to either idea may be they have a
connotation that has yet to be fulfilled. See II. 79, VI. 27, 70,
VIII. 54, IX. 41.

35

Le feu estaint, les vierges trahiront	The fire put out, the virgins will betray the greater part of the new band; lightning in sword, lances alone will guard the king, Tuscany and Corsica, by night throats slit.
La plus grand part de la bande nouvelle:	
Fouldre à fer, lance les seulz Roi garderont	
Etrusque & Corse, de nuict gorge allumelle.	

During the Empire, Tuscany and Corsica were both bothered
by the French as Tuscany was an ally and Genoa owned Corsica.

36

Les jeux nouveau en Gaule re-
    dressés,
Après victoire de l'Insubre[1] cham-
    paigne:
Monts d'Esperie, les grands liés,
    troussés:
De peur trembler la Romaigne
    & l'Espaigne.
	New games are set up in Gaul, after the victory of the Insubrian campaign. The mountains of Hesperia, the great ones tied and bound. Romania and Spain will tremble with fear.

If *Romaigne* in line 4 stands for the Roman Empire, i.e. Germany, the best interpretation of France's victories in Spain and the north would be the Napoleonic campaigns.

37

Gaulois par saults, monts viendra
    penetrer:
Occupera le grand lieu de
    l'Insubre:
Au plus profond son ost fera en-
    trer,
Gennes, Monech pousseront classe
    rubre.
	The Gauls will penetrate the mountains in leaps and occupy the great seat of Insubria. He will make his army go deep (into the land), Genoa and Monaco will repulse the red fleet.

MAY 1800. NAPOLEON

In the year 1800, Genoa was besieged by Austria, and surrendered on 4th June. The British fleet which had been helping with a blockade attacked Monaco on 23rd May. Earlier that month Napoleon made his incredible crossing of the St Bernard pass with an army of 40,000 men, and took Milan (Insubria) on 2nd June. A very satisfactory quatrain.

38

Pendant que Duc, Roy, Royne
    occupera,
Chef Bizant du captif en Sa-
    mothrace:
Avant l'assault l'un l'autre man-
    gera,
Rebours ferré suivra du sang la
    trace.
	While the Duke occupies the King and Queen, the Byzantine leader is held captive in Greece. Before the attack one will devour the other. The metalled reverse will follow the trail of blood.

[1] *Insubre* = Italy, around Milan, Lombardy.

MACHINE?

Does the 'metalled reverse' indicate a type of machine similar to a Geiger counter, that will be able to follow a man's tracks?

39

Les Rhodiens demanderont se-cours,	The people of Rhodes will demand help, abandoned by the neglect of their heirs. The Arab Empire will assess its course, its cause revived again by the West.
Par le neglect de ses hoirs de-laissée:	
L'Empire Arabe revalera son cours,	
Par Hesperies la cause redressée.	

USA AND MIDDLE EAST

At a time of unrest in Greece, which could refer to the present régime, the UAR will reassess its position and be helped in some way by the West, probably by America. The Camp David talks come to mind. The last line may well refer to the complicated issues now being brought to bear by the USA on the Middle East, Iran, Iraq and Afghanistan in particular.

40

Les forteresses des assiegés serrés,	The fortress of the besieged shut up by gunpowder sunk into its depths; the traitor will be entombed alive, never did so pitiful a schism happen to the sextons.
Par poudre à feu profondés en abisme:	
Les proditeurs seront tous vifs serrés,	
Onc aux sacristes n'advint si piteux scisme.	

HITLER'S BUNKER AT BERLIN

The clue to this verse lies in the last line. *Sacristes* normally translates as sextons, which is meaningless in this context. However, if Nostradamus meant Saxons, the Germans, and this is associated with a schism, a breaking up of a party, it could refer to Hitler and those pitiful few of his followers who remained in the fortified bunker to be shelled by the Allies. See I. 34, II. 24, III. 35, 53, 58, 61, 94, IV. 68, VI. 7, 51, VIII. 29, IX. 90.

41

Gymnique[1] *sexe captive par hostage,*
Viendra de nuit custodes decevoir:
Le chef du camp deçeu par son langage:
Lairra à la gente, sera piteux à voir.

A female (sex) captive as a hostage will come by night to deceive the guards. The leader of the camp deceived by her language will leave her to the people, it will be pitiful to see.

An unknown woman who is abandoned to a mob after tricking the guards; very general.

42

Geneve & Langres par ceux de Chartres & Dole,
Et par Grenoble captif au Montlimard:
Seysset, Losanne par fraudulente dole
Les trahiront par or soixante marc.

Geneva and Langres through the people of Chartres and Dôle and Grenoble, captive at Montelimar: Seysel, Lausanne, through a fraudulent trick will betray them for sixty gold marks.

There are too many scattered place-names in both Switzerland and France to make this quatrain clear. A mark was 8 oz. of gold.

43

Seront ouis au ciel les armes battre:
Celui an mesme les divins ennemis:
Voudrant loix sainctes injustement debatre,
Par foudre & guerre bien croyans à mort mis.

Weapons will be heard fighting in the skies: in the same year the divine are enemies: they will want unjustly to query the holy laws, through lightning and war many believers put to death.

A HOLY WAR AND AERIAL WARFARE

When the 'divine' are enemies, which implies religious sects, at the same time weapons will be heard fighting in the skies

[1] *Gymnique*—Misprint for Greek, *gynique* = female.

which helps place this quatrain in the 20th century. I had said initially that this was hard to decipher but the implication of putting many believers to death does give rise yet again to thoughts of Islam. See I. 63, 64.

44

Deux gros de Mende, de Roudés & Milhau,	The two large ones of Mende, of Rodez and Milhau, Cahors
Cahours, Limoges, Castres malo sepmano	and Limoges, Castres a bad week: by night the entry; from
De nuech l'intrado de Bourdeaux un cailhau,	Bordeaux an insult, through Perigord at the peal of the
Par Perigort au toc de la campano.	bell.

A quatrain of mixed Provençal and French phrases. Unfortunately they seem to disguise little more than the names of a series of towns in south-west France.

45

Par conflit Roi, regne abandonnera,	Through a battle the king will abandon his kingdom, the
Le plus grand chef faillira au besoing:	greatest leader will fail in time of need. Dead, ruined, few
Mors profligés peu en rechapera,	will escape it all cut down,
Tous destranchés, un en sera tesmoing.	save one who will be a witness.

This quatrain is suggested as suitable for Napoleon I at Waterloo, Napoleon III at Sédan or Kaiser Wilhelm II. The reader can take his choice. A typical prophecy.

46

Bien defendu le faict par excellence,	The deed, through its excellence, strongly forbidden,
Garde toy Tours de ta proche ruine:	Tours, beware of your approaching ruin. London and
Londres & Nantes par Reims fera defense	Nantes will make a defence through Reims. Do not go
Ne passe outre au temps de la bruine.	further afield at the time of the fog.

47

Le noir farouche quand aura es-
sayé
Sa main sanguine par feu, fer,
arcs tendus:
Trestout le peuple sera tant ef-
frayé,
Voir les plus grans par col &
pieds pendus.

When the ferocious king will
have exercised his bloody hand
through fire, the sword and
the bended bow. All the nation will be so terrified seeing
the great ones hanging by
their neck and feet.

MASSACRE OF ST BARTHOLEMEW
24th AUGUST, 1572

In line 1 *noir* is the usual anagram for *roi*, King. The savage
king was the mad Charles IX, who was reputed to kill for the
sake of blood when out hunting, decapitating animals which
came across his path. The fear of the people refers to the
massacre of St Bartholomew, of the French Huguenots on
24th August 1572, when Admiral Coligny was killed by the
mob and hung from a gibbet by one foot. This took place
some eight years after Nostradamus' death.

48

Planure Ausonne fertile, spa-
cieuse,
Produira taons si tant de sauter-
elles:
Clarté solaire deviendra nubi-
leuse,
Ronger le tout, grand peste venir
d'elles.

The plains of Ausonia, rich
and wide, will produce so
many gadflies and grasshop-
pers, that the light of the sun
will be clouded over. They
will devour everything and a
great pestilence will come from
them.

Perhaps *sauterelles* could be translated as locusts in this context.
But have they ever been found as far north as Naples (Ausonia)?

49

Devant le peuple, sang sera res-
    pandu,
Que du haut ciel ne viendra es-
    loigner:
Mais d'un long temps ne sera en-
    tendu,
L'esprit d'un seul le viendra tes-
    moigner.
	Blood will be spilt in front of
	the people, which will not go
	far from the high heavens.
	But for a long time it will not
	be heard, the spirit of a single
	man will bear witness to it.

Line 2 probably implies that the spilt blood was calling to the heavens for vengeance, but the bloody deed which caused it is not clarified.

50

Libra verra regner les Hesperies,
De ciel & terre tenir la monar-
    chie:
D'Asie forces nul ne verra peries,
Que sept ne tiennent par rang la
    hierarchie.
	Libra will be seen to reign in
	the West, holding the rule
	over the skies and earth. No
	one will see the strength of
	Asia destroyed until seven
	hold the hierarchy in succes-
	sion.

AMERICA AND ASIA

This is a very interesting quatrain and reads quite differently from what I thought it did at first. According to this prediction, when Libra the Balance rules over America, that country will be at the height of its powers but will start to decline, possibly after the seventh decade—after Nixon and Watergate, Chappaquiddick and President Carter's vaccilations this may not be an unsurprising reading. Nostradamus does not envisage a pleasant 80th decade for the world.
It may alternatively mean that trouble comes with the seventh ruler in Asia—we are on the fifth, having just got rid of the 'Gang of Four'. It may equally mean that war between East and West would break out during the seventh decade of this century, and Vietnam, Cambodia and Thailand were certainly examples of this. See II. 89. IV. 95. V. 78. VI. 21, 33.

51

Un Duc cupide son enemi en-suivre,	A Duke eager to follow his enemy will enter in, hinder-ing the phalanx. Hurried on foot they follow so closely that the day of the battle is near Ganges.
Dans entrera empeschant la phalange:	
Hastez à pied si pres viendront poursuivre,	
Que la journee conflite pres de Gange.	

Ganges may be understood as a town in France near Montpellier, or the River Ganges. The former is more likely.

52

En cité obsesse aux murs hommes & femmes,	In the besieged city men and women at the walls, the en-emy without, the leader ready to surrender; the wind will be strong against the armed men, they will be driven off by lime, dust and cinders.
Ennemis hors le chef prest à soi rendre	
Vent sera fort encontre les gen-darmes,	
Chassez seront par chaux, pous-iere, & cendre.	

53

Les fugitifs & bannis revoquez,	The fugitives and the ban-ished are recalled, fathers and sons strengthening the deep wells. The cruel father and his followers suffocated; His most wicked son drowned in the well.
Peres & fils grand garnissant les hauts puits:	
Le cruel pere & les siens suffo-quez,	
Son fils plus pire submergé dans le puits.	

54

Du nom qui onques ne fut au Roy Gaulois,	Of a name which never held by a French king, never was there so fearful a thunder-bolt. Italy, Spain and the Eng-lish tremble; he will be greatly attentive to foreign women.
Jamais ne fut un fouldre si crain-tif:	
Tremblant l'Italie, L'Espaigne & les Anglois,	
De femme estrangiers grande-ment attentif.	

NAPOLEON I

This is a fascinating quatrain. Napoleon brought the new name of Bonaparte to the line of French kings, for most kings had shared the same names, i.e. Louis (6), Henri (2), Charles (2), Francis (1), since Nostradamus' time. Napoleon's was the great reshaping of the map of Europe and he was very enamoured of his two foreign wives, Josephine the Créole, Marie Louise the Austrian, and possibly it also refers to his Polish mistress, Marie Walewska. The reference to his name being dreadful as a thunderbolt should be compared with IV. 82, where Nostradamus calls him the Destroyer. See I, 76. IV, 82. VIII, 1.

55

Quant la corneille sur tout de brique joincte,
Durant sept heures ne fera que crier:
Mort presagee de sang statue taincte,
Tyran meutri, aux Dieux peuple prier.

When the crow on a tower made of brick will do nothing but croak for seven hours; it foretells death, a statue stained with blood, a tyrant murdered, people praying to their Gods.

Both the crow, and the statue weeping blood are common omens of evil, the latter has been recorded even in this country. But the results of these omens are too general to pinpoint the stanza.

56

Apres victoire de rabieuse langue,
L'esprit tempté en tranquil & repos:
Victeur sanguin par conflict faict harangue,
Roustir la langue & la chair & les os.

After the victory of the raging tongue, the spirit tempted in tranquil rest. Throughout the battle the bloody victor makes speeches, roasting the tongue, the flesh and the bones.

57

Ignare envie au grand Roi sup- portee, *Tiendra propos deffendre les escripitz:* *Sa femme non femme par un autre tentee,* *Plus double deux ne fort ne criz.*	Ignorant envy supported by the great king, will propose forbidding the writings. His wife, not his wife, tempted by another, no longer will the double dealing couple protest against it.

It has been suggested that Nostradamus is here referring to
his own writings and Henri II's cool reception of the Prophecies. The mistress would be Diane de Poitiers. There is a
similar reference in VII. 9. The last line is very difficult to
translate.

58

Soleil ardent dans le gosier coller, *De sang humain arrouser terre Etrusque:* *Chef seille[1] d'eaue, mener son fils filer,* *Captive dame conduicte en terre Turque.*	To swallow the burning sun in the throat, the Tuscan land sprinkled with human blood, the leader leads his son away, the pail of water, a captive lady led into Turkish lands.

59

Deux assiegez en ardente ferveur, *De soif estaincts pour deux plaines tasses:* *Le fort limé, & un vieillart res- veur,* *Au Genevois de Nira monstra trasse.*	Two besieged in a burning heat, killed by thirst for want of two full cups; the fort filed, and an old dreamer will show the tracks of Nira to the Ge- nevans.

IRAN

Nira is a simple anagram for Iran. The old dreamer is
probably the Ayatollah.

[1]*seille*—O.F. = pail, bucket.

60

Les sept enfans en hostaige laissés,	The seven children left in
Le tiers viendra son enfant tru-	hostage, the third will come
cider:	to slaughter his child. Two
Deux par son filz seront d'estoc	will be pierced by a hook be-
percés,	cause of his son, he will come
Gennes, Florence, los viendra en-	to strike against Genoa and
cunder.[1]	Florence.

It is not clear whether these seven children are the Valois children of Catherine de' Medici; the rest of the quatrain does not clarify the position.

61

Le vieux mocqué & privé de sa	The old man, mocked and
place,	deprived of his position by
Par l'estrangier qui le subornera:	the foreigner who will suborn
Mains de son filz mangées devant	him. The hands of his sons
sa face,	are devoured before his face,
Le frere à Chartres, Orl. Rouen	he will betray his brother at
trahira.	Chartres, Orléans and Rouen.

MARSHAL PÉTAIN, 1940–4

Marshal Pétain's nickname during the Vichy régime was *Le Vieux*, and nothing could describe his position more clearly than line 2. The hands which are devoured in front of him are the forces of his régime which are destroyed. The brothers are the Allies who simultaneously reached the three towns here mentioned, Chartres, Orleans and Rouen on 19th August 1944. They were betrayed by Pétain to the Germans, who was deported to Sigmariggen on the very day of their liberation.

62

Un coronel machine ambition,	A colonel intrigues through
Se saisira de la plus grand armée,	ambition, he will seize the
Contre son prince fainte inven-	greater part of the army.
tion,	Against his Prince a false in-
Et descouvert sera soubz sa ramée.	vention; he will be discovered
	under his flag.

[1] *encunder*—Probably from the Latin, *incutiere* = to strike against.

OLIVER CROMWELL

Most commentators accept this as a general quatrain about Oliver Cromwell, who took over the greater part of Charles I's armies and fought with them under the British flag. He certainly connived in the plotting and accusations laid against the king at his trial and execution. However it would apply very neatly to Colonel Gadaffi who overthrew King Idris of Libya in 1971.

63

L'armée Celtique contre les montaignars,	The Celtic army against the mountaineers, who will be revealed and caught in a trap.
Qui seront sceus & prins à la lipee:	The fresh bracken will soon be pressed by the peasants,
Paysans fraisz pousseront tost faugnars,	they will all perish on the sword's blade.
Precipitez tous au fil de l'espee.	

FRANCE 1702–4

This probably refers to Marshal Villar's fight against the Camisard rebels of the Cevennes who practised a very competent form of guerrilla warfare (1702–4).

64

Le deffaillant en habit de bourgeois,	The defaulter, dressed as a citizen will come to try the king with his offence; Fifteen soldiers, for the most part outlaws, the end of his life and the greater part of his estate.
Viendra le Roi tempter de son offence:	
Quinze souldartz la plupart Ustagois,	
Vie derniere & chef de sa chevance.	

65

Au deserteur de la grand forteresse,	To the deserter of the great fortress, after he will have abandoned his post, his adversary will display such prowess that the Emperor will soon be condemned to death.
Apres qu'aura son lieu abandonné:	
Son adversaire fera si grand prouesse,	
L'Empereur tost mort sera condamné.	

NAPOLEON III

Napoleon III, while still Louis Napoleon, was condemned to life detention in the fortress of Ham by the French, but on 25th May 1846 escaped from the castle to England. Louis Philippe abandoned his position as king of France in the 1848 Revolution and Louis Napoleon was voted Prince-President in December of the same year. He did not, however, display great skills as an Emperor, and his policies were responsible for the Franco-Prussian war and the consequent disaster to France. He died soon afterwards in 1873. The adversaries who are so powerful are, of course, the Prussians.

66

Soubz couleur faincte de sept testes raseés	Under the false colours of seven shaven heads several
Seront semés divers esplorateurs:	spies will be scattered. The
Puys & fontaines de poisons arrousées,	wells and springs will be sprinkled with poisons, at the
Au fort de Gennes humains devorateurs.	fort of Genoa, they devour human flesh.

Shaven heads is sometimes used by Nostradamus to describe Cromwell's roundheads.

67

L'an que Saturne & Mars esgaux combuste,	In the year that Saturn and Mars are equally fiery, the air
L'air fort seiché longue trajection:	is very dry, a long meteor. From hidden fires a great
Par feux secrets, d'ardeur grand lieu adust	place burns with heat, little rain, a hot wind, wars and
Peu pluie, vent chault, guerres, incursions.	raids.

21st MARCH 1986

The configuration of Saturn and Mars is a common one, so further information is needed to understand this quatrain. The dating of the comet or meteor is probably the key, Halley's comet, due next in 1986.

68

En lieu¹ bien proche non esloigné de Venus,	At a nearby place not far from Venus, the two greatest ones of Asia and Africa will be said to have come from the Rhine and Hitler; cries and tears at Malta and the ligurian coast.
Les deux plus grans de l'Asie & d'Affrique	
Du Rhin & Hister qu'on dira sont venus,	
Cris, pleurs à Malte & costé ligustique.	

TRIPARTITE PACT. HITLER AND MUSSOLINI

The word Venus is the clue to this quatrain. It probably stands for Venice, thus linking Italy with Hitler. The two dictators met not far from the city at the Brenner Pass to seal the Tripartite Pact with Asia, that is, the Japanese. The last line refers to the blockade of Malta by the Italians, and the trouble on the Ligurian coast, to the Allied bombing of Genoa, and to the bombardments by British battleships operating from Gibraltar. See I. 34. II. 24. III. 35, 53, 58, 61. IV. 40. V. 29, 94. VI. 7, 51. IX. 90., and for Mussolini, III. 32, 68. IV. 68.

69

La cité grande les exiles tiendront,	The exiles will hold the great city, the citizens are dead, murdered and driven out. The people of Aqualeia will promise Parma to show them the entrance by untrodden paths.
Les citadins morts meurtris & chassés:	
Ceulx d'Aquilee à Parme promettront,	
Monstrer l'entree par les lieux non trassés.	

Aqualeia was a great city in ancient times, but nothing more than a village by the 16th Century. Parma belonged to the Papacy and became an hereditary duchy for the Pope's bastard in 1545.

¹alternative reading—*l'an* = year.

70

Bien contigue des grans monts Pyrenees,	Very near the great mountains of the Pyrenees, a man
Un contre l'aigle grand copie adresser:	will raise a great army against the Eagle. Veins will be
Ouvertes veines, forces exterminees,	opened, strength disappears;
Comme jusque à Pau le chef viendra chasser.	the leader will chase them as far as the Pau.

WELLINGTON'S CAMPAIGN IN THE PENINSULAR WAR

This describes Wellington's approach to France through Portugal and Spain where he is to confront the Eagle, Napoleon. The opened veins probably indicate the lost supply lines of the French when they were driven back as far as the Pau, despite the French victory at Toulouse, which was of uncertain value to Napoleon.

71

En lieu d'espouse les filles trucidées,	Instead of a bride the girls are slaughtered, murder with such
Meurtre à grand faulte ne sera superstile:[1]	wickedness, there will be no survivors. The vestals are
Dedans le puys vestules inondées,	drowned in the wells, and the
L'espouse estraincte par hauste d'Aconile.[2]	bride killed by a draught of Aconile.

Aconite is a classical poison distilled from monkshood and wolfsbane. Otherwise the quatrain seems completely obscure.

72

Les Artomiques par Agen & l'Estore,	The Artomiques through Agen & Lectoure will hold
A sainct Felix feront leur parlement:	their parliament at St Felix. Those of Bazas will come at
Ceux de Basas viendront à la mal'heure,	an unfortunate time to seize Condon & Marsan promptly.
Saisir Condon & Marsan promptement.	

[1]*superstile*—Misprint for *superstite* = survivor.

[2]Aconile—misprint for Aconite.

What the Artomiques are is not certain. Artos in Greek means bread, but there is also a resemblance to the modern word atomic.

73

Le nepveu grand par forces prouvera, Le pache[1] faict du coeur pusillanime: Ferrare & Ast le Duc esprouvera, Par lors qu'au soir sera le pantomime.	The nephew shall prove by great strength the crime committed by a cowardly heart. The Duke will try Ferrara and Asti; then when the comedy takes place in the evening.

ASSASSINATION OF THE DUKE DE BERRY, 1820

This event is described vividly by Nostradamus in I. 84 and III. 96 in which quatrain he gives the date as well. The Duke de Berry was killed leaving the Opéra on the evening of 13th February 1820. The nephew who benefits from this is Napoleon III who later succeeds to the throne because of the assassination of the male heir.

74

Du lac liman & ceux de Brannonices,[2] Tous assemblez contre ceux d'Aquitaine Germains beaucoup, encor plus Souisses, Seront defaictz avec ceux d'Humaine.[3]	The people of Lake Geneva and of Mâcon, all gathered against the people of Aquitaine; many Germans, even more Swiss will be routed together with those of Maine.

It is just possible that by *Humaine* in the last line Nostradamus is referring to the Humanists whom he would regard as responsible for the Protestants Reformation in Switzerland.

[1] *pache*—O.F. = treaty. Variant, *peche* = crime.
[2] *Brannonices*—Latin = people from around Mâcon.
[3] *Humaine*—Variant, *ceux du Maine*.

75

Prest à combatre fera defection.	He who was ready to fight will
Chef adversaire obtiendra la vic-	desert, the chief adversary
toire.	will win the victory. The rear
L'arriere garde fera defension,	guard will make a defence,
Les deffaillans mort au blanc ter-	those faltering, dying in a
ritoire.	white country.

WATERLOO, 1815

Marshal Grouchy is the deserter in the first line. He was commander of the French cavalry whose orders from Napoleon were delayed for twelve hours, but even when he received them, Grouchy did not do as asked. Wellington is the great adversary of the French who is victorious. The famous stand of Napoleon's Imperial Guard who fought to the last man is described in the following line, while the white country may be an indirect reference to Napoleon's retreat from Moscow in 1812, and is a direct one to the sign of the white cockade of the Bourbons. It was said that after Napoleon's capture there were so many white cockades that Paris looked as though there had been a fall of snow.

76

Les Nictobriges[1] par ceux dè Per-	The people of Agen by those
igort,	of Perigord will be troubled
Seront vexez tenant jusques au	as far as the Rhône. The as-
Rosne:	sociation of Gascons & Bi-
L'associé de Gascons & Begorne,	gorre, betrays the Church,
Trahir le temple, le prebstre estant	the priest giving his sermon.
au prosne.	

Both Agen and Perigord are about two hundred miles west of the Rhône. Bigorre was a Gascon town, but also a rallying cry of Henri de Navarre's Huguenots, and the verse is probably hinting at the Protestant/Catholic conflict in France in the 16th Century.

[1]*Nictobriges* = the people around Agen.

77

SELIN monarque l'Italie paci-
fique,
Regnes unis Roi chrestien du
monde:
Mourrant voudra coucher en terre
blesique[1]
Apres pirates avoir chassé de
l'onde.

SELIN king, Italy peaceful,
kingdoms united by the
Christian king of the world.
When he dies, he will want to
lie in Blois territory, having
chased the pirates from the
sea.

This is the quatrain upon which many 19th Century royalists
built their hopes of a great French king who would come and
change the face of Europe. The key to the quatrain is the word
SELIN; it comes from the Greek *Selene*, the Moon or Diana.
There is a strong possibility that Nostradamus went completely
off the rails with this series of quatrains and intended them
for Henri II and his mistress Diane de Poitiers. Henri II also
adopted the moon as his device, but nevertheless these verses
were not understood by his contemporaries. Perhaps they are
a good example of retroactive history, as I explain in the introduction, of something that seems unlikely now ever to take
place. The notion of a Christian king governing the world
seems impossible, particularly when compared with the quatrains which describe the situation envisaged by Nostradamus
between America and the Far East.

78

La grand armee de la pugne civ-
ile,
Pour de nuict Parme à l'estrange
trouvée,
Septante neuf meurtris dedans la
ville,
Les estrangiers passez tous à
l'espee.

The great army of the civil
war, Parma taken at night by
foreigners. Seventy-nine
murdered in the town, the
foreigners all put to the sword.

Parma was an Italian duchy and an ally of the French, so the
Spanish army is the most likely interpretation for line 2.

[1]*blesique*—Med. Latin, *Blesa* = Blois.

79

Sang Royal fuis, Monhurt, Mas, Eguillon,	Flee, royal blood, Monheurt, Mas, Aiguillon, the Landes
Remplis seront de Bourdelois les landes,	will be full of people from Bourdeaux. Navarre, Bigorre, points and spurs, deeply
Navarre, Bigorre poinctes & eguillons,	gorre, points and spurs, deeply hungry they devour acorns of
Profondz de faim vorer de liege glandes.	the cork oak.

All these places are in South-west France and have probably some connection with IV. 76, the struggle of the Huguenots and Henri of Navarre against the Catholics. As mentioned before, Bigorre was the rallying cry of the Protestants.

80

Pres du grand fleuve, grand fosse, terre egeste,	Near the great river, a great trench, earth excavated, the
En quinze pars sera l'eau divisee:	water will be divided into fifteen parts. The city taken,
La cité prinse, feu, sang, cris conflict mettre	fire, blood, cries and battle given, the greater part con-
Et la plus part concerne au collisee.[1]	cerned with the collision.

THE MAGINOT LINE

James Laver suggests that this is the quatrain which persuaded the Abbé Torné to insist that France erected the infamous Maginot line, which fell so quickly to the Germans. The River in line 1 is the Rhine. Hitler partially ignored the Maginot line and advanced from other directions thus fulfilling lines 3 and 4. The collision becomes the series of battles fought in France during the Second World War.

[1]*collisee*—Latin, *collisus* = clash.

81

Pont on fera promptement de na-
*   celles,*
Passer l'armee du grand prince
*   Belgique:*
Dans profondres¹ & non loing de
*   Brucelles,*
Outre passés, detrenchés sept à
*   picque.*

A bridge will quickly be built
from boats, to cross the army
of a great Belgian Prince.
Poured forth inside not far
from Brussels, having passed
over, seven will be cut down
by a pike.

When Nostradamus wrote, the word Belgian was archaic and
could only have referred to Philip II, who had been given the
territory in 1554 by the Emperor Charles V. An attack on
Northern France, crossing the River Scheldt was made in the
1560s.

82

Amas s'approche venant d'Escla-
*   vonie,*
L'Olestant vieux cité ruinera:
Fort desolee verra sa Romanie.
Puis la grand flamme estaindre
*   ne sçaura.*

A mass of men will draw near,
coming from Slavonia, the
Destroyer will ruin the old
city; he will see his Romania
quite desolated, then will not
know how to extinguish the
great flame.

NAPOLEON'S RETREAT FROM MOSCOW, 1812–13

The Grand Armée retreated from Moscow during the bitter
winter of 1812/13. The word Olestant means Destroyer and
Nostradamus refers to Napoleon as this in IV. 54 when he
calls him the dreadful thunderbolt. The old city is Moscow
which was razed to the ground by fire. The word Romanie
cannot refer to Rumania which did not exist in Nostradamus'
time, but may well refer to Rome, as Napoleon's young son
had just been made king of Rome, and his empire would not
continue for much longer. The great flame is probably a metaphor for the war which Napoleon started and which gathered
in momentum to finally defeat him. See I. 76, IV. 54, VIII.
1.

¹*profondres*—Latin, *profondatus* = poured forth.

83

Combat nocturne le vaillant cap-
itaine,
Vaincu fuira peu de gens pro-
fligé:
Son peuple esmeu, sedition non
vaine,
Son propre filz le tiendra assiegé.

In a night battle the brave
captain is overcome and flees,
ruined by a few men. His people are moved, they agitate
successfully, his own son will
hold him besieged.

84

Un grand d'Auxerre mourra bien
miserable,
Chassé de ceux qui soubs lui ont
esté:
Serré de chaines, apres d'un rude
cable,
En l'an que Mars, Venus, & Sol,
mis en esté.

An important man from Auxerre will die very wretchedly,
driven out by the people who
were under him. Bound in
chains, then with a strong
rope, the year that Mars, Venus and the Sun are in conjunction in the summer.

This is a very rare conjunction but has not brought forth an
important man from Auxerre to date, so this quatrain may
apply to the future.

85

Le charbon blanc du noir sera
chassé,
Prisonnier faicte mené au tom-
bereau:
More[1] Chameau sus piedz entre-
lassez,
Lors le puisné sillera l'aubereau.

The white coal is driven out
by the black, made a prisoner,
led to the tumbril: his feet are
tied together like a rogue,
when the last born will let slip
the falcon.

LOUIS XVI AND THE FRENCH REVOLUTION, 1793

Charbon is an anagram for Bourbon, *noir* the usual anagram
for king and white the colour of the Bourbon standard. Louis
XVI was the last Bourbon king before the Revolution. He was
imprisoned in the Temple and dragged on a tumbril, with his
feet tied, to his death on 27th January 1793. The last line

[1]*more*—Latin, *mos, moris* = custom, practice.

probably implies that his heir, Louis XVII, about whom there has been so much speculation and doubt, may have escaped from the Temple and have lived quietly in Europe. Nostradamus refers to this theme elsewhere in the Prophecies. Louis was the second son, the last born son of the family. His elder brother Charles died in 1795.

86

L'an que Saturne en eau sera conjoinct,
Avecques Sol, le Roi fort & puissant:
A Reims & Aix sera reçeu & oingt,
Apres conquestes meutrira innocens.

In the year Saturn is in conjunction with Aquarius, and with the Sun, the very powerful king will be received and anointed at Reims & Aix. After conquests he will murder innocent people.

The astrological conjunction of lines 1 and 2 is again reasonably rare. Reims is the traditional coronation site for the French Kings and Aix that of the German and Holy Roman Emperors. No king has been crowned in both places since Nostradamus' time. This is another of the quatrains used by French Royalists to predict the return of the French royal line.

87

Un filz du Roi tant de langues aprins,
A son aisné[1] au regne different:
Son pere beau[2] au plus grand filz comprins
Fera perir principal adherent.

The son of a king, having learnt many languages, different from his elder in the kingdom. His father-in-law understanding well the elder son, will cause the main adherent to perish.

The quatrain implies that the younger son of a king will take over the kingdom, the elder, legitimate heir having been removed by his father (in law?).

[1]*aisné* = elder or predecessor.
[2] *pere beau* = father-in-law or handsome father.

88

Le grand Antoine du nom de faicte sordide
De Phthiriase¹ à son dernier rongé:
Un qui de plomb voudra estre cupide,
Passant le port d'esleu sera plongé.

Anthony, great in name, in his actions base, at the end will be devoured by lice. One who is eager for lead, passing the harbour will be drowned by the elected one.

A difficult prophecy for someone named Anthony. Phthiriasis, pediculosis, is an illness caused by lice.

89

Trente de Londres secret conjureront,
Contre leur Roi sur le pont² entreprinse,
Lui, satalites la mort degousteront.
Un Roi esleu blonde, natif de Frize.

Thirty Londoners will secretly conspire against their king, the enterprise on the sea. He and his courtiers will not like death, a fair king elected, native of Friesland.

WILLIAM III OF ENGLAND

This is a good prediction of the Glorious Revolution of 1688–9. William III insisted that those lords who supported him in England should sign a document. There were certainly a number of conspirators crossing the seas to Holland and back before William sailed with his fleet. The ones who dislike death are James II and his supporters who decide to flee rather than fight the matter out once the Duke of Marlborough, who led the army, deserted their cause. It is not certain whether William III was fair-haired but he did come from Friesland. What makes this prophecy so interesting is that there was no possible Dutch candidate for the English throne while Nostradamus was alive.

¹*Phthiriase—Phthisis* = consumption, Phthiriasis = suffering from lice.
²*pont*—Latin, *pontus* = sea, not a bridge in this context.

90

Les deux copies aux murs ne pourront joindre.	The two armies cannot join up at the walls. At that time Milan and Pavia tremble. Hunger, thirst and doubt will weigh upon them so much, they will not have a scrap of meat, bread nor supplies.
Dans cest instant trembler Milan, Ticin:[1]	
Faim, soif doubtance si fort les viendra poindre,	
Chair, pain, ne vivres n'auront un seul boucin.[2]	

91

Au duc Gauloise contrainct battre au duelle,	For the French duke compelled to fight in a duel, the ship Mellele will not approach Monaco. Wrongly accused in perpetual prison his son will attempt to reign before his death.
La nef Mellele monech n'approchera,	
Tort accusé, prison perpetuelle,	
Son fils regner avant mort taschera.	

Mellele may be a corruption of Melilla, a Moroccan sea port, but it does not fit into context very well. Perhaps this quatrain has some connection with IV. 83? The last lines are very similar.

92

Teste tranchee du vaillant capitaine,	The head of the brave captain cut off it will be thrown down in front of his adversary. His body hung from the masts of the ship, confused, he will flee using oars in a contrary wind.
Sera gettee devant son adversaire:	
Son corps pendu de la classe à l'antenne,	
Confus fuira par rames à vent contraire.	

RADIO OR RADAR EQUIPMENT?

It is interesting that Nostradamus used the word *antenne* here instead of *mât* for the ship's mast. Perhaps he was using

[1] *Ticin*—Latin, *Ticinum* = Pavia.
[2] *boucin*—Provençal = mouthful, morsel.

this word to indicate complex equipment with which he was
not familiar but which he recognized to be scientific, such as
a radio mast or radar equipment?

93

Un serpent veu proche du lict royal,	A serpent will be seen near the royal bed by a lady at
Sera par dame nuict chiens n'abayeront:	night, the watchdogs will not bark; Then will be born in
Lors naistre en France un Prince tant royal,	France a Prince so royal, that all the princes will see him as
Du ciel venu tous les Princes verront.	a gift from heaven.

THE COUNT DE CHAMBORD, 1820–83

A very important quatrain. The Duchesse de Berry gave
birth to a son in 1820, seven months after her husband's assassination. The legitimacy of the birth was contested by the
Duke of Orléans, the snake, who had right of entry as a member of the family and so the watchdogs were not alerted. This
birth of a grandson to Charles X was the cause of great re-
joicing to French monarchists. The child was nicknamed 'Dieu-
donné', a gift from heaven, as Nostradamus so aptly puts it.

94

Deux grans freres seront chassez d'Espaigne,	Two great brothers will be driven out of Spain, the elder
L'aisné vaincu sous les monts Pyrenees:	is beaten under the Pyrenean mountains. The sea is red-
Rougir mer, rosne, sang lemam d'Alemaigne,	dened, the Rhône, blood in Lake Geneva from Germany,
Narbon, Blyterre, d'Agath[1] con-taminees.	Narbonne and Beziers con-taminated by Agde.

A detailed but unconvincing quatrain. It contains five separate predictions.
1 Exile for two Spanish leaders.
2 Defeat for one of them near the Pyrenees.
3 A bloody naval battle.
4 An attack against Geneva from Germany.

[1]*Agath*—Latin = Agde.

5 A possible plague spreading from Agde, see also VIII. 21
to local towns.
None of these apart from 1, 2 and 3 which are very general
can have much relevance. If we could understand the other
two the quatrain could probably be put into context.

95

La regne à deux laissé bien peu tiendront,	The rule left to two, they will hold it a very short time.
Trois ans sept mois passés feront la guerre.	Three years and seven months having passed they will go to war. The two vestals will rebel against them; the victor then born on American soil.
Les deux vestales contre rebelle-ront,	
Victor puis nay en Armorique terre.	

VICTORY FOR AMERICA

If in this quatrain the two powers are understood to be
world powers, it implies that 3 years and 7 months after the
Russian/American alliance, which Nostradamus predicts elsewhere, has taken place they will go to war against Asia. *Vestales*
in line 3 is probably a corruption of *vassals*—two smaller countries disagree with this decision and perhaps stay neutral. The
final victory lies in the West, with America. Nostradamus' references to war in the 80s connected with Halley's comet in
1986 seem to make this just probable. See I. 91, II. 41, 46, IV. 32,
V. 78.

96

La soeur aisnée de l'isle Britan-nique,	The elder sister of the island of Britain will be born fifteen years before her brother. Be-cause of his promise proving to be true, she will succeed to the kingdom of the Balance.
Quinze ans devant le frere aura naissance:	
Par son promis moyennant ver-rifique,	
Succedera au regne de balance.	

WILLIAM AND MARY

Mary was the elder sister of James III, who never came to
the English throne, but she was in fact twenty-six, not fifteen
years older than her brother. Mary acceded to the throne

through her own, and her husband William of Orange's, promises to the English Parliament. The Balance is Libra, the zodiacal sign, which Nostradamus seems here to apply to England although many astrologers apply it to Austria and Savoy. It also governs a trading nation, which the British certainly are. Note that again Nostradamus speaks of the British Isles and not of England which immediately dates the quatrain later than 1603.

97

L'an que Mercure, Mars, Venus, retrograde,
Du grand Monarque la ligne ne faillit:
Esleu du peuple l'usitant¹ pres de Gagdole,²
Qu'en paix & regne viendra fort envieillir.

In the year that Mercury, Mars and Venus are retrograde, the family line of the great King will not fail. Elected by the Portuguese people near Cadiz, who in peace will grow very old in his kingdom.

This quatrain seems to describe the Portuguese succession and is limited in time by the conjunction of line 1. It seems also to imply that the Portuguese king is elected in Spain, which never happened. But Philip II of Spain seized the Portuguese throne and ruled it until 1621, followed by his son Philip III, until the Portuguese revolted against the Spanish in 1640. However, Nostradamus did appear to understand the Spanish seizure of the Portuguese throne.

98

Les Albanois passeront dedans Rome,
Moyennant Langres demipler³ affublés,
Marquis & Duc ne pardonnes à homme,
Feu, sang, morbilles⁴ point d'eau, faillir les bleds.

The people of Alba will cross into Rome, by means of Langres the multitude are weakened. The Marquis and the Duke will spare no man, fire, blood and smallpox, no water, the crops will fail.

¹usitant—Misreading for Lusitans = Portuguese.
²Gagdole—Probable misprint for Gades = Cadiz, as the present reading doesn't even rhyme and is obviously incorrect.
³demipler—A word invented by Nostradamus, probably from the Greek, demi-pleres = mob-full or multitude.
⁴morbilles—O.F. = smallpox.

The word *Albanois* is hard to interpret. It probably stands for the troops of the Duke of Alba, but Albania is a possibility. The many disasters are obscure. *Langres* is in Champagne, so possibly it is the same person as in VII. 4?

99

L'aisné vaillant de la fille du Roy,	The brave eldest son of a king's daughter will drive the Celts back very far. He will use thunderbolts, so many in such an array, few and distant, then deep into the West.
Repoussera si profond les Celtiques:	
Qu'il mettra foudres, combien en tel arroi	
Peu & loing puis profond és Hesperiques.[1]	

MISSILES OR ROCKETS.

The Celts referred to here are the French who are driven back by an unidentified leader. He fights with such fearful and far-reaching weapons that they can even penetrate as far as Spain or America, implying either mortar shells, missiles or possibly rockets with warheads. See VI. 34.

100

De feu celeste au Royal edifice,	Fire will fall from the sky on to the royal building when the light of war is weakened. For seven months a great war, people dead through evil, Rouen and Evreux will not fail the king.
Quant la lumiere de Mars defaillira:	
Sept mois grand guerre, mort gent malefice,	
Rouen, Eureux au Roi ne faillira.	

FRANCO-PRUSSIAN WAR, 1870–71

During the siege of Paris the royal palace, the Tuileries, was destroyed by cannon fire. The glory of the Bonaparte family was weakened and almost ended by this war. Napoleon III was to die two years later, and France remained a republic from then on. The Franco-Prussian war did last for seven months, July 1870 to February 1871, an accurate prediction. The last line refers to towns in Normandy, which part of France remained loyal to the king and wanted to restore the monarchy through the National Assembly.

[1]*Hesperiques*—As always, either the Western lands of Spain and Portugal, or the USA.

CENTURY V

231

1

Avant venu de ruine Celtique,
Dedans le temple deux parlemen-
*   teront*
Poignard coeur, d'un monté au
*   coursier & pique,*
Sans faire bruit le grand enter-
*   reront.*

Before the ruin of France,
there will be parliamentary
discussions about the second.
Stabbed to the heart by one
riding on a charger with a
lance, they will bury the great
one secretly.

THE MURDER OF LOUIS XVII (1785–95?)

There has always been much speculation about the fate of
Louis XVII, the second son and heir of Louis XVI and Marie
Antoinette. The King and his family were housed in the Temple in 1792, when the Revolutionary mobs appeared to be
getting out of hand. The fate of the whole family was debated
by the newly formed French Legislative Assembly (*parlemen-
teront*). It is not known how Louis XVII died but Nostradamus
indicates clearly that he was killed in line 4. The third line
describes his killer as an unidentified soldier. He was appall-
ingly ill-treated in prison, separated from his mother and sis-
ters and kept in the dark for months on end, like a wild beast.
In May 1795 he was declared to be seriously ill and his death
was announced on 8th June. Several pretenders came forward
during the next forty years claiming to be the young Prince,
but if Nostradamus is correct he was buried at the Church of
St Marguerite on 10th June, as was officially announced, without even a stone to mark the spot, *'sans faire bruit'*.

2

Seps conjurés au banquet feront
*   luire,*
Contre les trois le fer hors de na-
*   vire:*
L'um des deux classes au grand
*   fera conduire*
Quand par le mail. Denier au
*   front lui tire.*

Seven conspirators at a banquet will cause their weapons
to flash against the three who
come from the ship. One of
the two will take the fleet to
the leader when the other will
shoot him in the forehead
through his armour.

3

Le successeur de la Duché vien-
dra,
Beaucoup plus outre que la mer
de Tosquane:
Gauloise branche la Florence
tiendra,
Dans son giron d'accord nautique
Rane.[1]

The successor to the Duchy
will come from far beyond the
sea of Tuscany. A French
branch will hold Florence, in
its wake a nautical agreement
(with the frog?).

DUKE OF LORRAINE, 1737

Florence was the capital of the Duchy of Tuscany from the
rule of Alessandro de Medici in 1531 until the death of Gian
Gastone in 1737 when the Duchy was assigned to Francis, Duke
of Lorraine, a Frenchman, and remained in the Lorraine family until 1859, except during the French Revolution. The reference to a nautical agreement and a frog is unclear. It may
refer to the myth in which the earliest inhabitants of Tuscany
were turned into frogs by Bacchus.

4

Le gros mastin de cité deschassé,
Sera fasché de l'etrange alliance,
Apres aux champs avoir le cerf
chassé
Le loup & l'Ours se donront de-
fiance.

The great mastiff is driven
out of the city, angered by the
foreign alliance. Later having
chased the stag to the field,
the wolf and the bear will defy
each other.

SECOND WORLD WAR

The other name for a mastiff in French is *le dogue anglais*,
and England is probably intended in line 1. Angered by a
foreign treaty England chases the stag to the battlefield where
the wolf (Italy) and the Bear (Russia) are defying each other.
This appears to refer to the Second World War when the
Russians entered the war as British Allies.

---

[1]*Rane*—Latin, *rana* = a frog, possible misprint for *rame* = oar,
which is more suitable.

5

Souz ombre faincte d'oster de servitude,
Peuple & cité l'usurpera lui mesmes:
Pire fera par fraux de jeune pute,
Livré au champ lisant le faux proesme.

Beneath the faint pretext of removing servitude, the people and the city will themselves usurp power. He will do worse because of the trickery of the young whore, delivered in the field, reading the false promise.

LOUIS XVI AND MARIE ANTOINETTE, 1792

An important quatrain. This describes the French Revolution, which replaced Louis XVI's rule with one just as autocratic. The people of Paris took over government of their city, after the revolt of the Bastille, 14th July 1789. The woman who makes things worse by her double dealing is Marie Antoinette, by her general extravagance and in particular by the affair of the diamond necklace from which her popularity never recovered. When she and Louis were later caught trying to go to St Cloud in 1792, the family were turned back by the crowds who said to Louis XVI, 'we love you alone'. The false promises were those given by the king when he promised not to try to escape from the Temple where he and his people had been placed to protect them from the people. They fled to Varennes in 1792 and were caught. See IX. 20, and IX. 34. Varennes is a comparatively small town even now.

6

Au roi l'Augur sur le chef la main mettre,
Viendra prier pour la paix Italique:
A la main gauche viendra changer le sceptre
De Roi viendra Empereur pacifique.

The Augur will put his hand on the king's head and pray for peace in Italy. The sceptre will be changed to his left hand, from king he will become a peaceful Emperor.

NAPOLEON III

The Pope was godfather by proxy to the son of Louis Napoleon, later Napoleon III. He was not too successful in his

dealings with Italy and the Vatican because the Roman Revolutionaries felt he was too accommodating. The changing of
the sceptre probably refers to Napoleon III's underhand ma-
nipulation of the Revolution in France of 1848 and to the fact
that he declared himself Emperor on 2nd December 1851.
Nostradamus views him as a peaceful monarch, which ties in
well with the famous statement Napoleon III made on ac-
quiring power, *'L'empire, c'est la paix.'* "The art of Empire is
peace."

7

Du Triumvir seront trouvé les os,	The bones of the Triumvir
Cherchant profond thresor aenig- *matique:*	will be found by those search- ing for a deep and enigmatic
Ceux d'alentour ne seront en re- *pos.*	treasure. Those around will not be peaceful. This hollow-
Ce concaver marbre & plomb *metallique.*	ing of marble and metallic lead.

LOUIS PHILIPPE

This describes Louis Philippe's attempt to revive his waning
popularity when he brought back Napoleon's ashes from St
Helena and interred them in the Invalides. *Triumvir* is the
key word; after the *coup d'etat* of 18th Brumaire Napoleon
reduced the five members of the Directory to three, and made
himself first Consul. The treasure Louis Philippe was searching
vainly for was Napoleon's popular appeal, some of which he
hoped to gain by honouring Napoleon's ashes. The restless
people are the Bonapartistes who were politically encouraged
by this and insisted on helping in the task of burying the ashes.
The coffin itself was of lead.

8

Sera laissé le feu vif, mort caché,	There will be let loose living
Dedans les globes horrible espou- *vantable,*	fire and hidden death, fearful inside dreadful globes. By
De nuict à classe cité en poudre *lasché,*	night the city will be reduced to rubble by the fleet, the city
La cite à feu, l'ennemi favorable.	on fire, helpful to the enemy.

BOMBS

The dreadful object Nostradamus visualizes here is certainly no cannonball but some sort of bomb containing explosive material. Ships appear to bombard a city which, once on fire, is a landmark probably helpful to enemy aircraft.

9

Jusques au fonds la grand arq demolue,
Par chef captif, l'ami anticipé:
Naistra de dame front face chevelue,
Lors par astuce Duc à mort attrapé.

At the foot of the great fallen arch, the friend is captured forestalled by the leader. A woman will bear a son whose face and forehead are covered with hair; then through cunning the Duke escapes death.

ASSASSINATION ATTEMPT ON NAPOLEON III, 1858

The first two lines are thought to refer to Napoleon III who had been involved in the Italian revolutionary movement when a young man. After some years of power in France the Italians felt he had betrayed their cause and four of them attempted to assassinate him as he left the Opéra on the night of 14th January 1858. The plot was led by Count Orsini—the building was damaged but did not collapse as Nostradamus describes it, although several bystanders were killed. The captured friend was Pieri, a friend of Orsini's, who was arrested before the explosion. Napoleon III was only slightly hurt. The third line is obscure but the last implies that Napoleon III escaped death through foreknowledge, probably due to Pieri's arrest. This quatrain appears to lead straight on to the next one, presumably Nostradamus forgot to separate them.

10

Un chef Celtique dans le conflict blessé,
Aupres de cave voyant siens mort abbatre:
De sang & plaies & d'ennemis pressé,
Et secourus par incognus de quatre.

A French leader wounded in the struggle sees his subjects struck dead near the theatre. Hustled by enemies with bloody wounds, he will be saved from the four by unknown people.

ASSASSINATION ATTEMPT, NAPOLEON III
(*continued*)

As stated in V. 9, Napoleon III was slightly wounded when Italian revolutionaries attempted to kill him with a bomb outside the Opéra. (*Cavea* is the Latin word for theatre.) The ordinary people standing around him saved him by shielding him from the blast. The four conspirators were Orsini, Pieri, Gomez and Rudio.

11

Mer par solaires seure ne passera,	Those of the sun will not cross
Ceux de Venus tiendront toute l'Affrique:	the sea in safety, the people of Venus will hold the whole
Leur regne plus Saturne n'occupera,	of Africa. Then Saturn occupies their kingdom no
Et changera la part Asiatique.	longer and the part of Asia will change.

SECOND WORLD WAR. ITALY AND THE EAST, 1941–3

Japan's flag is a sun; her ships will not be safe once she has entered the war, and caused Asian politics to change, as China then joined with the Allied Powers in 1941. The people of Venice (Venus is a common corruption for this city throughout the Prophecies) which stands for Italy, are fighting with Rommel in North Africa. The malign influence of Saturn on Italian affairs causes them to withdraw from the war in 1943.

12

Aupres du lac Leman sera conduite,	Near Lake Geneva he will be led by a foreign woman who
Par garse estrange cité voulant trahir:	wants to betray the city. Before her death a great retinue
Avant son meutre à Auspourg la grande suitte,	will come to Augsburg. They will come to invade the people
Et ceux du Rhin la viendront invahir.	of the Rhine.

THIRTY YEARS WAR, 1636

The Battle of Augsburg, during the Thirty Years War forced the retreat of Bernhard, Duke of Saxe Wiemar, across

the Rhine. This left Southern and Central Germany exposed
to the attacks of the Hapsburg armies of the Holy Roman
Emperor, Ferdinand II. Augsburg fell to Ferdinand as did
other towns along the Rhine near the Swiss border. The use
of the word Auspourg by Nostradamus is probably a typical
pun, containing the two key words of the Hapsburg and Augs-
bourg. The only puzzle is the young woman.

13

Par grand fureur le Roi Romain Belgique	In a great rage the Roman king will wish to trouble Bel-
Vexer vouldra par phalange barbare:	gium with barbarian warriors. In a gnashing fury he will
Fureur grinsseant chassera gent Libyque	chase the Libyan peoples from Hungary as far as Gilbraltar.
Despuis Pannons[1] jusques Hercules la hare.[2]	

THIRTY YEARS WAR

The Holy Roman Emperor Ferdinand II and Philip of
Spain were allied together against Denmark, Norway and Sweden. In 1648 the Treaty of Westphalia recognized the republic
of the United Netherlands, part of which is now modern Belgium. The barbarian warriors are the German Protestant powers. The Thirty Years War started as a revolt in Bohemia and
spread as far as Gibraltar when Spain and France refused to
recognize the 1648 treaty and continued to fight until the
Treaty of the Pyrenees in 1659.

14

Saturne & Mars en leo Espagne captifve,	Saturn and Mars in Leo, Spain is captive, taken in battle by
Par chef Libyque au conflict attrapé,	a Libyan leader. Near when Malta and (the knights of)
Proche de Malthe, Heredde prinse vive,	Rhodes are captured alive, and the Roman power smit-
Et Romain sceptre sera par coq frappé.	ten by the cock.

[1]*Pannons*—Latin, *Pannonia* = now Hungary.
[2]*hare*—Misprint for *bare* = pillars of Hercules, or Gibraltar.

NAPOLEON'S CAMPAIGNS, 1797–1807/8

The only time that Spain can be considered as captive is during the Peninsular War of 1807/8, when Napoleon's troops occupied both Spain and Portugal. The resistance of Spanish patriots led the British to send in an army under General Sir Arthur Wellesley, who succeeded in driving out the French after five years of fighting. The rest of the quatrain refers to events ten years earlier. In 1797 the first action of Napoleon's Egyptian campaign was the capture of Malta held by the Knights of Rhodes, Heredde being an anagram. Finally at the Treaty of Tolentino the Pope ceded part of the Vatican and Church states to the cock, the symbol of France.

15

En navigant captif prins grand pontife,	While sailing, the great Pope will be captured; great preparations by the troubled clerics fail. The second elected absent, his power declines, his favourite bastard, put to death.
Grans aprets faillir les clercz tumultuez:	
Second esleu absent son bien debise,	
Son favori bastard à mort tué.	

PIUS VII AND NAPOLEON, 1808

Pius VII was taken prisoner by the French in 1808 having travelled to crown Napoleon in Paris in 1804. He is the second Pope to be materially hurt by Napoleon, the first was Pius VI who died in exile at Valence. The trouble among the clergy describes the great religious discontent in France after the abolition of the established Church. The bastard of the final line is usually interpreted as Napoleon inheriting a crown that was not rightfully his, who having received the favours of the Pope, sacks Rome in 1808 and imprisons the Pope, although he doesn't kill him.

16

A son hault pris plus la lerme sabee,	The Sabine tears will no longer be of value, human flesh through death is burnt to ashes; the island of Pharos disturbed by (man of) the cross, when at Rhodes a dreadful sight is seen.
D'humaine chair par mort en cendre mettre,	
A l'isle Pharos par croisars perturbee,	
Alors qu'à Rodes paroistra dur espectre.	

SECOND WORLD WAR. AFRICA AND GREECE

This quatrain seems to implicate Italy with the appalling deaths of Jews and others in the German concentration camps. It is important to remember that cremation was anathema to a 16th-Century man such as Nostradamus, and condemned not only by the Church but also socially. Pharos is an island opposite Alexandria and is probably used by Nostradamus to indicate Tobruk which is not far from there. It was disturbed several times by the men of the Cross, the Nazis, as the battles in the African desert between the Allies and Rommel waged back and forth. The dreadful sight at Rhodes would be the invasion of Greece by Mussolini in 1940, followed by the Germans in 1941. Despite British evacuations, the Germans claimed 270,000 prisoners. In fact about 70,000 people were believed to have died.

17

De nuict passant le roi pres d'une Andronne,	The king, passing at night through a narrow lane, the man from Cyprus is the main guard; the king dies, the hand flees the length of the Rhône: the conspirators will put him to death.
Celui de Cypres & principal guette:	
Le roi failli la main fuict long du Rosne,	
Les conjurés l'iront à mort mettre.	

Cyprus belonged to Venice until 1571, but the place of this conspiracy is obscure.

18

De deuil mourra l'infelix profligé,	The wretched man, destroyed, will die of grief. His victorious consort will celebrate the ceremonies. Former laws, free edicts drawn up, both the Prince and the wall fall on the seventh day.
Celebrera son vitrix l'hecatombe:	
Pristine loi franc edict redigé,	
Le mur & Prince au septiesme jour tombe.	

This quatrain implies that a man is destroyed by his actions, whereas his wife celebrates his death and brings an end to an oppressive régime. The wall may refer to the legal repressions, or may be understood literally. There is a hint that the wife

may have helped towards his death. The seventh day means
either a Sunday or, more literally, that the Prince took seven
days to die.

19

Le grand Royal d'or, d'aerain augmenté,	The great golden Royal, augmented by brass breaks the covenant; war is started by a young man. The people are afflicted by a lamented leader, the land will be covered with barbarian blood.
Rompu la pache,[1] par jeune ouverte guerre:	
Peuple affligé par un chef lamenté,	
De sang barbare sera converre terre.	

20

Dela les Alpes grand armée passera,	A great Army will cross over the Alps. A short while before a wretched monster will be born. In a strange way, suddenly, the great Tuscan will return to his native land.
Un peu devant naistra monstre vapin:	
Prodigieux & subit tournera,	
Le grand Tosquan à son lieu plus propin.	

NAPOLEON III, 1859

Napoleon III crossed the Alps against Austria in 1859. The
evil monster is the Italian Revolution; it is interesting to note
that one of the first results of the 1859 campaign was to drive
the Grand Duke of Tuscany, Leopold II, from Florence. He
was a Hapsburg and retired to Austria to escape the Italians,
thus fulfilling line 4 in retiring to his native land. The wretched
monster is understood to refer to Garibaldi.

21

Par le trespas du monarque latin,	By the death of a Latin king, those people whom he will have assisted during his reign; the fire glows, the booty is shared out; public death for the bold incursors.
Ceux qu'il aura par regne secouruz:	
Le feu luira, divisé le butin,	
La mort publique aux hardis incoruz.	

---

[1]*pacha*—Provençal = treaty, covenant.

The Latin monarch is difficult to interpret. If it stands for the ruler of Latium it means the Pope. It could possibly refer to Mussolini and the Fascists.

22

Avant qu'à Rome grand aie rendu
    l'ame,
Effrayeur grande à larmée es-
    trangere:
Par Esquadrons, l'embusche pres
    de Parme,
Puis les deux rouges ensemble fer-
    ont chere.

Before the great man gives up his soul at Rome, there is much fear among the foreign army. The ambush by the squadrons takes place near Parma, then the two red ones will feast together.

While a Pope lies dying some trouble occurs in Parma, in Northern Italy. At the same time two revolutionary leaders will be meeting each other in a festive way. It may continue in the next quatrain.

23

Les deux contens seront unis en-
    semble,
Quand la pluspart à Mars seront
    conjoinct.
Le grand d'Affrique en effrayeur
    & tremble:
DUUMVIRAT par la classe des-
    joinct.

The two contented men are united together when most (planets) are conjunct with Mars. The African leader trembles in terror. THE TWIN ALLIANCE scattered by the fleet.

TWO ALLIES

If the two mentioned here are a continuation of the two warmongers of V. 22, they are very soon involved in war with most other nations. Africa is troubled by the alliance which is finally broken through naval strength.

24

Le regne & lois souz Venus es-
    levé,
Saturne aura sus Jupiter empire:
La loi & regne par le Soleil levé,
Par Saturnins endurera le pire.

The kingdom and law raised under Venus, Saturn will dominate Jupiter. Law and empire raised by the Sun, will endure the worst through those of Saturn.

This verse is similar to V.11, but the meanings of Saturn and Venus are unclear. Nostradamus is probably using a configuration for dating purposes. The Sun could also stand for Charles V, or the Catholic Church. It is a very difficult quatrain to decipher.

25

Le prince Arabe Mars, Sol, Venus, Lyon,	The Arab Prince, Mars, the Sun, Venus and Leo, the rule
Regne d'Eglise par mer succombera:	of the Church will succumb to the sea. Towards Persia
Devers la Perse bien pres d'un million,	very nearly a million men will invade Egypt and Byzantium,
Bisance, Egypte, ver. serp.[1] invadera.	the true serpent.

WAR IN 1987

When Mars, the Sun and Venus are in conjunction with Leo, the following predictions are forecast about a new Arabian Empire. It will attack Persia, Egypt, Constantinople (Byzantium) and the navies of Christendom. According to the commentator Lee McCann (1942) this conjunction will take place on 21st August 1987. This must therefore in some way link up with the quatrains about the uprising in Asia.

26

La gent esclave par un heur martial,	The Slav people, through fortune in war, will become elevated to a high degree. They
Viendra en haut degré tant esleuee:	will change their Prince, one
Changeront prince, naistre un provincial,	born a provincial; an army raised in the mountains to
Passer la mer copie aux monts levee.	cross over the sea.

KING CONSTANTINE OF GREECE, 1917–20

The world *esclave* may mean either slave or Slav. The Russians were not regarded as Slavs in Nostradamus' day, this word was used to describe the Balkan peoples. The Greeks, partially Slav, rose against the Turks and landed troops at

---

[1] *ver. serp.*—Suggested interpretation, *vera serpens* = true serpent.

Smyrna in 1919 and stayed there until 1922. They also
changed their king at this time as Nostradamus predicted.
King Constantine, who was exiled in 1917, was recalled in 1920
but exiled again in 1922. Although of German origins Constantine was born in Athens. His rival was Premier Venizelos
from Crete.

27

Par feu & armes non loing de la marnegro,	With fire and weapons, not far from the Black Sea, he will
Viendra de Perse occuper Trebisonde:	come from Persia to occupy Trebizond. Pharos and Mytilene tremble, the Sun is bright,
Trembler Phatos Methelin, Sol alegro,	the Adriatic sea covered with Arab blood.
De sang Arabe d'Adrie couvert onde:	

IRAN—THE MAN WITH THE BLUE TURBAN

The first two lines are self explanatory. The power of Persia
will extend as far as Egypt and Greece. Presumably the Arabs
come off worse in the end as the Adriatic Sea is covered with
Arabian blood. See II.2, VI.80.

28

Le bras pendu & la jambe liée,	His arm hung and his leg bound, with pale face and a
Visage pasle au seing poignard caché:	dagger hidden in his breast:
Trois qui seront jurez de la meslee,	Three who will be sworn in the scuffle, against the great
Au grand de Gennes sera le fer lasché.	one of Genoa will the blade be drawn.

ASSASSINATION OF KING UMBERTO
OF ITALY, 1900

King Umberto was assassinated on 29th July 1900 by an
unemployed smith called Acciarito. Genoa belonged to Savoy
after 1815. Nostradamus seems to imply that the assassin had
an arm in a sling, which was not the case in this instance. It
is therefore possible that another assassination is referred to
here. It has not yet taken place but it seems unlikely.

29

La liberté ne sera recouvree,
L'occupera noir fier vilain inique:
Quand la matiere du pont sera
*   ouvree,*
D'Hister, Venise fasché la repub-
*   lique.*

Liberty will not be regained;
it will be occupied by a black,
proud, villainous and unjust
man. When the matter of the
Pope is opened by Hitler, the
republic of Venice will be
vexed.

HITLER, THE VATICAN AND MUSSOLINI

This quatrain describes Mussolini's intrigues to secure an
alliance with Hitler between the years 1934–8. Hitler and
Mussolini met at Venice—by this time a republic with Mussolini
as its dictator. Note how accurate Nostradamus' details are.
The adjective black probably refers to the Fascisti—the black-
shirts. The matter of the Pope (Pontifex) refers to the Con-
cordat drawn up between Mussolini and the Pope in 1928,
which line 4 infers will bring trouble or war to Italy, as indeed
it did. We must also consider Pope Pius' extremely ambiguous
attitude towards the Nazis and the help that the Vatican gave
them to escape at the end of the war. A disgraceful ending to
any Papacy. See I. 34, II. 24, III. 35, 53, 58, 61, IV. 40, 68,
V. 29, 94, VI. 7, 51, IX. 90.

30

Tout à l'entour de la grand Cité,
Seront soldats logez par champs
*   & villes:*
Donner assaut Paris, Rome in-
*   cité,*
Sur le pont lors sera faicte grande
*   pille.*

All around the great City soldiers will be billeted in fields
and towns. Paris will make the
assault, Rome incited: there
will be great pillage made
against the Pont(iff).

SACK OF ROME, 1797/1808

This verse describes Rome being sacked by the French
which occurred twice, in 1797 and 1808. The great pillage
refers to the fact that the Pope was made to cede part of the
Papal States in 1797, and in 1809 they were incorporated into
the republic of France.

31

Par terre Attique chef de la sap-
  ience,
Qui de present est la rose du
  monde:
Pont ruiné & sa grand preem-
  inence,
Sera subdite & naufrage des
  undes.

From the land of Attica, source
of all wisdom which at the
present is the rose of the
world: the Pont(iff) ruined,
its great pre-eminence will be
subjected and wrecked be-
neath the waves.

PRESIDENT MAKARIOS AND ENOSIS

If the word Pont in line 4 refers to the Pope of the Cypriot
Church, President Makarios makes sense in this verse. Attica
means South Eastern Greece, North of the Peloponnesus. It
is Makarios' assassination that ruins the Papacy, i.e. accelerates
the problems between Cypriots and Turks.

32

Oú tout bon est tout bien Soleil
  & Lune,
Est abondant sa ruine s'approche:
Du ciel s'advance vaner ta for-
  tune,
En mesme estat que la septiesme
  roche.

Where all is good, all well
abundant, in Sun and Moon
its ruin approaches. It comes
from heaven as you boast of
your fortune, in the same
state as the seventh rock.

FRANCO-PRUSSIAN WAR, 1870–1

James Laver suggests that this refers to the Franco-Prussian
war. The use of *ta fortune*, the second person singular, is applied only to France by Nostradamus. When Paris is at the
height of her fortune, the Exposition Universelle of 1867, etc;
then the Prussians will declare war, as they did on 19th July
1870. The seventh rock is understood as a reference to the
desolation of the seventh rock in the Apocalypse.

33

Des principaux de cité rebellee
Qui tiendront fort pour liberté
ravoir:
Detrencher masles, infelice mes-
lee,
Cris hurlemens à Nantes piteux
voir.

Some of the principal citizens of the rebellious city who will try hard to regain their liberty; the men are cut up, unhappy confusion; Cries, groans at Nantes pitiful to see.

ATROCITIES AT NANTES, 1793

During the excesses of the Revolution, Nantes suffered a series of appalling atrocities known as the Noyades. In 1793 its principal citizens had allied themselves with neighbouring districts and declared a Central Assembly of Resistance to Oppression. The National Convention quickly broke this counter-Revolution. Over 1,000 citizens were guillotined (cut up); others were tied, two together, face to face, naked, and placed in boats which were rowed to the middle of the river Loire and scuttled. The wretched victims were watched by their executioners as they drowned in a threshing mob of bodies.

34

Du plus profond de l'occident
Anglois.
Où est le chef de l'isle Britan-
nique:
Entrera classe dans Gironde par
Blois,
Par vin & sel, feux cachez aux
barriques.

From the deepest part of the English West where is the leader of the British Isles; a fleet will enter Gironde through Blois, through wine and salt, fires hidden in casks.

It is unlikely that this quatrain refers to the West of England although these are the traditional lands of the heir to the English throne, i.e. the Prince of Wales and the Duchy of Cornwall. Some interpret it as suggesting the Anglicization of North America, or even the Hundred Years War when the English held the West Coast of France for some decades. The wine and salt are suggested as metaphors for taxation, like the *gabelle* or salt tax. The fires in casks may be weapons. This quatrain is possibly still to be fulfilled.

35

Par cité franche de la grand mer Seline,	For the free city of the great crescent sea, which still carries the stone in its stomach, an English fleet will come in under the mist to seize a branch, war opened by the great one.
Qui porte encores à l'estomac la pierre:	
Angloise classe viendra soubs la bruine	
Un rameau prendre, du grand ouverte guerre.	

This quatrain may connect with the preceding one and refer to a series of protracted encounters with English invaders. The crescent sea may have the usual meaning of Genoa, but is a rare theatre of operations for a British fleet.

36

De soeur le frere par simulte faintise,	The sister's brother through feigned deceit will come to mix dew into the mineral. On the cake given to the slow old woman who dies tasting it, she will be simple and rustic.
Viendra mesler rosee en mineral:	
Sur la placente¹ donne à vielle tardifve,	
Meurt, le goustant sera simple & rural.	

The only information I can offer here is that the *rosee*, dew, in the second line may stand for a Latin poison, *rosarius*, which was extracted from the laurel rose.

37

Trois cents feront d'un vouloir & accord,	Three hundred will be of one agreement and accord to come to the execution of their end; twenty months later, after all remembrance, their king is betrayed pretending a feigned hatred.
Que pour venir au bout de leur attaincte:	
Vingt mois apres tous & records,	
Leur Roi trahi simulant haine saincte.	

¹*placente*—Latin, *placenta* = a cake.

38

Ce grand monarque qu'au mort succedera,	He who succeeds upon the death of a great king will lead an illicit and debauched life. Through carelessness he will give way to all so that in the end Salic law will fail.
Donnera vie illicite & lubrique,	
Par nonchalance à tous concedera,	
Qu'à la parfin faudra la loi Salique	

LOUIS XV

Louis XV succeeded his great grandfather Louis XIV (great in both senses) and led a life of great debauchery and irresponsibility. An example of this was his famous *seraglio* at the Parc des Cerfs, and, of course, the influence of Madame de Pompadour. The *Encyclopaedia Britannica* says that it is difficult to find a European king whose life shows such a record of vulgar vice. His carelessness in state affairs was partially responsible for the troubles which were to come to a head under the Revolution. Salic law forbade the accession of women to the throne. Louis was succeeded by his son. Could the line possibly mean that France was effectively ruled by the mistresses and wives of both these men—Mme de Pompadour, Mme du Barry and finally (Louis XVI) by Marie Antoinette? Some historians would accept this view.

39

Du vrai rameau de fleur de lys issue	Issued from the true branch of the fleur de lis, placed and lodged as heir to Etruria: his ancient family line woven by many hands, will make the armorial bearings of Florence flower.
Mis & logé heretier de Hetrurie:	
Son sang antique de longue main tissu	
Fera Florence florir en l'armoirie.	

COMTE DE CHAMBORD

The Comte de Chambord was the heir to Charles X and his legitimacy was questioned by the Duke of Orléans at his birth (see IV. 93). His mother, the Duchess of Berry, took her son into exile with her to Venice, Etruria standing for Italy. Here in 1846 he married the daughter of Duke Francis IV of Florence. The fleur de lis is part of the coat of arms of the house of Florence as well as the French royal line, and their marriage caused their united family lines to flower.

40

Le sang royal sera si tresmeslé,	The Royal blood will be very
Contrainct seront Gaulois de	mixed, the French will be re-
l'Hesperie:	strained by the West. They
On attendra que terme soit coulé,	will wait until his term of of-
Et que memoire de la voix soit	fice has ended, and the mem-
perie.	ory of his voice has perished.

COMTE DE PARIS, PRETENDER TO FRENCH THRONE

The first line probably indicates that the Royal blood in France is no longer truly royal, i.e. is not a ruling power, which brings the quatrain into the 20th Century. The restraint put on France by America (*Hesperie*) may well refer to the pressures to allow England to join the Common Market. Once de Gaulle's term of office has ended through his death, his policy, the famous '*Non*', is soon forgotten.

41

Nay souz les umbres & journée	Born beneath the shadows on
nocturne	a dark day, he will be sover-
Sera en regne & bonté souver-	eign in ruling and in good-
aine:	ness. He will cause his blood
Fera renaistre son sang de	to revive the ancient urn, re-
l'antique urne,	newing the century of gold
Renouvellant siecle d'or pour	for one of brass.
l'ærain.	

42

Mars esleue en son plus haut be-
*   froi,*[1]
Fera retraire les Allobrox[2] *de*
*   France:*
La gent Lombarde fera si grand
*   effroi,*
A ceux de l'aigle comprins souz
*   la balance.*

A warlike man raised to the
heights will bring about the
return of Savoy to France.
The people from Lombardy
will cause such great fear to
those of the Eagle included
under the Balance.

THE RETURN OF SAVOY TO FRANCE, 1860

Napoleon III and Cavour of Italy agreed between them
that in return for French assistance for driving the Austrians
(the Eagle) out of Italy (Libra), Savoy should be returned to
France, which occurred on 22nd March 1860.

43

La grande ruine des sacrez ne
*   s'esloigne,*
Provence, Naples, Sicille, Seez
*   & Ponce:*
En Germanie, au Rhin & la Col-
*   ogne,*
Vexez à mort par ceux de Ma-
*   gonce.*[3]

The great ruin of the clergy
is not far off, Provence, Naples, Sicily, Sees and Pons. In
Germany at the Rhine and
Cologne, vexed to death by
those of Maine.

UNSUCCESSFUL QUATRAIN

In this far-reaching quatrain Nostradamus is probably in-
ferring that Mainz and the other places would turn Protestant,
possibly because Mainz was the centre of Gutenberg's city and
the original centre of printing with all its inherent dangers. If
so, a totally unsuccessful quatrain.

[1]*befroi*—Literally a belfry.
[2]*Allobrox*—The Allobroges were a tribe that occupied what is present
day Savoy.
[3]*Magonce* Maguntiacum = Mainz or Mayenze.

44

Par mer le rouge sera prins de pirates,	On the sea the red one will be taken by pirates and because
La paix sera par son moyen troublee:	of him peace will be troubled. He will reveal anger and greed
L'ire & l'avare commettra par fainct acte	through a false act; the army of the great Pontiff will be
Au grand Pontife sera l'armee doublee.	doubled.

UNSUCCESSFUL QUATRAIN

This prophecy was probably a contemporary one because it implies that a Cardinal (*le rouge*) will be captured by pirates— probably the corsairs of the Mediterranean. During the 16th Century Popes still had real armies. There is no record of its being fulfilled.

45

Le grand Empire sera tost desolé	The great Empire will soon
Et translaté pres d'arduenne silve:	be desolated and changed near
Les deux bastardz par l'aisné decollé,	the forest of Ardennes. The two bastards will be beheaded
Et regnera Aenodarb, nez de milve.	by the oldest, Aenodarb, will rule, the hawk-nosed one.

BATTLE OF SEDAN, 1940

The whole of the French empire was lost to the Germans in 1940 and there were great battles around the Ardennes forests, both then and in 1944/5. The two bastards may be the two 'unworthy' French generals who let the German advance through after the Battle of Sedan, André Georges Corap of the French 9th Army and the second-in-command, Henri Giraud, who was taken prisoner. The commander-in-chief, Maxime Weygand (*l'aisné*) then took over, but the battle was already lost for the Allies. The hawk-nosed man may refer to General de Gaulle. He was the only French general who, with the 4th Armoured Division, put up any real opposition to the Germans at Montcornet May 17th–19th. Dunkirk followed upon this crushing defeat.

46

Par chapeaux rouges querelles & nouveaux scismes	Quarrels and new schisms by the red hats when the Sabins will have been elected. They will produce great sophisms against him and Rome will be injured by those of Albania.
Quand on aura esleu le Sabinois:	
On produira contre lui grans sophismes,	
Et sera Rome lesee par Albanois.	

AFGHANISTAN?

Could Nostradamus be thinking of the strong Communist influence in Albania which helped lead to the capture of Afghanistan? See V.49.

47

Le grand Arabe marchera bien avant,	The great Arab will march well to the fore, he will be betrayed by the Byzantians: ancient Rhodes will come forward to meet him and greater harm through the other Hungarians.
Trahi sera par les Bisantinois:	
L'antique Rodes lui viendra au devant,	
Et plus grand mal par autre Pannonois.	

The Byzantines are the Turks, since their capital was originally Byzantium. Nostradamus seems to imply that Rhodes in Greece will be the base for an operation against the Arabs. The Turkish conquest of Hungary is referred to in the final line. Probably a retroactive prophecy.

48

Apres la grand affliction du sceptre,	After the great affliction of the sceptre two enemies will be defeated by them. A fleet from Africa will come forth to the Hungarians; dreadful deeds will occur on land and sea.
Deux ennemis par eux seront defaictz:	
Classe d'Afrique aux Pannons viendra naistre,	
Par mer & terre seront horribles faictz.	

This is almost certainly a continuation from the last quatrain. The fleet may be going to Fiume, now *Rijeka*, which used to belong to the Holy Roman Empire.

49

Nul de l'Espaigne mais de l'antique France	Not from Spain but from ancient France will he be elected for the trembling ship. He will make a promise to the enemy who will cause great plague during his reign.
Ne sera esleu pour le tremblant nacelle,	
A l'ennemi sera faicte fiance,[1]	
Qui dans son regne sera peste cruelle.	

FUTURE POPE

Since Nostradamus' day there have only been Italian Popes so this prediction may lie in the future. It indicates that there will be two main candidates for the Papacy, one Spanish and one French, when the Church is doing badly, 'trembling ship'. The French candidate may be elected and will try to compromise with his enemy, presumably Communism, with remarkably little success. See V. 46, VI. 12.

50

L'an que deux freres du lys seront en aage,	The year that the brothers of the lily come of age one of them will hold great Romania. The mountains tremble, a Latin passage is opened; a treaty to march against the fort of Armenia.
L'un d'eux tiendra la grand Romanie:	
Trembler les monts, ouvert Latin passage	
Pache macher, contre fort d'Armenie.	

The brothers of the lily are presumably sons of the French royal house. Romania is probably the Holy Roman Empire, and the mountains, the Alps crossing to Rome. Armenia is difficult to interpret. In V. 94 it connects with Hitler and the Second World War and is generally believed to refer to Russia.

[1] *fiance*—O.F. = assurance, promise.

51

La gent de Dace,[1] *d'Angleterre & Polonne*	The people of Dacia, England and Poland and Czechoslovakia will form a new alliance. In order to pass beyond the straights of Gibraltar the Spanish and the Italians will hatch a cruel plot.
Et de Boesme[2] *feront nouvelle ligue:*	
Pour passer outre d'Hercules la colonne,	
Barcins,[3] *Tyrrens*[4] *dresser cruelle brique.*	

ALLIED ALLIANCE. SECOND WORLD WAR, 1939

One of Nostradamus' most interesting predictions. In March 1939 Britain allied with the Balkan countries. Her support of Poland started the war in September 1939. It was essential to keep the Mediterranean open for shipping for allied troops and supplies. The Italians were allied to Germany and the Spanish were technically neutral, their plot presumably the aid given to Hitlerian Germany.

52

Un Roi sera qui donra l'opposite,	There will be a king who will give opposition, the exiles elected over the kingdom. The chaste, poor ones swim in blood and he will flourish for a long time under this standard.
Les exilez esleuez sur le regne:	
De sang nager la gent caste[5] *hyppolite,*[6]	
Et florira long temps soubs telle enseigne.	

53

La loi du Sol, & Venus contendens,	The law of the Sun contending with Venus, appropriating the spirit of prophecy. Neither the one nor the other will be understood; the law of the great Messiah retained through the Sun.
Appropiant l'esprit de prophetie:	
Ne l'un ne l'autre ne seront entendus,	
Par Sol tiendra la loy du grand Messie.	

[1]*Dace* = Dacia—Now part of modern Rumania.
[2]*Boesme*—Modern Czechoslovakia.
[3]*Barcins* –Latin, *Barcino* = Barcelona; therefore Spanish.
[4]*Tyrrens*—Latin, *Tyrrheni* = the ancestors of the Tuscans and therefore Italians.
[5]*castus*—Latin = chaste, pure.
[6]*hyppolite*—Greek, *hypolitos* = poor, mean, little.

CHRISTIANITY AND ISLAM

The Sun here stands for Christianity and Venus for Islam. This is yet another repetition of Nostradamus' belief that eventually Christianity would rule the world, a prophecy which seems unlikely to reach fulfillment.

54

Du pont Euxine, & la grand Tartarie,	From beyond the Black Sea and great Tartary, there will
Un roi sera qui viendra voir la Gaule	be a king who will come to see France. He will pass through
Transpercera Alane & l'Armenie,	Alania and Armenia and leave
Et dans Bisance lairra sanglante Gaule.	his bloody rod in Byzantium.

MAN FROM THE EAST. 3RD ANTICHRIST?

Nostradamus says elsewhere that the Third Anti-Christ of this century will come from Asia, and this quatrain seems to confirm this view, as he will come from beyond Tartary, probably from China. His route to France lies through Alania, Southern Russia, and Armenia round the Balkan peninsula to Constantinople. The mention of a bloody rod occurs also in connection with a man from the East and France in II. 29. It may be intended as a weapon of some sort. See VI. 80.

55

De la felice Arabie contrade,[1]	In the fortunate country of Arabia will be born one pow-
Naistra puissant de loi Mahome-tique:	erful in the laws of Mahomet.
Vexer l'Espaigne conquester la Grenade,	He will trouble Spain and conquer Grenada and most of
Et plus par mer à la gent Ligustique[2]	the Ligurian nation from the sea.

Nostradamus seems to envisage a reconquest of Spain and Grenada by the Arabs who will extend their rule into Italy. Grenada was lost to the Moors in 1492.

[1]*contrade*—Provençal, *contrada* = country.
[2]*Ligustique*—The Ligurians come from around Genoa.

56

Par le trespas du tres vieillart pontife,	Through the death of the very old Pope will be elected
Sera esleu Romain de bon aage:	a Roman of good age. It will
Qu'il sera dict que le siege debisse,	be said of him that he weak-
Et long tiendra & de picquant ouvrage.	ens the (Holy) Seat, but he will hold it long and with stinging effort.

NEW POPE. CARDINAL BASIL HUME?

It is just possible that the next Pope will be the youngest Benedictine Cardinal, Basil Hume. This was also predicted by Malachy, who said that the next Pope would be of this order, Olivacians, and to date Cardinal Hume is the only one.

57

Istra du Mont Gaulfier & Aventin,	There will go forth from Montgaulfier and the Aven-
Qui par trou avertira l'armée:	tine one, who through a hole
Entre deux rocs sera prins le butin,	will warn the army. The booty will be taken between two
De SEXT. mansol faillir le renommee.	rocks. The renown of Sextus the celibate will fail.

MONTGOLFIER BALLOON AND THE BATTLE OF FLEURUS, 1794

The hot air balloon was invented by the Montgolfier brothers in 1783 and was used on a scouting party at the Battle of Fleurus, 1794. The French victory at Fleurus was the turning point in the first coalition phase of the Revolutionary Wars paving the way for the sack of Rome and the Aventine. The word *mansol* is derived from *manens solus*—he who remains alone. Elsewhere, Nostradamus calls monks and priests *les seuls.* *Sext.* is short for Sextus, and Pius VI, who was captured by Napoleon, is the only Pope since Nostradamus' day, apart from Paul VI, to have this number. By the Treaty of Tolentino 1797, the Pope was deprived of much of his lands, the rocks on which his power was based.

58

De l'acqueduct d'Uticense,[1] *Gardoing,*	By the aqueduct of Uzès by Gard, through the forest and
Par la forest & mont inaccessible,	inaccessible mountain; in the
En mi du pont sera tasché au poing,	middle of the bridge he will be cut in the hand, the chief
Le chef nemans[2] *& qui tant sera terrible.*	of Nîmes who will be very terrible.

1627

There is a famous Roman aqueduct in France which extended from Uzès to Nîmes. In 1627 the Duke de Rohan tried to support his fellow Calvinists who were besieged at Nîmes. He moved his artillery in by means of the aqueduct. Line 3 is interpreted as some of his soldiers cutting some of the supports of the bridge at Gard to widen the path for the cannons to be brought up. When Rohan arrived at Nîmes he was put in command. An impressive quatrain. See II. 32. III. 19.

59

Au chef Anglois à Nîmes trop sejour,	The English chief stays too long at Nîmes, towards Spain
Devers l'Espaigne au secours Aenobarbe:	Aenobarbe to the rescue. Many will die through war
Plusieurs mourrant par Mars ouvert ce jour,	started on that day, when a bearded star falls in Artois.
Quand an Artois faillir estoille en barbe.[3]	

See IX. 6.

60

Par teste rase viendra bien mal eslire,	Through the shaven heads he will be seen to have been
Plus que sa charge ne porte passera:	wrongly elected. Burdened with a load he cannot carry.
Si grand fureur & raige fera dire,	He will be made to proclaim with such great fury and rage
Qu'à feu & sang tout sexe trenchera.	that all one sex will be cut to pieces by fire and blood.

[1]*Uticense*—Castrum Uceciense, Uzès.
[2]*nemans*—Nemansus = Nîmes.
[3]*estoille en barbe* = comet or meteorite.

CROMWELL

Although many commentators interpret this verse as applying either to Napoleon or to the Popes, whose heads were shaven as monks, I think it is more appropriately applied to Cromwell. Nostradamus says that Cromwell is elected to power, he did not rule by divine right. The fury and rage that cover Britain refers to the Civil War between Cavaliers and Roundheads (*testes rases*) which was a war both of politics and religion. A great number of men (*tant un sexe*) lost their lives during this time. There were comparatively few atrocities committed on women and children. See footnotes.

61

L'enfant du grand n'estant à sa naissance,	The child of the great man, not through his birth, will
Subjugera les hauts monts Apennis:	subjugate the high Apennine mountains. He will make all
Fera trembler tous ceux de la balance,	those under the Balance tremble, fire from the moun-
Et de monts feux jusques à mont Senis.	tains as far as Mount Cenis.

EUGÈNE DE BEAUCHARNAIS

The nearest person to fulfil this quatrain to date is Eugène de Beaucharnais, the son of Josephine. It states that the adopted son of a French ruler will vex the Hapsburgs (Libra) in Spain and Italy and conquer Italy. Unfortunately it was Napoleon who conquered. Eugène only acted as ruler.

62

Sur les rochers sang on les verra plouvoir,	Blood will be seen to rain on the rocks, Sun in the East,
Sol Orient, Saturne Occidental:	Saturn in the West. War near
Pres d'Orgon guerre, à Rome grand mal voir,	Orgon, a great evil seen near Rome, ships sunken and the
Nefs parfondrees & prins le Tridental.[1]	trident taken.

One of Nostradamus' detailed but unintelligible quatrains. The Sun is probably Christianity and Saturn the Antichrist. Tridental refers to general sea power. See II. 32. III. 19.

[1]*Tridental* = One who holds the trident: i.e. power of the seas.

63

De vaine emprise l'honneur indue plaincte,
Galiotz errans par latins froit, faim, vagues
Non loing du Timbre de sang la terre taincte.
Et sur humains seront diverses plagues.

From the useless enterprise honour and undue complaint, boats wandering among the Latins, cold, hunger, waves; Not far from the Tiber the land stained with blood and there will be several plagues upon mankind.

64

Les assemblés par repos du grand nombre,
Par terre & mer conseil contremandé:
Pres de l'Autonne Gennes, Nice de l'ombre
Par champs & villes le chef contrebandé.

Those assembled through the calm of the great number, countermanded by land and sea; near Autonne, Genoa, the shadow of Nice, revolution against the leader through fields and towns.

UNSOLVED ANAGRAM

Autonne is one of Nostradamus' unsolved anagrams, written Antonne in some editions. The nearest equivalents phonetically are Nentone or Antibes (Antipolis) but do not clarify the meaning.

65

Subit venu l'effrayeur sera grande,
Des principaux de l'affaire cachés:
Et dame en braise plus ne sera en veue
Ce peu à peu seront les grans fachés.

Suddenly appeared, the terror will be great, hidden by the ringleaders of the affair. The women on the charcoal will no longer be seen; thus, little by little, the great ones will be angered.

66

Soubs les antiques edifices vestaulx,	Under the ancient buildings of the vestals not far from the ruin of the aquaduct. There will be the glittering metals of Sun and Moon, the golden lamp of Trojan burning, pillaged.
Non esloignez d aqueduct ruine:	
De Sol & Lune sont les luisans metaulx,	
Ardante lampe Traian d'or burine.	

It has been suggested by Jaubert that the convent of St Sauveur-de-la-Fontaine at Nîmes was built on the site of a temple of Diana and that a lamp of gold and silver will eventually be dug up.

67

Quand chef Perouse n'osera sa tunique	When the great head of Perugia dare not risk his tunic, without any cover and strip himself quite naked. The seven aristocrats will be taken, father and son dead through a wound in the throat.
Sens au couvert tout nud s'expolier:	
Seront prins sept faict Aristocratique,	
Le pere & fils mors par poincte au colier.	

VATICAN AND FRANCE, 1585–9

The head of Perugia was the Pope, in this case Sixtus V who, in 1585, had excommunicated Henri de Navarre and was therefore reluctant to do the same to Henri III and risk losing France (stripping himself naked). When he was eventually forced to do so in 1589, he did not release his Catholic subjects from their oath of allegiance, because the Papacy had already lost the revenues of England and Northern Europe. The seven are again the children of Catherine de' Medici. Their father was already dead from a wound in the throat and his last ruling son, Henri III was to die from stab wounds, not in the throat but in the stomach in 1589. Possibly Henri's assassin Jacques Clément meant to get the king in the throat but missed.

68

Dans le Danube & du Rhin vien-
dra boire,
Le grand Chameau ne s'en re-
pentira:
Trembler du Rosne & plus fort
ceux de Loire,
Et pres des Alpes coq le ruinera.

The great Camel will come to drink of the Danube and the Rhine, and will not repent of it. Those of the Rhône tremble and even more so those of the Loire; near the Alps the cock will ruin him.

SHAH OF IRAN

By the great Camel Nostradamus probably means an Arabian leader, possibly the Shah of Iran. The connection with Germany is not clear, but he certainly gets his comeuppance from France through the Ayatollah. See I. 70, III. 47, 95.

69

Plus ne sera le grand en faux
sommeil,
L'inquietude viendra prendre re-
poz:
Dresser phalange d'or, azur, &
vermeil,
Subjuger Affrique la ronger jus-
ques oz.

The great one will no longer be in a false sleep; unease will take the place of repose. The phalanx of gold, blue and vermilion to subdue Africa and gnaw it down to the very bone.

1830. ACCESSION OF LOUIS PHILIPPE

Louis Philippe usurped his nephew's French crown in 1830, having waited for an opportune moment, line 2. He was the first legitimate Bourbon to accept the tricolour of red, white and blue. The French conquest of Algeria took place in the same year that he snatched the throne. Nostradamus says the flag is gold, red and blue. James Laver makes a charming comment, 'the old eyes of the prophet may be pardoned for being slightly colour blind'.

70

Des regions subjectes à la Bal- *ance,* *Feront troubler les monts par* *grande guerre.* *Captifz tout sexe deu & tout Bis-* *ance,* *Qu'on criera à l'aube terre à terre.*	Some of the regions subject to the Balance will trouble the mountains with a great war. The entire sex will be captured, enthralled, and all Byzantium, so that at dawn they will call from land to land.

The Balance, Libra, as always is astrologically either Austria and Savoy, and sometimes England by Nostradamus' own reckoning. It appears that this country will overthrow the Ottoman empire. Possibly Austria's troubles in the Balkans in the early 1900s are hinted at in this verse?

71

Par la fureur d'un qui attendra *l'eau,* *Par la grand raige tout l'exercite* *esmeu:* *Chargé des nobles à dix sept ba-* *teaulx,* *Au long du Rosne, tard messagier* *venu.*	By the fury of one who will wait for the water, by the great rage that moves all the army; seventeen boats loaded with nobles, the messenger comes too late along the Rhône.

This quatrain has been tentatively applied to every would-be invader of Britain. Napoleon, Hitler etc.

72

Pour le plaisir d'edict volup- *tueux,* *On meslera la poison dans l'aloy:* *Venus sera en cours si vertueux,* *Qu'obfusquera du soleil tout à* *loy.*	For the pleasure of an edict of vice, poison will be mixed with the law. At Court, Venus will be so virtuous, that all the glory of the sun will be obscured.

EDICT OF POITIERS, 1577

Nostradamus considered that the edict of Poitiers encouraged vice because it allowed the clergy to marry and legalized Calvinism. Henri III's court was very depraved; his openly flaunted homosexuality offended the country and his minions were notorious for the fantastic wealth they acquired. The King was reputed to be a sorcerer with a familiar named Tarragon. Is the reference to the sun an oblique reference to the Roi Soleil, Louis XIV of the next century?

73

Persecutee sera de Dieu l'eglise,
Et les sainctz temples seront ex-
poliez:
L'enfant la mere mettra nud en
chemise,
Seront Arabes aux Polons raliez.

The Church of God will be persecuted, and the holy temples will be pillaged; the mother will put out the child, naked in a shift. The Arabs will ally with the Poles.

74

De sang Troyen[1] naistra coeur
Germanique
Qu'il deviendra en si haute puis-
sance:
Hors chassera gent estrange Ar-
abique
Tournant l'Eglise en pristine pre-
eminence.

Of Trojan blood he will be born with a German heart and will rise to very great power. He will drive out the foreign, Arabic nation and return the Church to her early glory.

75

Montera haut sur le bien plus à
dextre,
Demourra assis sur la pierre
quarree:
Vers le midi posé à la fenestre,
Baston tortu en main, bouche ser-
ree.

He will rise high over his wealth, more to the right, he will remain seated on the square stone, towards the south placed at the window, a crooked staff in his hand, his mouth sealed.

A typically convoluted Nostradamus quatrain. A crooked staff normally refers to a bishop's crook.

[1]*sang Troyen*—Refers to the myth by which the French royal line were descended from Francus, son of Priam of Troy.

76

En lieu libere tendra son pavillon,	In a free place he will pitch his tent, he will not want to stay in the cities. Aix, Carpentras, L'Ile Vaucluse, Montfavet, Cavaillon, in all these places he will abolish his trace.
Et ne voudra en citez prendre place:	
Aix, Carpen l'isle volce, mont Cavallon,	
Par tous ses lieux abolira sa trasse.	

All these places are quite close to Salon in Provence.

77

Tous les degrez d'honneur Ecclesiastique	All degrees of ecclesiastical honour will be changed to Jupiter and Quirinus. A priest of Quirinus in martial guise then a king of France will make him a man of Vulcan.
Seront changez en dial¹ quirinal.²	
En Martial quirinal flaminique,	
Puis un Roi de France le rendre vulcanal.	

78

Les deux unis ne tiendront longuement,	The two will not remain allied for long; within the thirteen years they give in to barbarian power. There will be such a loss on both sides, that one will bless the bark (of Peter) and its leader.
Et dans treize ans au Barbare Satrappe:	
Au deux costez seront tel perdement,	
Qu'un benira le Barque & sa cappe.	

SHAH'S CONNECTION WITH USA AND USSR

The alliance between the USSR and the USA, created because of Eastern developments will not last for more than thirteen years, maybe less. Then the barbarian hordes will cause them to fight. The scale of modern warfare makes Nostradamus' comment quite mundane, but it is interesting to see that he expects a Pope to play a singular and important part towards world peace. The prophecies of Malachy give four

¹*dial*—Latin, *Dialis* = of Jupiter.
²*Quirinus*—Sabine = Mars, identified with Romulus.

more Popes until the end of the world, and the name for the third is Gloria Olivae—the olive branch, which is traditionally a sign of peace. Most Popes are old men when elected. If we allow each an average of ten years this would bring us to the 1990s. The alliance should therefore occur in the late 1970s or early 1980s. The Shah did go to the USA in 1979 although not under the pomp and circumstance he might have expected but as a sick refugee. See IV. 32, 50, 95. VI, 21.

79

La sacree pompe viendra baisser les aisles, *Par la venue du grand legislateur:* *Humble haulsera vexera les rebelles,* *Naistra sur terre aucun aemulateur.*	The sacred pomp will come to lower its wings at the coming of the great law giver. He will raise the humble and trouble the rebellious; his like will not again appear on earth.

NAPOLEON

This is a general quatrain but the generalities do apply particularly well to Napoleon. He treated the Church and the Popes with arbitrary power. He originated the Code Napoléon, France's legal system. He made aristocrats from the lowly, and stamped out rebellion brutally. Line 4 may be an exaggeration, but he was a great man.

80

Logmion¹ grande Bisance approchera, *Chasse sera la barbarique ligne:* *Des deux loix l'une l'estinique² lachera,* *Barbare & franche en perpetuelle brigue.*	Ogmios will approach great Byzantium, the barbarian league will be driven out. Of the two laws the pagan one will fail, barbarian and freeman in perpetual struggle.

¹*L'Omigon* was the Celtic Hercules.
²*l'estinique*—Latin, *ethnicus* = pagan.

81

L'oiseau royal sur la cité solaire,	The royal bird over the city
Sept mois devant fera nocturne augure:	of the sun will give a nightly warning for seven months;
Mur d'Orient cherra tonnerre esclaire,	the wall in the East will fall, thunder and lightning, in
Sept jours aux portes les ennemis à l'heure.	seven days the enemies directly to the gates.

FRANCE. BERLIN WALL?

The royal bird is probably an eagle which flying over Paris or Rome will warn of a disaster to come. The wall in the East has been identified with the fall of France, the Maginot line and the Blitzkrieg, the seven days being 5th–11th June 1940. However, it may refer to the Berlin wall, and indicate that it will come down eventually, although other disasters will follow in its wake.

82

Au conclud pache hors de la forteresse,	At the conclusion of the treaty outside the fortress he will not
Ne sortira celui en desespoir mis:	go who is overcome with despair. When the people of
Quand ceux d'Arbois, de Langres, contre Bresse,	Arbois, Langres, against Bresse, will have an enemy
Auront monts Dolle, bouscade[1] d'ennemis.	ambush at the mountains of Dôle.

83

Ceux qui auront entreprins subvertir,	Those who will have an undertaking to subvert an un-
Nompareil regne puissant & invincible:	paralleled kingdom, powerful and invincible. They will
Feront par fraude, nuictz trois advertir,	deceive, warn of three nights, when the greatest one is read-
Quant le plus grand à table lira Bible.	ing his Bible at the table.

The propaganda mentioned here could have many applications in this century.

[1]*bouscade*—embuscade = ambush.

84

Naistra du gouphre & cité im-
  mesuree,
Nay de parents obscurs & tene-
  breux:
Qui la puissance du grand roi
  reveree,
Voudra destruire par Rouen &
  Evereux.
	Born of the gulf and the im-
	measurable city, born of par-
	ents both obscure and dark.
	He who will wish to destroy
	the power of the great, re-
	vered king through Rouen
	and Evereux.

Rouen and Evereux are linked also in IV. 100 as loyal to
Napoleon III and the monarchy.

85

Par les Sueves[1] & lieux circon-
  voisins,
Seront en guerre pour cause des
  nuees:
Gamp marins locustes & cousins,
Du Leman fautes seront bien des-
  nuees.
	Through the Swiss and sur-
	rounding areas they will war
	because of the clouds. A swarm
	of marine locusts and gnats,
	the faults of Geneva will be
	laid quite bare.

LEAGUE OF NATIONS AND THE
SECOND WORLD WAR

This quatrain describes very accurately the failure of the
League of Nations and the commencement of the Second
World War. See also I. 47.

86

Par les deux testes, & trois bras
  separés,
La cité grande par eaux sera
  vexee:
Des grands d'entre eux par exile
  esgarés,
Par teste perse Bisance fort pres-
  see.
	Divided by the two heads and
	three arms, the great city will
	be troubled by water. Some
	of the great men among them,
	wandering in exile; Byzan-
	tium is hard pressed by the
	leader of Persia.

---

[1]*Sueves*—Latin, Suevi = ancestors of German Swiss.

PARIS, PERSIA AND TURKEY
17th AND 18th CENTURIES

This probably describes Paris flooded by the Seine, which occurred reasonably frequently during the early 17th Century when the Turks (Byzantium) were hard pressed by Persia. There was further fighting in the East during the first half of the 18th Century.

87

L'an que Saturne hors de servage,
Au franc[1] terroir sera d'eau in-
undé:
De sang Troyen[2] sera son mar-
iage,
Et sera ceur d'Espaignols cir-
cundé.

In the year that Saturn is freed from servitude the Frankish territory will be inundated by water. His marriage will be of Trojan blood and he will be closely encircled by the Spaniards.

The only clear factor here is that a French prince (or princess) will marry a Spaniard at the time of a great flood.

88

Sur le sablon par un hideux del-
uge,
Des autres mers trouvé monstre
marin:
Proche du lieu sera faict un ref-
uge,
Tenant Savone esclave de Turin.

Through a dreadful flood on the sand a marine monster will be found from other seas. A refuge will be made near the place, holding Savona the slave to Turin.

1815

In 1815 Savona, which was part of the State of Genoa, was given to the House of Savoy to whom Turin also belonged. The sea monster was not recorded.

[1]*franc*—Either Frank, probably *Franche Comté*, or free.
[2]*sang Troyen*—Again the reference to the French royal line and its mythical descent from Francus, son of Priam.

89

Dedans Hongrie par Boheme,
Navarre,
Et par banniere fainctes sedi-
tions:
Par fleurs de lys pays portant la
barre,
Contre Orleans sera emotions.

Into Hungary through Bo-
hemia, Navarre and by the
banner feigned sedition. The
country of the fleur de lis carrying the bar; they will cause
disturbances against Orléans.

The fleur de lis with a diagonal bar to each corner was the
arms of the Bourbon family. The junior branches such as the
Vendômes, who got the throne, and the Condés, just had a
diagonal bar in the centre. It appears that Nostradamus is
describing an expedition into Bohemia and Hungary led by
one of the French royal line, possibly a Bourbon Vendôme of
Navarre? It is all very obscure, and appears to be unfulfilled.

90

Dans les cyclades, en perinthe
& larisse,
Dedans Sparte tout le Pellopon-
nesse:
Si grand famine, peste par faux
connisse,[1]
Neuf mois tiendra & tout le cher-
ronesse.

In the Cyclades, in Perinthus
and Larissa, in Sparta and all
of the Peloponnesus; a very
great famine, plague through
false dust: it will last nine
months throughout the whole
peninsula.

CHEMICAL WARFARE IN GREECE
AND THE BALKANS?

It is possible that by the words 'false dust' Nostradamus is
trying to imply that the plague and famine described here are
artificially induced? It appears to be a widespread disaster
throughout the whole of Greece and the southern Balkans.
This quatrain may tie in with the ones that predict trouble in
the Middle East.

[1]*connisse*—Difficult, possibly Greek, *Konis* = dust, or Latin, *connissus*
= exerted.

91

Au grand marché qu'on dict des mensongiers,	At the great market, called that of the liars, of all Torrent
Du tout Torrent[1] & champ Athenien:	and the field of Athens: they will be surprised by the light
Seront surprins par les chevaux legiers,	armed horses, by the Albanians, when Mars is in Leo, and
Par Albanois Mars, Leo, Sat. un versien.[2]	Saturn in Aquarius.

Again a reference to an attack from the Albanians with vague chronological dating.

92

Apres le siege tenu dix sept ans,	After the See has been held
Cinq changeront en tel revolu terme:	seventeen years, five will change within the same pe-
Puis sera l'un esleu de mesme temps,	riod of time. Then one will be elected at the same time who
Qui des Romains ne sera trop conforme.	will not be too agreeable to the Romans.

THE VATICAN AND ITS FUTURE

Nostradamus says that after a Pope rules for seventeen years there will be five Popes within the next seventeen years. If he is slightly out in his calculations this could apply to Pius XII who reigned for nineteen years. It is interesting to note that the Irish prophet, Malachy, with whom Nostradamus seems to agree to a remarkable degree, gives only another five Popes before the Final Coming. John XXIII ruled for five years. Pope John Paul I reigned for less than a month, Pope John Paul II is not a young man so a third Pope within this period may just be possible.

[1]*Torrent*—It is unclear whether this is a proper name or not.
[2]*versien*—*Verseau* = Aquarius.

93

Soubs le terroir du rond globe lu-
  naire,
Lors que sera dominateur Mer-
  cure:
L'isle d'Escosse fera un lumi-
  naire,
Qui les Anglois mettra à decon-
  fiture.

Under the land of the round moonlike globe, when Mercury is at the height of his powers. The island of Scotland will produce a leader, who will put the English into confusion.

THE YOUNG PRETENDER

Most commentators apply this to Charles I, because he was born in Scotland in 1600 before the Stuarts came to the throne. But it seems more applicable to Bonnie Prince Charlie who did put the English into confusion for a while when he marched as far south as Derby.

94

Translatera en la grand Ger-
  manie,
Brabant & Flandres, Gand,
  Bruges & Bolongne,
La traifue fainte, le grand duc
  d'Armenie,
Assaillira Vienne & la Coloigne.

He will change into the Greater Germany, Brabant and Flanders, Ghent, Bruges and Boulogne. The truce feigned, the great Duke of Armenia will assault Vienna and Cologne.

HITLER AND RUSSIA, 1939/40

The Greater Germany is, of course, the Third Reich. Hitler assimilated all of the places mentioned in the quatrain during his march across Europe. The feigned truce probably describes the invasion of Poland under the guise of help, which Nostradamus elsewhere calls *'similé secours'*. The Duke of Armenia stands for Russia, who moved troops southwards into Germany. See I. 34. II. 24. III. 35, 53, 58, 61. IV. 40, 68. V. 29. VI. 7, 8. IX. 90.

95

Nautique rame invitera les umbres	The nautical oar will invite
Du grand Empire lors viendra	the shadows and then come
conciter:	to provoke the great Empire.
La mer Aegee des lignes les en-	In the Aegean sea the re-
combres,	mains of (bits of) wood, ob-
Empeschant l'onde Tirrene def-	struct the Tyrrhenian sea and
flotez.	impede it.

This seems to describe a few ships 'nautical oars', which grow in power into a mighty fleet and trouble the Empire, whether French or Roman is not clear. The end result is a devastating sea battle and great destruction in Italy.

96

Sur le milieu du grand monde la	The rose upon the middle of
rose,	the world, because of new
Pour nouveaux faicts sang public	deeds, public blood is shed;
espandu:	to speak the truth they will
A dire vrai on aura bouche close,	have closed mouths, then, at
Lors au besoing viendra tard	time of need the awaited one
l'attendu.	will come late.

97

Le nay difforme par horreur suf-	One born deformed, suffo-
foqué,	cated through horror in the
Dans la cité du grand Roi hab-	city inhabited by the great
itable:	king. The severe edict of the
L'edict severe des captifs revoqué,	captives is revoked, hail and
Gresle & tonnere, Condon ines-	thunder, Condon too great.
timable.	

THE MAN IN THE IRON MASK

It has been suggested that the first two lines refer to the man in the Iron Mask, reputed son of the Queen and Cardinal Mazarin. Line 3 is taken as a reference to the Edict of Nantes, 1685.

98

A quarante huict degré climate- rique, *A fin de Cancer si grande seich- eresse:* *Poisson en mer, fleuve, lac cuit hectique,* *Bearn, Bigorre par feu ciel en destresse.*	At the forty-eighth degree of the climacteric, the end of Cancer there is a very great drought. Fish in the sea, river and the lake boiled hectic, Bearn and Bigorre in distress from fire in the sky.

The 48° of the climacteric may mean 48° latitude, which runs
through France near Rennes, Orléans and Langres. The
drought is predicted as occurring after 22nd July when the
sun leaves the sign of Cancer; there is another reference to
fish cooking in the heat in II. 3. Fire in the sky is probably
some form of freak electrical storm or an attack by bombs or
rockets.

99

Milan, Ferrare, Turin & Aquil- leye, *Capne Brundis vexés par gent Celtique:* *Par le Lion & phalange aquilee* *Quant Rome aura le chef vieux Britannique.*	Milan, Ferrare, Turin & Aquileia, Capua and Brindisi vexed by the Celtic nation: by the lion and his eagle-like phalanx, when Rome will have the old British chief.

NAPOLEON AND THE LAST OF THE STUARTS, 1807
The cities mentioned cover all regions of Italy showing how
complete was Napoleon's conquest. It is specifically dated to
the time of Napoleon because it was in 1807 that Cardinal
York, the last of the Stuarts, died in Rome.

100

Le boutefeu par son feu attrapé, *De feu du ciel à Carcas & Com- inge:* *Foix, Aux, Mazere, haut veillart eschappé,* *Par ceux de Hasse, des Saxons & Turinge.*	The incendiary trapped in his own fire; fire from the sky at Carcassonne and Com- minges: Foix Auch & Ma- zeres, the important old man escaped, through those of Hesse and Thuringia and some Saxons.

Yet another reference to fire in the sky, perhaps a battle, this time in South-western France. Not many Germans got as far South as this even during the Second World War, so this verse may still be unfulfilled.

CENTURY VI

1

Autour des monts Pyrenees grans amas,
De gent estrange secourir roi nouveau:
Pres de Garonne du grant temple du. Mas,
Un Romain chef le craindra dedans l'eau.

Around the Pyrenean mountains a great throng of foreign people will help the new king. Near the great temple of Mas by the Garonne, a Roman leader will fear him on the water.

Le Mas d'Agenais has many famous Roman antiquities which Nostradamus would have seen when he lived at Agen. The Roman chief is unclear.

2

En l'an cinq cens octante plus & moins,
On attendra le siecle bien estrange:
En l'an sept cens, & trois cieux en tesmoings.
Que plusieurs regnes un à cinq feront change.

In the year five hundred and eighty more or less one will await a very strange century. In the year seven hundred and three, the skies as witness that several kingdoms, one to five, will make a change.

1580 AND 1703

A daring quatrain with two dates, both of which seem accurate. In 1580, Nostradamus nearly always leaves out the thousand for reasons of scansion, France was torn by the Civil War called the Seventh War and had little to look forward to. But by 1703 Louis XIV was defying Europe and fighting the war of the Spanish Succession. The five kingdoms were probably the Two Sicilies, Milan, the Netherlands, the Americas and Spain which were inherited by the French grandson of Louis XIV, Philip V.

3

Fleuve qu'esprouve le nouveau
nay Celtique,
Sera en grande de l'empire discord:
Le jeune prince par gent ecclesiastique,
Ostera le sceptre coronel de concorde.

The river that the newborn
French heir attempts; there
will be great discord among
the empire. The young prince,
because of the ecclesiastics
will remove peace from crown
and sceptre.

There is a legend that in former times new-born heirs to
the French throne were put on a target and made to swim up
to the Rhine to see if they were lawfully begotten or not.
(Garancières.)

4

Le Celtiq fleuve changera de ri-
vaige,
Plus ne tiendra la cité
d'Agripine:[1]
Tout transmué ormis le vieil lan-
gaige,
Saturne, Leo, Mars, Cancer en
rapine.

The French river will change
course and no longer sur-
round the city of Agrippina;
all changed except the old
language, Saturn in Leo, Mars
plundering in Cancer.

CHANGES OF FRENCH BORDER

After the Franco-Prussian war and the surrender of Alsace
and Lorraine to the Germans the Rhine—the French river—
was no longer the border between France and Germany. The
old language that remained was German; everything else will
be changed by war.

5

Si grand famine par unde pestifere.
Par pluie longue le long du polle
arctique,
Samarobrin cent lieux de
l'hemisphere,
Vivront sans loi exempt de polli-
tique.

A very great famine (caused)
by a pestilent wave will extend
its long rain the length of the
Arctic pole. Samarobrin one
hundred leagues from the
hemisphere; they will live
without law, exempt from
politics.

[1]Agripine—Colonia Agrippina = Cologne.

MANNED SPACE STATION? FALLOUT OR
BACTERIAL WARFARE

This quatrain has caused more comment than most in the Prophecies. It seems to indicate that a great pestilence, caused perhaps by fallout or bacterial warfare, will cover the Northern pole of the earth, and that it appears to come from the unidentified Samarobrin which is circling above at a height of approximately two hundred and seventy miles. Could Nostradamus possibly have foreseen a manned space station? The word Samarobrin may be the nearest he can get to its name. This quatrain may well fit the decade of the 1980s. Already there have been space stations manned for long periods sent up by both Russia and the USA.

6

Apparoistra vers la Septentrion,	He will appear towards the
Non loin de Cancer l'estoille chevelue:	North, not far from the bearded star in Cancer; Susa,
Suze, Sienne, Boece, Eretrion,	Siena, Boetia, Eretria, the
Mourra de Rome grand, la nuict disperue.	great man of Rome will die, the night dispersed.

POPE LEO XIII

The great man of Rome was Puis IX who died in February 1878. He was succeeded by Pope Leo XIII whose family arms have a comet, a bearded star, and who is also called Lumen in Caelo, Light in the Sky, by the prophet Malachy.

7

Norneigre & Dace, & l'isle Britannique,	Norway and Dacia and the British Isles, will be troubled
Par les unis freres seront vexeés:	by the united brothers. The
Le chef Romain issue de sang Gallique,	Roman leader, came from French blood; the forces thrust
Et les copies au forestz repoulsées.	back into the forests.

HITLER AND MUSSOLINI

This quatrain is similar to V. 51. Hitler and Mussolini are the united brothers or allies who trouble Norway, Dacia (Rumania) and Great Britain during the Second World War. The forces in the forests are the famous Resistance Movements, which so troubled the Nazis. This cannot refer to the Kennedy brothers because of their lack of connection with Norway, Rumania and Great Britain. For Mussolini, see III. 32, 68, IV. 68. For Hitler, I. 34, II. 24, III. 53, 58, 61, IV. 40, 68, V. 29, 94, VI. 51, IX. 90.

8

Ceux qui estoient en regne pour scavoir,
Au Royal change deviendront apouvris:
Uns exilez sans appui, or, n'avoir,
Lettrez & lettres ne seront à grand pris.

Those who were in the kingdom for knowledge will become impoverished by a royal change. Some exiled without support, having no gold, neither learning nor the learned will be held of much value.

A general comment on Nostradamus' belief that learning would decline during a period after his death.

9

Au sacrez temples seront faicts escandales,
Comptez seront par honneurs & louanges.
D'un que on grave d'argent, d'or les medalles,
La fin sera en torments bien estranges.

In the sacred temples scandals will be committed, they will be thought of as honours and praiseworthy. By one whom they engrave on silver, gold and medals; the end will be in very strange torments.

10

Un peu de temps les temples des couleurs
De blanc & noir des deux entremeslée:
Rouges & jaunes leur embleront les leurs
Sang, terre, peste, faim, feu, d'eau affollée.

In a short time the colours of temples; with black and white, the two will be intermingled. The red and yellow ones will carry off their (possessions), blood, earth, plague, hunger, fire, maddened by thirst.

11

Des sept rameaux à trois seront reduicts,	The seven branches will be reduced to three, the elder ones will be surprised by death.
Les plus asinez seront surprins par mort,	
Fraticider les deux seront seduicts,	Two will be attracted towards fratricidal (strife): the conspirators will die while asleep.
Les conjurez en dormans seront morts.	

FRANCE 1575–88

A good quatrain. When Catherine de' Medici's seven children have been reduced to three, which occurred in 1575 when only Henri III, François d'Alençon and Marguerite of Navarre were alive, then Henri and his brother were involved in a series of complicated plots. François allied himself with the Leaguers, led by the Duc de Guise, and hoped to succeed to the throne. Both the de Guise brothers were murdered at Blois in the early morning on Henri's orders. See II. 18, III. 51, VI, 12.

12

Dresser copies pour monter à l'Empire,	To raise forces to ascend to Empire from the Vatican the Royal blood will hold fast. Flemish, English, Spain with Aspire: he will fight against France and Italy.
Du Vatican le sang Royal tiendra:	
Flamans, Anglois, Espaigne avec Aspire,[1]	
Contre l'Italie & France contendra.	

EUROPE?

This is interesting because Europe is visualized in modern, not medieval, terms. Italy did not exist as such until 1870, and the Flemings were a Hapsburg dependency until modern Belgium was created. The prophecy states three main points. The first will be an attempt to gain the Imperial throne. The second, a French Pope (possibly of Royal Blood). The third, the Hapsburgs and English will ally against France and Italy, which

---

[1]*Aspire*—Uncertain, possibly Speyer or Spires?

occurred during the Napoleonic wars, as did the first point.
We have not yet had a French Pope who occurs also in V. 49,
and V. 46.

13

Un dubieux ne viendra loing du regne,	A doubtful one will not come far from the kingdom the
La plus grand part le voudra soustenir.	greater part will wish to support him. A Capitol will not
Un Capitole[1] ne voudra point qu'il regne,	want him to reign: he will not be able to bear his great bur-
Sa grande charge ne pourra maintenir.	den.

This has been generally applied to the fall of the House of
Savoy, the rulers of Italy.

14

Loing de sa terre Roy perdra la bataille,	Far from his country, a king will lose the battle; quickly
Prompt eschappé poursuivi sui- vant prins,	escaped, he is followed and taken. The ignorant one taken
Ignare prins soubs la doree maille.	under the golden chain-mail under a false garment, and
Soubs fainct habit & l'ennemy surprins.	the enemy surprised.

KING SEBASTIAN I OF PORTUGAL, 1578

Here is another quatrain to support a romantic theory, such
as V. 1. King Sebastian of Portugal decided to raise a Crusade
despite the objections of the Pope and the Spanish king. He
crossed to Morocco in 1578 and attacked the Army of the King
of Fez and was obliterated at the Battle of Kasr Al-Kabir. He
was reported killed but there were persistent rumours that he
had escaped. Nostradamus seems to believe that he did so by
changing armour with one of his followers. Although the
Moors discovered this they did not reveal the news for political
reasons. Nostradamus gives us a new slant on history!

[1] *Capitole*—Probably the Pope, as the Capitol was the Roman citadel.

15

Dessoubs la tombe sera trouvé le
 Prince,
Qu'aura le pris par dessus Nu-
 remberg:
L'Espaignol Roi en Capricorne
 mince,
Fainct & trahi par le grand
 Uvitemberg.

Under the tomb will be found
a Prince, who will have taken
him above Nuremberg. The
Spanish king, Capricorn thin,
deceived and betrayed by the
great Wittemberg.

16

Ce qui ravi sera du jeune Milve,
Par les Normans de France &
 Picardie:
Les noirs du temple du lieu de
 Negrisilve
Feront aulberge & feu de Lom-
 bardie.

That which the young hawk
will carry off, by the Normans
of France and Picardy. The
black ones of the temple at
the Black wood will make an
inn and fire at Lombardy.

The black ones are almost certainly the Benedictines, sometimes known as the Black monks, who had a monastery at
Harrenalb in the Black Forest. The rest is obscure.

17

Apres les limes[1] brusler les asi-
 niers,[2]
Contraints seront changer habits
 divers:
Les Saturnins bruslez par les
 meusniers,
Hors la plupart qui ne sera con-
 vers.

After the penances are burned
the ass drivers will be forced
to change into different cloth-
ing. Those of Saturn burnt by
the millers, except the greater
part which will not be covered.

[1]limes—O.F. = penance.
[2]asniers—Some texts have rasniers but both readings are doubtful.

18

Par les phisiques le grand Roy
    delaissé,
Par sort non art de l'Ebrieu est
    en vie,
Lui & son genre au regne hault
    poussé.
Grace donnee à gent qui Christ
    envie.

The great king deserted by the physicians lives through chance not the skill of the Jew. He and his people placed high in the realm, pardon given to the race which denies Christ.

JEWISH INFLUENCES

An interesting quatrain which unfortunately does not seem to have occurred. But it is worth remembering Nostradamus' Jewish background and beliefs. It does not sound as though he had relinquished them in this verse.

19

La vraie flamme engloutira la
    dame,
Que voudra mettre les Innocens
    à feu:
Pres de l'assaut l'exercite
    s'enflamme,
Quant dans Seville monstre en
    bouef sera veu.

The true flame will swallow up the woman who will want to put the Innocents to the fire. Near the assault, the army is inflamed, when in Seville a monstrous ox will be seen.

The ox and Seville are probably a reference to bull fighting, although the fanatic queen's identity is not clear.

20

L'union faincte sera peu de durée,
Des uns changés reformés la plus-
    part:
Dans les vaissaux sera gent en-
    durée,
Lors aura Rome un nouveau lie-
    part.

The feigned union will last a short time, some changed, the greater part reformed. People will be suffering in the vessels, then when Rome has a new Leopard.

POPE JOHN XXIII

In heraldry a leopard is a lion walking to the left with its head turned left towards the spectator. Pope John XXIII had a leopard in his coat of arms, at a time when it was predicted there would be great changes. There may also be here an oblique reference to the Lion of St Marks. See VI. 26.

21

Quant ceux du polle artiq unis ensemble,	When those of the Northern pole are united together in the East will be great fear and dread. A new man elected, supported by the great one who trembles, both Rhodes and Byzantium will be stained with Barbarian blood.
En Orient grand effrayeur & crainte:	
Esleu nouveau, soustenu le grand tremble,	
Rhodes, Bisance de sang Barbare taincte.	

ALLIANCE OF USA AND USSR

This quatrain must be linked with VI. 5 which describes the people of the northern pole as devastated by a possibly man-induced plague. Nostradamus does seem to indicate that the USA and USSR will finally unite to form a new geopolitical group and that this will cause the East, China, to worry at the shift in the balance of power. This is followed by war, particularly in the Middle East. See IV. 32, 95, V. 78, VI. 80.

22

Dedans la terre du grand temple celique,	In the land of the great heavenly temple, a nephew at London is murdered through a false peace. The ship will then be schismatic, false liberty will be shouted abroad.
Nepveu à Londres par paix faincte meutri:	
La barque alors deviendra scismatique,	
Liberté faincte sera au corn & cri.	

The above quatrain appears to describe England as the land of the great heavenly temple. The nephew of a ruler is asked to come to London on a peace treaty, and then murdered, so this rules out the two Pretenders. At the same time there will

be trouble and schism in the Vatican. Some commentators
have seen the death of Darnley, Mary Queen of Scots' second
husband, in this verse. It is one of the most frustrating in all
the Prophecies.

23

D'esprit de regne munismes des-
criées,
Et seront peuples esmuez contre
leur Roi:
Paix, faict nouveau, sainctes loix
empirées,
Rapis onc fut en si tres dur arroi.

Defences undermined by the
spirit of the kingdom people
will be stirred up against their
king. A new peace is made,
holy laws become worse, never
was Paris in such great trouble.

FRENCH REVOLUTION

Rapis is Nostradamus' standard anagram for Paris. This
verse is full of generalities which best apply to the French
Revolution, new peace and new laws, with religious observa-
tions being controlled by the state, and Paris in a state of
anarchy.

24

Mars & le sceptre se trouvera
conjoinct,
Dessoubz Cancer calamiteuse
guerre:
Un peu apres sera nouveau Roi
oingt,
Qui par long temps pacifera la
terre.

Mars and the sceptre will be
in conjunction, a calamitous
war under Cancer. A short
time afterwards a new king
will be anointed who will bring
peace to the earth for a long
time.

WAR DURING 1980's? JUNE/JULY.

The sceptre here stands for Jupiter. This may be another
prediction concerning the war Nostradamus foresees during
the 1980s which will be followed by an era of peace.

25

Par Mars contraire sera la mon-
  archie,
Du grand pecheur en trouble ruineux:
Jeune noir[1] rouge prendra la
  hierarchie,
Les prodigeurs iront jour brui-
  neux.

With Mars adverse the monarchy of the great fisherman
will be in ruinous trouble.
The young red king will take
over the government. The
traitors will act on a misty day.

VICTOR EMMANUEL AND ITALIAN REVOLUTION

The Vactican will be in trouble when its troops are defeated.
This happened in 1796–1815 against Napoleon and again in
1860–70. The young king with politically socialist leanings
probably stands for Victor Emmanuel and the Italian Revolution.

26

Quatre ans le siege quelque bien
  peu tiendra,
Un surviendra libidineux de vie:
Ravenne & Pise, Veronne sous-
  tiendront,
Pour eslever la croix de Pape envie.

For four years the seat will be
held for some little good, one
will acceed to it who is libidi-
nous in life: Ravenna and
Pisa, Verona will support him,
desirous of elevating the Papal Cross.

JOHN XXIII

A good Pope will die after four years to be succeeded by
a worldly one. This might possibly refer to John XXIII who
was Pope for just under four and a half years. He was probably
a more popular Pope than any for several centuries. Paul VI
appeared more sophisticated and withdrawn. See VI. 20.

[1]noir = Anagram for king as elsewhere.

27

Dedans les isles de cinq fleuves
  à un,
Par le croissant du grand Chyren
  Selin:
Par les bruines de l'aer fureur de
  l'un,
Six eschapés, cachés fardeaux de
  lin.

Within the islands of five rivers to one, by the crescent of
the great Chyren Selin.
Through the mists in the air
the fury of one; six escaped,
hidden in bundles of flax.

Although connected with the other Chyren Selin quatrains
this remains undeciphered.

28

Le grand Celtique entrera dedans
  Rome,
Menant amas d'exilés & bannis:
Le grand pasteur mettra à mort
  tout homme,
Qui pour le coq estoient aux Alpes
  unis.

The great Celt will enter
Rome, leading a crowd of ex-
iled and banished. The great
Pastor will put to death every
man who was united over the
Alps for the Cock.

PIUS VII

The Great Celt may refer to Napoleon's conquering of
Rome and the subsequent return of the Pope Pius VII with
his clergy who had been imprisoned in France. But the third
line is totally incorrect as Pius VII was extraordinarily kind to
his ex-captors and their adherents until his death in 1823.

29

La veuve saincte estendant les
  nouvelles,
De ses rameaux mis en perplex
  & trouble:
Qui sera duict appaiser les quer-
  elles,
Par son pourchas des razes fera
  comble.

The holy widow hearing the
news of her offspring in trouble and distress: He who will
be led to calm the quarrels by
his pursuit will make the
shaven heads pile up.

CATHERINE DE' MEDICI AND HER SONS
Catherine de' Medici will learn of the problems and troubles of her children, in particular the massacre of St Bartholomew and the murder of the Duke de Guise and of his brother by her son, Henri III. These actions all increased civil unrest and led to the eventual civil war between the Leaguers and the Huguenots.

30

Par l'apparence de faincte saincteté,
Sera trahi aux ennemis le siege:
Nuict qu'on cuidoit dormir en seureté,
Pres de Braban marcheront ceux de Liege.

By the appearance of fake holiness, the seat will be betrayed to the enemies, in the night when they thought to sleep safely; the people of Liège will march near Brabant.

Liège was a province east of Brabant in the Netherlands. Normally the word seat in Nostradamus indicates the Vatican but here it is difficult to be sure.

31

Roi trouvera ce qu'il desiroit tant,
Quand le Prelat sera reprins à tort.
Responce au duc le rendra mal content,
Qui dans Milan mettra plusieurs à mort.

The King will find that which he desires so greatly; when the Prelate will be wrongfully taken. The reply to the Duce will make him angry; in Milan he will put several to death.

MUSSOLINI
The king of Italy, gets what he desires when he angers the Duce, Mussolini. The executions at Milan probably refer to the deaths of Ciano and others. The Pope being wrongfully taken is understood as the Vatican, a neutral city, being completely surrounded by a hostile Fascist Italy. See III. 22, 68, IV. 68.

32

Par trahison de verges à mort
   battu,
Prins surmonté sera par son de-
   sordre:
Conseil frivole au grand captif
   sentu,
Nez par fureur quant Berich
   viendra mordre.

Beaten to death by rods for treason; captured he will be overcome because of his disorder. Frivolous advice is handed to the great captive, when Berich comes to bite his nose in a rage.

The name of Berich, possibly an anagram, remains unsolved to this day.

33

Sa main derniere par Alus san-
   guinaire
Ne se pourra par la mer guar-
   entir:
Entre deux fleuves craindre main
   militaire,
Le noir[1] l'ireux le fera repentir.

His hand finally through the bloody Alus, he will be unable to protect himself by sea. Between two rivers he will fear the military hand, the black and angry one will make him repent of it.

NAME OF THIRD ANTICHRIST?

Alus is another unsolved mystery. I wonder whether it connects with the fearsome Mabus of II. 62? There is the repetition of the word 'main' in connection with both. It may be an approximation of name of the third Antichrist tying up with the cryptic quatrain (II. 28) where Nostradamus seems to be trying to spell the letters of his name. See II. 5, 62, 89, IV. 50, VII. 77.

34

Du feu volant la machination,
Viendra troubler au grand chef
   assiegez:
Dedans sera telle sedition,
Qu'en desespoir seront les profli-
   gez.

The machine of flying fire will come to trouble the great, besieged chief. Within there will be such sedition that those abandoned will be in despair.

[1]noir—Possible anagram for king—roi.

BOMBING OR ROCKETS

A general quatrain describing the situation of any place besieged by modern weapons. However, the first line is very striking. See IV. 99.

35

Pres de Rion[1] *& proche à la blanche laine,*	Near the Bear and close to the white wool, Aries, Taurus, Cancer, Leo, Virgo, Mars, Jupiter the Sun will burn the great plain, woods and cities; letters hidden in the candle.
Aries, Taurus, Cancer, Leo, la Vierge,	
Mars, Jupiter, le Sol ardra grand plaine,	
Bois & citez, lettres cachez au cierge.	

The white wool is probably the Milky Way, but Nostradamus has produced too many constellations for one to be sure what he intended apart from a drought on a great plain.

36

Ne bien ne mal par bataille terrestre,	Neither good nor evil from the earthly battle will come to the borders of Perugia. Pisa to rebel, Florence seen to be in bad (times): a king on a mule, wounded by night, to the black covering.
Ne parviendra aux confins de Perousse:	
Rebeller Pise, Florence voir mal estre,	
Roi nuict blessé sur mulet à noire house.	

37

L'oeuvre ancienne se parachevera,	The ancient work will be accomplished and from the roof evil ruin will fall on to the great man. Being dead, they will accuse an innocent of the deed, the guilty one hidden in the misty woods.
Du toict cherra sur le grand mal ruine:	
Innocent faict mort on accusera:	
Nocent caiché taillis à la bruine.	

[1]*Rion*—Misprint for *Trion*, from Latin, Triones = the Bear Constellation.

Although this is a detailed prophecy and seems likely to have occurred, I do not know of its ever having been fulfilled.

38

Au profligez de paix les ennemis,	The enemies of peace, the
Apres avoir l'Italie superee:	dissolute ones, having over-
Noir¹ sanguinaire, rouge sera commis,	come Italy the bloody black one, red will be seen, fire,
Feu, sang verser, eaue de sang couloree.	bloodshed, water coloured with blood.

The exposure of the colour red presumably means revolution although the colour did not contain this sense until the late 18th Century. Before and since then has referred to the Spanish or to Cardinals of the Church. Some of Nostradamus' concepts are surprisingly modern.

39

L'enfant du regne par paternelle prinse,	The child of the kingdom, through his father's capture,
Expolié sera pour delivrer:	will be deprived to deliver
Apres du lac Traismen l'azur prinse,	him; near Lake Trasimene that azure captive, in order
La troupe hostaige pour trop fort s'enivrer.	that the hostage troop may become very drunk.

40

Grand du Magonce² pour grand soif estaindre,	To quench the great thirst the great one of Mainz will be
Sera privé de sa grand dignité:	deprived of his great dignity.
Ceux de Cologne si fort le viendront plaindre,	Those from Cologne will come to complain so strongly that
Que le grand groppe³ au Rin sera getté.	the great rump will be thrown into the Rhine.

¹*Noir*—either black or king, the usual anagram.
²*Magonce*—Latin, *Maguntiacum* = Mainz or Mayence.
³*groppe*—Low Latin, *groppa* = haunches, rump.

HOLY ROMAN EMPIRE, 1806

The Archbishop of Mainz was one of the Electors of the Empire. Mainz was captured by the French during the Revolution and ceded by the Treaty of Campoformio to the French. However, the Elector held his title until the formal end of the Holy Roman Empire in 1806. The Archbishop of Cologne was also an elector, whose office was abolished three years earlier in 1803, so he had the right to complain.

41

Le second chef du regne d'Annemarc,	The second leader of the kingdom of Annemarc,
Par Ceux de Frise & l'isle Britannique,	through those of Frisia and the British Isles, will spend
Fera despendre plus de cent mille marc,	more than one hundred thousand marks, attempting in
Vain exploicter voyage en Italique.	vain a voyage to Italy.

PRINCESS ANNE AND MARK PHILIPS

A difficult quatrain made interesting by the fact that when Nostradamus wrote, England and Frisia had the same ruler, Philip of Spain, husband to Mary of England and ruler of all the Netherlands. In IV. 89, Nostradamus foresees William of Orange, a Frisian, attaining to the English throne. A problem remains in the uninterpreted Annemarc. An unlikely interpretation but one that has been made by many people as relating to Princess Anne and Mark Philips. 'Annemarc'. See IV. 27.

42

A lomygon¹ sera laissé le regne,	To Ogmios the kingdom of
Du grand Selin qui plus fera de faict:	the great Selin will be left, who will do even more. He
Par les Italies estendra son enseigne,	will extend his banner throughout Italy and it will be
Regi sera par prudent contrefaict.	ruled by careful forgery.

---

¹*lomygon*—Misprint for Ogmios, the Celtic Hercules.

Ogmios also appears in V. 80, VIII. 44, IX. 89, but his identity is not certain.

43

Long temps sera sans estre habitée,	For a long time it will remain uninhabited around where the Seine and Marne come to gush forth. Tried by Tamise and soldiers, the guards deceived in believing it rebuffed.
Où Signe & Marne autour vient arrouser:	
De la Tamise & martiaux tentée,	
Decevez les gardes en cudant repouser.	

Paris is the city between the Seine and Marne which Nostradamus seems to envisage here as uninhabited. The Tamise can mean the river Thames in London, or a town of that name near Antwerp.

44

De nuict par Nantes L'Iris apparoistra,	By night the rainbow will appear near Nantes, the marine arts will raise up rain. In the Arabian Gulf a great fleet will flounder: in Saxony a monster will be born of a bear and a sow.
Des artz marins susciteront la pluie:	
Arabique goulfre grand classe parfondra,	
Un monstre en Saxe naistra d'ours & truie.	

20th CENTURY

This quatrain may apply to the 20th Century. In 1947 the scientists discovered how to produce artificial rain (line 2). At a time when a rainbow appears at Nantes a fleet will meet disaster either in the Red Sea, since there is no actual Gulf of Arabia, or in the Arabian sea, which lies to the south, or the Persian Gulf to the east. It seems to indicate a strong naval presence in this area—could this be a confrontation between the Ayatollah and President Reagan?

45

Le gouverneur du regne bien sca- vant, *Ne consentir voulant au faict* *Royal:* *Mellile classe par le contraire* *vent,* *Le remettra à son plus desloyal.*	The very learned governor of the kingdom does not wish to consent to the Royal deed. The fleet at Melilla, by a con- trary wind, will deliver him back to his most disloyal one.

Melilla is in Spanish Morocco; from this some commentators apply the quatrain to the Spanish Civil War.

46

Un juste sera en exile renvoyé, *Par pestilence aux confins de* *Nonseggle,* *Response au rouge le fera des-* *voyé,* *Roi retirant à la Rane & à* *l'aigle.*	A just one will be sent back into exile through pestilence to the confines of Nonseggle. His reply to the red one will mislead him, the king with- drawing to the Frog and the Eagle.

Nonseggle remains an unsolved proper name or anagram. The
frog reappears here as in quatrains V. 3, and V. 95. The first
line may refer to Louis XVIII during the Hundred Days but
the rest is completely obscure.

47

Entre deux monts les deux grans *assemblés* *Delaisseront leur simulté[1] se-* *crette:* *Brucelle & Dolle par Langres* *acablés,* *Pour à Malignes executer leur* *peste.*	The two great ones, assem- bled between two mountains will give up their secret quar- rel. Brussels and Dôle over- come by Langres in order to execute their pestilence at Malines.

[1]*simulté*—O.F. = quarrel.

Brussels and Dôle and Malines were all in the Spanish Netherlands. This quatrain may therefore predict their being conquered by France, Langres. Note that lines 2 and 4 do not rhyme correctly. Unusual in the Prophecies.

48

La saincteté trop faincte & seductive,	The holiness, too false and too attractive accompanied by
Accompaigné d'une langue diserte.	an eloquent tongue: The old city, Parma too hasty, they will
La cité vieille & Parme trop hastive,	make Florence and Siena even more deserted.
Florence & Sienne rendront plus desertes.	

49

De la partie de Mammer[1] grand Pontife,	The great Pontiff by the warlike party who will subjugate
Subjugera les confins du Danube:	the borders of the Danube. The cross pursued by hook or
Chasser les croix par fer raffe ne riffe,	by crook; captives, gold, jewels, more than one hundred
Capitfz, or, bagues plus de cent mille rubes.	thousand rubies.

THE SWASTIKA

The cross is described as *ne raffe ne riffe*, an expression which can mean by hook or by crook, but also, by extension, crooked. The crooked cross can only be the swastika. Hitler's party originated in Austria, the Danube. The last line is horribly reminiscent of the millions of pounds of personal jewellery, gold and possessions the Nazis stole from their victims, most of whom ended up in the concentration camps. The position of the Pope in the verse is not clear but Pius XII was criticized for not taking a stronger line against the Nazis and for allowing them refuge in the Vatican city after the war.

[1]*Mammer* = (*a*) Mamers, Sabine name for Mars. (*b*) Mamertini, People of Messina, Sicily.

50

Dedans le puys seront trouvés les
oz.
Sera l'incest conmis par la mar-
atre:[1]
L'estat changé on querra bruict
& loz,
Et aura Mars attendant pour son
astre.

The bones will be found inside the wells; it will be incest
committed by the step-
mother. The state changed he
will seek renown and praise
and will have Mars attendant
as his star.

51

Peuple assemblé, voir nouveau
expectacle,
Princes & Rois par plusieurs as-
sistans:
Pilliers faillir, murs, mais comme
miracle
Le Roi sauvé & trente des in-
stans.

The people gathered to see
a new sight; Princes and Kings
among many onlookers. The
pillars, walls, fall, but as if by
a miracle the King and thirty
of those present are saved.

HITLER, KRAFFT QUATRAIN 1939

This is probably the verse that caused Ernst Krafft, who
worked on Nostradamus for Goebbels' Propaganda Ministry,
to warn Hitler against an assassination attempt that was made
upon him in November 1939. The bomb was hidden in a pillar
behind the rostrum and it was by sheer chance that Hitler and
some of his Party members left for Berlin unexpectedly early.
The notoriety gained by Krafft after this was to eventually cost
him his life. See I. 34, II. 24, III. 35, 53, 61, IV. 40, 68, V. 29,
94, VI. 7, X. 90.

52

En lieu du grand qui sera con-
demné,
De prison hors son ami en sa
place:
L'espoir Troien en six mois joinct,
mort nay,
Le Sol à l'urne seront prins fleuves
en glace.

In the place of the great one
who will be condemned he is
outside prison, his friend in
his place. The Trojan hope
for six months joined, the
born, dead; the Sun in Aquarius, the rivers will be frozen.

[1]maratre—more likely stepmother than mother-in-law because of
the incest theme.

LOUIS XVII's POSSIBLE ESCAPE

Another tantalizing quatrain in which Nostradamus contradicts the little that is known of an historical mystery, the fate of Louis XVII, see V.I. Here he implies that another child dies in prison in 1795 in his place, the Trojan blood always referring to French royal blood because of the legend of Francus, son of Priam of Troy. Line 3 is difficult to interpret. Does it refer to the death of the fake king after six months, or to the death of the real king six months after his escape? The Sun in Aquarius applies from mid February to mid-March. The Dauphin was reported dead on 8th June 1795, but this prophecy must refer to the earlier months.

53

Le grand Prelat Celtique à Roi suspect,	The great French Prelate suspected by the king by night
De nuict par cours sortira hors du regne:	will flee from his realm; through a Duke fertile to his
Par duc fertile à son grand Roi, Bretaigne,	great King, Britain, Byzantium to Cyprus and Tunis un-
Bisance à Cipres & Tunes insuspect.	discovered.

This quatrain appears to indicate that a French Cardinal or Bishop will flee to England and from there to Tunis via Constantinople and Cyprus. Very confused.

54

Au poinct du jour au second chant du coq,	At daybreak at second cock-crow, those of Tunis, Fez and
Ceulx de Tunes, de Fez, & de Bugie,	of Bougie; the Arabs captured by the king of Morocco
Par les Arabes captif le Roi Maroq,	in the year sixteen hundred and seven by the Liturgy.
L'an mil six cens & sept, de Liturgie.	

FAILED QUATRAIN 1607

This quatrain seems to be one of Nostradamus' total failures. He appears to see the fall of the Ottoman Empire through a new European king, and also in Asia through new

Persian and Arab Empires in the year 1607. The only point
in Nostradamus' favour is that no commentator can agree
about what is meant by 'the Liturgy'. This may alter the date
as it now appears, but how is not clear. It could simply be an
equivalent of Anno Domini, but Nostradamus was usually
more convoluted than that.

55

*Au chalmé Duc, en arrachant
　l'esponce,
Voile Arabesque voir, subit des-
　couverte:
Tripolis Chio, & ceux de Tra-
　pesonce,
Duc prins, Marnegro & la cité
　deserte.*

The calmed duke drawing up
the contract, the Arabian sail
is seen, a sudden discovery.
Tripolis, Chios and those of
Trabzon; the Duke captured,
the Black Sea and the city deserted.

All one can say with certainty about this verse is that the action
takes place in Asia Minor, the Black Sea and the Aegean
(Chios).

56

*Le crainte armee de l'ennemi
　Narbon,
Effrayera si fort les Hesperiques;*[1]
*Parpignan vuide par l'aveugle
　darbon,*[2]
*Lors Barcelon par mer donra les
　piques.*

The dreaded army of the
Narbonne enemy will greatly
terrify the Hesperians. Perpignan empty, through the
blind one of Arbon, then Barcelona by sea will take up her
weapons.

SIEGE OF PERPIGNAN, 1597

In this quatrain it appears that the Spaniards are being
terrified by the French from Narbonne. Narbonne was only
forty miles north of Perpignan, while Barcelona, sending supplies and relief, lies about one hundred miles to the south.
Perpignan was besieged for a short while by the French in
1597.

[1]*Hesperiques*—(*a*) Spanish or Western. (*b*) American.
[2]*Arbon* (?) may be geographical. If so either in France or Switzerland.

57

Celui qu'estoit bien avant dans le regne,	He who was well to the front in the kingdom, having a red chief close to the seat of power. Harsh and cruel he will make himself most greatly feared; he will succeed to the sacred monarchy.
Ayant chef rouge proche à la hierarchie:	
Aspre & cruel, & se fera tant craindre,	
Succedera à sacré monarchie.	

A cruel cardinal will succeed to the Papacy. It is difficult to know if Nostradamus had any particular one in mind. The quatrain is very general.

58

Entre les deux monarques esloinguez,	Between the two distant monarchs when the clear Sun is lost by Selin; great enmity between two indignant ones, so that liberty is restored to the Islands and to Siena.
Lors que Sol par Selin clair perdue:	
Simulté grande entre deux indignez,	
Qu'aux Isles & Sienne la liberté rendue.	

PHILIP II AND HENRI II

This was a quatrain contemporary with Nostradamus' lifetime. The sun and the chariot of Apollo were the devices of Philip II of Spain. The moon was that of Henri II of France, partly to honour his mistress, Diana of Poitiers, *Selin* meaning the Moon, line 2. Nostradamus seems to think France will conquer the Hapsburgs. Siena was held by the French at this time and they were also trying to conquer Corsica. Does the restoration of Liberty mean the coming or the withdrawal of the French? Nostradamus is usually more patriotic than this.

59

Dame en fureur par rage d'adultere,	The lady, furious, in an adulterous rage, will come to conspire not to speak to her Prince. But the culprit will soon be known so that seventeen will be martyred.
Viendra à son Prince conjurer non de dire:	
Mais bref cogneu sera le vitupere,	
Que seront mis dix sept à martyre.	

60

Le Prince hors de son terroir Celtique
Sera trahi, deceu par l'interprete:
Rouan, Rochelle par ceux de
  l'Armorique
Au port de Blaue deceus par
  moine & prebstre.

The Prince, outside his French
territory will be betrayed, deceived by the interpreter.
Rouen, La Rochelle, by those
of Brittany at the port of
Blaye deceived by monk and
priest.

61

Le grand tappis plié ne mon-
  strera,
Fois qu'à demi la pluspart de
  l'histoire:
Chassé du regne loing aspre apparoistra
Qu'au faict bellique chascun le
  viendra croire.

Folded, the great carpet will
not show except by halves, the
greater part of its history.
Driven far out of the kingdom he will appear harsh, so
that each one will believe in
his warlike act.

62

Trop tard tous deux les fleurs seront perdues,
Contre la loi serpent ne voudra
  faire:
Des ligueurs forces par gallots[1]
  confondues,
Savone, Albinque par monech
  grand martyre.

Too late both of the flowers
will be lost, the snake will not
want to act against the law;
the forces of the leaguers con-
founded by the French, Savona, Albenga through Monaco great martyrdom.

AN ERRONEOUS QUATRAIN

Nostradamus seems to intend a league against the French
in this verse in which the French triumph. But Monaco was
bound to the Spanish by treaty and Savona and Albenga belonged to Genoa. Nostradamus probably had one of the 16th-
Century Italian leagues in mind, but in this case, wrongly.

[1]gallots—O.F., gallot = Gallic or French.

63

La dame seule au regne demuree,	The lady left alone in the
L'unic estaint premier au lict d'honneur:	kingdom, her only (spouse) first dead on the bed of honour. For seven years she will
Sept ans sera de douleur exploree,	be weeping with grief, then
Puis longue vie au regne par grand heur.	a long life for the good fortune of the kingdom.

CATHERINE DE' MEDICI

Nostradamus may have been prejudiced in this quatrain when he describes Catherine de' Medici as living for the good of her kingdom. Equally, knowing the prophet's writings she may have gone out of her way to fulfil the prediction. Catherine left off mourning for her husband on 1st August 1566, seven years after his death. She lived on until 1589 as Regent under Francis II and Charles IX, but lost most of her power under Henri III.

64

On ne tiendra pache aucune arresté,	They will not keep any peace agreed upon, all the receivers
Tous recevans iront par tromperie:	will go through deceit. In peace and truce, land and sea
De paix & trefve, terre & mer protesté'.	having protested, the fleet is seized with skill by Barcelona.
Par Barcelone classe prins d'industrie.	

65

Gris & bureau¹ demie ouverte guerre,	Grey and brown in half declared war, at night they will
De nuict seront assaillis & pillez:	be besieged and pillaged. The
Le bureau prins passera par la serre²	captured brown one will pass through the prison, his temple opened, two slipped in the
Son temple ouvert, deux au plastre grillez.	plaster.

¹*bureau*—variant of *burel*. O.F. = brown.
²*serre*—Literally lock, or saw.

It is likely that Nostradamus was describing a feud between two monastic orders. The Franciscans wore grey habits, although some were brown in subsidiary orders.

66

Au fondement de la nouvelle secte,	At the founding of a new sect the bones of the great Roman will be found. A sepulchre covered in marble will appear: the earth will quake in April, badly buried.
Seront les oz du grand Romain trouvés,	
Sepulchre en marbre apparoistra couverte,	
Terre trembler en Avril, mal enfouetz.	

It appears that an April earth tremor may reveal the sepulchre of an important Roman, probably a Pope. This is also mentioned in III. 65. The sect is presumably Protestant. See IV. 11.

67

Au grand Empire parviendra tout un aultre	Quite a different man will attain to the great Empire, distant from kindness, more so from happiness. Ruled by one not long come from his bed, the kingdom rushes to great misfortune.
Bonté distant plus de felicité:	
Regi par un issue non loing du peaultre,	
Corruer regnes grande infelicité.	

There are two interpretations of the third line, either that the new Emperor is but a child having left the bed where he was born, or, that he leads a debauched life because *peaultre* can also mean a brothel. Possibly the Emperor Napoleon ruled by Josephine.

68

Lors que soldatz fureur seditieuse,	When the soldiers in a treacherous fury at night rise up and fight against their leader. The enemy of Alba with furious hand then troubles Rome and wins over the principals.
Contre leur chef feront de niuct fer luire:	
Ennemi d'Albe soit par main furieuse,	
Lors vexer Rome & principaux seduire.	

THE DUKE OF ALVA

This prediction was probably meant for the near future, i.e. 16th Century and the Duke of Alva (Alba). Nostradamus foresees him trying to suppress a revolt in the Spanish army, which he had to do soon afterwards in the Netherlands.

69

La pitié grande sera sans loing tarder,
Ceux qui donoiont seront contrains de prendre.
Nudz affamez de froit, soif, soi bander,
Les monts passer commettant grand esclandre.

The great pity will arrive before very long: those who gave will be forced to take. Naked, starving with cold and thirst, they band together to cross the mountains causing a great scandal.

DISBANDING OF THE CLERGY, *c.* 1792

Once France had declared the disestablishment of the Clergy in 1792 many priests found themselves in wretched circumstances. Instead of keeping themselves through their duties to their parishes they were constrained to beg to stay alive. Many did band together to cross the Alps and take refuge in the Vatican. Their plight naturally caused a scandal.

70

Au chef du monde le grand Chyren sera,
Plus oultre¹ apres aimé, craint, redoubté:
Son bruit & loz les cieuz surpassera.
Et du seul titre victeur fort contenté.

The great Chyren will be chief of the world, after '*Plus oultre*' loved, feared and dreaded. His fame and praise go beyond the heavens and he will be greatly satisfied with the sole title of victor.

HENRY KISSINGER?

The implication of line 2 is that the new hero Chyren will be greater in every way than the Emperor Charles V. It is tempting to equate Chyren with Henri IV of Navarre, the

---

¹'*Plus oultre Carol Quint*' was the device of Charles V. It is in capitals in the 1605 edition which clarifies the reading.

word being the obvious anagram from the old spelling of Henri, HENRYC. But the other Chyren quatrains will not bear this interpretation. Perhaps Nostradamus foresaw several great men named Henri? See IV. 34. Some commentators relate Henryc with Henry Kissinger or Henry K as he is popularly known. See II. 79, IV. 34, VI. 27.

71

Quand on viendra le grand roi parenter
Avant qu'il ait du tout l'ame rendue,
Celui qui moins le viendra lamenter,
Par Lions, d'aigles, croix, couronne vendue.

When they will come to give the last rites to the great king, before he has quite given up his soul, he who will come to lament him the last, through lions the cross and crown of the eagles sold.

This general description could apply to the deaths of many kings. Presumably the last line indicates the armorial bearings of those involved.

72

Par fureur faincte d'esmotion divine,
Sera la femme du grand fort violee:
Juges voulans damner telle doctrine,
Victime au peuple ignorant imolee.

Through feigned fury of a divine emotion the wife of the great one will be badly violated. The judges wishing to condemn such a doctrine, the victim is sacrificed to the ignorant people.

CZARINA ALEXANDRA AND RASPUTIN, 1912–17

Many modern commentators see in this verse a reference to the manner in which Rasputin dominated the wife of the Czar. The word violated should be taken metaphorically although rumours certainly went around the Russian Court that the Priest was the Czarina's lover. The whole family became victims of their ignorant people, when they refused to understand the doctrines of the times, which led eventually to their deaths.

73

En cité grande un moine & artisan, *Pres de la porte logés & aux murailles:* *Contre Modene secret, cave disant,* *Trahis pour faire souz couleur d'espousailles.*	In a great city a monk and an artisan are lodged near the gate and the walls; speaking vainly and secretly against Modena, betrayed for acting under the guise of a marriage.

74

La deschassee au regne tournera, *Ses ennemis trouvés des conjurés:* *Plus que jamais son temps triomphera,* *Trois & septante à mort trop asseurés.*	She who was cast out will return to reign, her enemies found among conspirators. More than ever will her time be triumphant, at three and seventy to death very sure.

ELIZABETH I

Elizabeth was certainly rejected during her childhood and was the victim of conspiracies during her sister's reign. England rose to new heights during her reign. She died in her seventieth year in 1603. Most commentators want to insert a comma between *trois et septante*, indicating the first number as the year she died, 1603, and the second as her age. I leave it to the reader to decide.

75

Le grand pilot par Roi sera mandé, *Laisser la classe pour plus haut lieu attaindre:* *Sept ans apres sera contrebandé,* *Barbare armée viendra Venise craindre.*	The great pilot will be commissioned by the King to leave the fleet to attain to higher rank. Seven years later he will be in rebellion, Venice will come to fear the barbarian army.

GASPARD DE COLIGNY

De Coligny was made Henri II's Admiral of the fleet (*grand pilot*) in 1552 and resigned the post seven years later, 1559, after the King's death to join up with the Calvinist party. He was one of the principal instigators of the Huguenot/Catholic wars in France. These events occurred at the same time that Venice was suffering the attacks of the Sultan Selim II, who took Cyprus from them in 1570.

76

La cité antique d'antenoree¹ forge.	The ancient city created by
Plus ne pouvant le tyran sup-	Antenor is no longer able to
porter:	support the tyrant; a false
Le manchet² fainct au temple cou-	one-armed man in the temple
per gorge.	will cut the throat, the people
Les siens le peuple à mort viendra	will come to put his followers
boucher.	to death.

Padua belonged to Venice which, as I have mentioned earlier, was governed by an hereditary office of podestas. But there does not seem to be any record of a murder in a church followed by the further killings of followers.

77

Par la victoire du deceu fraud-	Through the fraudulent vic-
ulente,	tory of the deceived, two fleets
Deux classes une, la revolte Ger-	in one, the German revolt.
maine:	The chief murdered with his
Le chef meurtri & son filz dans	son in the tent. Florence and
la tente,	Imola pursued into Romania.
Florence, Imole pourchassés dans	
Romaine.³	

During the 16th and 17th Centuries there were many revolts against the authority of the Emperor. *Romaine* is most likely to be Romagna because Imola is located there.

¹*antenoree*—Antenor was the legendary founder of Padua.
²*manchet*—O.F. = one armed.
³*Romania* = (*a*) Romagna, (*b*) The Holy Roman Empire, or (*c*) The Papal States.

78

Crier victoire du grand Selin croissant,[1]	To shout aloud the victory of the great crescent moon the
Par les Romains sera l'Aigle clamé,	Eagle will be proclaimed by the Romans. Pavia, Milan and
Ticcin, Milan, & Gennes n'y consent,	Genoa will not agree to it: then the great Lord is claimed
Puis par eux mesmes Basil[2] grand reclamé.	by themselves.

RETROACTIVE PROPHECY?

This quatrain obviously refers to the Ottoman and Holy Roman Empires whose particular emblems were the crescent moon and the Eagle. The Sultan was known in Europe as the Grand Seignior, but not one has been captured by the Roman Empire since Nostradamus' day. The last was the Sultan Jem in the 15th Century, so this is possibly a retroactive prophecy.

79

Pres du Tesin les habitans de Loire,	Near the Ticino the inhabitants of the Loire, Garonne
Garonne & Saonne, Seine, Tain, & Gironde:	and Saône, the Seine, Tain and Gironde. Beyond the
Outre les monts dresseront promontoire,	mountains they will build a promontory; conflict en-
Conflict donné Pau granci,[3] submergé onde.	gaged, Pau seized, submerged by the wave.

BATTLE OF LODI, 10th MAY 1796

Many interpreters accept the word Pau in the last line as a shortened form of Napoleon, see VIII. 1. If so, this is a very precise description of an accident which befell Napoleon at the Battle of Lodi. While the bridge over the Adda was being stormed, Napoleon fell into the water (submerged by the wave) but was pulled out before he could drown.

[1]croissant = (a) Growing. (b) Crescent moon.
[2]Basil—Greed, Basilous = Lord, king, captain.
[3]granci—Either grancito, Tuscan for snatched, seized; or erratum for grandi.

80

De Fez le regne parviendra à ceux
    d'Europe,
Feu leur cité, & lame trenchera:
Le grand d'Asie terre & mer à
    grand troupe,
Que bleux, pers,¹ croix, à mort
    dechassera.

From Fez the kingdom will
stretch out to those of Europe. The city blazes, the
sword will slash; the great
man of Asia with a great
troop by land and sea so that
blues, perse, he will drive out
the cross to death.

IRAN MID 1980's
DEATH OF CHRISTIANITY

Nostradamus stated in VI. 54 that the King of Fez might
be captured by the Arabs, but I think this quatrain fits into a
more modern context. There is constant repetition of the
theme of War in the Middle East, connected with the man
from Asia, who is tentatively identified with Nostradamus'
Third Antichrist. This man with the blue turban, 'Perse' seems
to be expected to put an end to the Ayatollah's power, though
not necessarily to be a better ruler. See II. 29, IV. 32, V. 54.

81

Pleurs, cris & plaincts, hurle-
    ment effrayeur,
Coeur inhumain, cruel, noir &
    transi:
Leman, les isles de Gennes les
    majeurs,
Sang epancher. frofaim² à nul
    merci.

Tears, cries and wailing, howls
and terror, an inhuman cruel
heart, black and cold. Lake
Geneva, the Islands, the main
people of Genoa; blood pours,
hunger for wheat, mercy to
none.

This may continue the horrors of the last quatrain, with the
war spreading to Switzerland, Italy and the Mediterranean
islands.

¹*perse*—A colour, either blue or blue green.
²*frofaim*—A Nostradamus word possibly from *froment-faim* meaning
hunger for wheat?

82

Par les desers de lieu, libre & far- *ouche,* *Viendra errer nepveu du grand* *Pontife:* *Assommé à sept avecques lourde* *souche,* *Par ceux, qu'apres occuperont le* *cyphe.*	Through the deserts of the free wild place, the nephew of the Great Pontiff will wander. Killed by seven with a heavy club, by those who will afterwards occupy the chalice.

83

Celui qu'aura tant d'honneur & *caresses* *A son entree de la Gaule* *Belgique:* *Un temps apres fera tant de ru-* *desses,* *Et sera contre à la fleur tant bel-* *lique.*	He who will have so much honour and affection at his entry into Belgian Gaul; a while after he will act so very crudely and will be very bellicose towards the flower.

PHILIP OF SPAIN, FRANCE AND THE NETHERLANDS

When Charles V abdicated, Philip of Spain was well received in the Netherlands until his bigotry alienated the people to such a degree that they revolted in 1558. Then Francis Duke of Alençon was invited by the Netherlands to be their Protector in 1580 but stupidly he attempted to regain control of Antwerp and lost the loyalty of his subjects. The flower in the last line is presumably the fleur de lis of France, against which Philip went to war during 1589–98, against Henri of Navarre.

84

Celui qu'en Sparte Claude[1] ne *peut regner,* *Il fera tant par voie seductive:* *Que du court, long, le fera ar-* *aigner,* *Que contre Roi sera sa perspec-* *tive.*	The lame man who could not rule in Sparta, he will do much seductive ways. That by the long and the short of it he will be accused of aiming his objectives against the king.

[1]*Claude*—Latin, *claudus* = lame.

The first line merely refers to the fact that the Spartans killed any children who were born imperfect. Then one must look for famous lame men in history; perhaps Talleyrand if one may read Emperor for king, or Lord Byron working with the Greek Freedom fighters?

85

La grand cité de Tharse par Gaulois
Sera destruite, captifz tous à Turban:
Secours par mer du grand Portugalois,
Premier d'esté le jour du sacre Urban.

The great city of Tarsus by the Gauls will be destroyed, all captured at Turban. Help from the sea from the great Portuguese; the first day of summer, Urban's consecration.

Nostradamus seems to envisage a French army capturing Tarsus in Asia Minor and continuing on into Asia. Portugal was one of the greatest sea powers in Nostradamus' day, and he envisages them as allies of the French. The dating of the last line is obscure. There are two main saints called Urban, one is celebrated on 25th May, the other on 23rd January: there are twelve other minor saints with this name but the first is most likely as summer begins on 21st June.

86

Le grand Prelat un jour apres son songe,
Interpreté au rebours de son sens:
De la Gascogne lui surviendra un monge,
Qui fera eslire le grand Prelat de sens.

One day the great Prelate, after his dream interpreted the opposite to its meaning; from Gascony a monk will come to him who will cause the great Prelate of Sens to be elected.

87

L'election faite dans Frankfort,	The election made in Frank-
N'aura nul lieu Milan s'opposera:	furt will not be valid, Milan
Le sien plus proche semblera si	will oppose it. The closest fol-
grand fort	lower will seem so very strong
Que outre le Rhin és mareschz	that he will drive him out be-
chassera.	yond the Rhine into the
	marshes.

EMPEROR FERDINAND, 1558–62

The election at Frankfurt probably refers to the coronation of Ferdinand as Holy Roman Emperor which took place there in 1558. Philip, who was Ferdinand's rival had been given Milan by his Uncle Charles V before his death in 1542. Philip tries to drive Ferdinand out of Germany, line 4, and into the Netherlands. In fact he was not at all successful in this, but he did continue to intrigue against Ferdinand for the succession until 1562.

88

Un regne grand demourra desolé,	A great kingdom will remain
Aupres del Hebro se feront assem-	desolate, near the Ebro they
blees:	will be gathered in assemblies.
Monts Pyrenees le rendront con-	The Pyrenean mountains will
solé.	console him when in May
Lors que dans Mai seront terres	there will be earth tremors.
tremblees.	

89

Entre deux cymbes¹ piedz & mains	Feet and hands bound be-
estachés,	tween two boats, the face
De miel face oingt & de laict sub-	anointed with honey and
stanté:	touched with milk. Wasps and
Guespes & mouches, fitine² amour	flies, fatherly love angered,
fachés.	the cupbearer lies, the goblet
Poccilateur³ faucer, Cyphe⁴ tempté.	tried.

¹*cymbe*—O.F. = boat.
²*fitine*— Gk., *phitus* – father.
³*Poccilateur*—Latin, *poccilator* = cup-bearer.
⁴*Cyphe*—Latin, *scyphus* = cup, goblet.

The fact that the face is anointed with milk and honey indicates
that the victim was a crowned king for these are part of the
Coronation service. The wasps may be an indirect reference
to Napoleon's emblem of bees.

90

L'honnissement puant abhomin-
   able
Apres le faict sera felicité,
Grand excusé, pour n'estre fa-
   vourable,
Qu'à paix Neptune ne sera incité.

The stinking and abominable
shame, after the deed he will
be congratulated. The great
one excused for not being favourable, that Neptune cannot be tempted towards peace.

Someone gets away with a deed of such skullduggery that it
is almost incredible; and yet he is unsuspected and congratulated despite the fact that he cannot arrange for a naval peace.
Presumably he was in communication with the enemy?

91

Du conducteur de la guerre na-
   vale,
Rouge effrené, severe horrible
   grippe,
Captif eschappé de l'aisné dans
   la baste:
Quant il naistra du grand un filz
   Agrippe.

Of the leader of the naval
war, the red one unbridled,
severe, horrible quarrel; captive escaped from the older
one in the saddle, when the
great Agrippa bears a son.

The Naval commanders in Nostradamus' time were the Baron
de la Garde, and M. de la Mole, but the rest of the quatrain
is obscure.

92

Prince de beauté tant venuste,
Au chef menee, le second faict
   trahi:
La cité au glaive de poudre face
   aduste,
Par le trop grand meutre le chef
   du Roi hai.

The Prince of such handsome
beauty, intrigues against his
person, betrayed to the second rank. The city put to the
sword, consumed with a powder that burns. By this, so
great a murder, the head of
the king is hated.

LOUIS XVI's DEATH

Louis XVI was considered to be very handsome as a youth. He finds intrigues (*menees*) directed against him and will be deposed to the second rank of a constitutional king. Then he is betrayed. The line '*poudre face aduste*' has been most interestingly interpreted by James Laver from the Latin, *fax*, a torch, and *adustus*, burned, as consumed by a powder that burns. It was into quicklime that the hated head of the King was thrown from the wicker basket after his execution on the guillotine. The third line '*cité au glaive*', is an excellent description of revolutionary Paris.

93

Prelat avare d'ambition trompé.	The greedy prelate deceived
Rien ne sera que trop viendra cuider:	by ambition, he will think that nothing is too great (for him).
Ses messagiers, & lui bien attrapé,	He and his messengers, completely trapped, the man who
Tout au rebours voir, qui le bois fendroit.	cuts the woods sees all in reverse.

94

Un Roi iré sera aux sedifragues,[1]	A king will be angry with the
Quant interdicts seront harnois de guerre:	sedifragues[1] when warlike arms are prohibited; the poi-
La poison taincte au succre par les fragues[2]	son tainted with sugar in the strawberries, murdered by
Par eaux meutris, mors, disant serre serre.	waters, death, saying, close, close.

The see breakers, if one has understood Nostradamus correctly, probably refer to the Protestants who broke up the unity of the See of Rome.

[1] *sedifragus*—A Nostradamus word possibly compounded from *sedem frangere*—which literally means to break a seat.
[2] *fragues*—Latin, *fraga* = strawberries.

95

Par detracteur calumnie à puis nay.	Calumny against the younger born by the detractor, when enormous, martial deeds will occur. The least part doubtful for the elder one, and soon in the kingdom there will be partisan actions.
Quant istront faicts enormes & martiaux:	
Le moindre part dubieuse à l'aisnay	
Et tost au regne seront faicts partiaux.	

96

Grande cité à soldatz abandonné,	A great city abandoned to the soldiers, there was never a mortal tumult so close. Oh, what a dreadful calamity approaches; except for one offence it will not be forgiven.
Onques n'y eust mortel tumulte si proche,	
O quel hideuse calamité s'approche,	
Fors une offense n'y sera pardonnée.	

SACK OF ST QUENTIN, 1557

This quatrain is so general that it could be applied to the sack of any city. Commentators are particularly fond of applying it to the sack of St Quentin (1557) or Paris during the Revolution.

97

Cinq & quarante degrés ciel bruslera,	The sky will burn at forty-five degrees, fire approaches the great New City. Immediately a huge, scattered flame leaps up when they want to have proof of the Normans.
Feu approcher de la grand cité neufve,	
Instant grand flamme esparse sautera,	
Quand on voudra des Normans faire preuve.	

BOMBING OF NEW YORK

New York county lies between 40° and 45° parallel in the USA. There are other references to it as the *cité neufve*. It appears that the attack is very widespread (scattered flame). The position of France when this occurs is unclear, but France is also involved in a similar quatrain, see X. 49 in particular and I. 91, IX. 92.

98

Ruine aux Volsques[1] de peur si
   fort terribles,
Leur grand cité taincte, faict pestilent:
Piller Sol, Lune & violer leurs
   temples:
Et les deux fleuves rougir de sang
coulant.

Ruin for the Volcae, so very
terrible with fear, their great
city stained by a pestilential
deed. To plunder the Sun
and Moon and violate their
temples and to redden the
two rivers running with blood.

The sun and moon plundered are gold and silver. The capital
city of Languedoc would probably be Toulouse.

99

L'ennemi docte se tournera con-
   fus,
Grand camp malade, & de faict
   par embusches,
Monts Pyrenees & Poenus[2] lui
   seront faicts refus
Proche du fleuve decouvrant antiques o cruches.

The learned enemy will turn
around confused, the great
camp sick and defeated by
ambushes. The Pyrenean
Mountains and the Pennines
will be refused to him, near
the river discovering ancient
urns.

100

LEGIS CANTIO CONTRA
INEPTOS CRITICOS
Quos legent hosce versus maturè
   censunto,
Profanum vulgus & inscium ne
   attrectato:
Omnesq; Astrologi Blenni,[3] Bar-
   bari procul sunto,
Qui alter facit, is ritè, sacer esto.

INCANTATION OF THE
LAW AGAINST INEPT
CRITICS.
May those who read this verse
think upon it deeply, let the
profane and ignorant herd
keep away. Let all astrologers,
idiots and barbarians stay far
off, he who does otherwise,
let him be priest to the rite.

[1]*Volsques*—People of Languedoc. Southern France.
[2]*Poenus*—Latin, *Alpes Poeninae* = the Pennine Alps.
[3]*Blenni*—Greek, *Blennos* = simpleton, idiot.

This verse is odd. Line 4 sounds vaguely like a threat or curse. If the verses were originally written in Latin, as I believe they were, this gives the reader a good idea of the type of construction and vocabulary used by Nostradamus. Why does Nostradamus include Astrologers among the people he damns? Is this yet another example of his trying to bluff the authorities?

CENTURY VII

1

L'arc du thresor par Achilles deçeu,	The arc of the treasurer deceived by Achilles, the quadrangule known to the procreators. The invention will be known by the Royal deed; a corpse seen hanging in the sight of the populace.
Aux procrées[1] sceu la quadrangulaire:	
Au faict Royal le comment sera sceu,	
Cors veu pendu au veu du populaire.	

There are only two well-known Achilles in French history. The first was Achille de Harlay, President of the Parlement de Paris who contributed to the downfall of the Queen Regent's favourite, Concini, who was assassinated in 1517. The other was Achilles Bazaine, a Marshal of France whose incapacity and defeatism led to the fall of France in 1870.

2

Par Mars ouvert Arles ne donra guerre,	Arles opened up by war will not offer resistance, the soldiers will be astonished by night. Black and white concealing indigo on land under the false shadow you will see traitors sounded.
De nuict seront les soldartz estonnés:	
Noir, blanc à l'inde dissimulés en terre,	
Sous la faincte umbre traistres verez & sonnés.	

3

Apres de France la victoire navale,	After the naval victory of France, the people of Barcelona the Saillinons and those of Marseilles; the robber of gold, the anvil enclosed in the ball, the people of Ptolon will be party to the fraud.
Les Barchinons, Saillinons,[2] les Phocens,	
Lierre d'or, l'enclume serré dedans la basle,	
Ceux de Ptolon[3] au fraud seront consens.	

[1]*procrées*—There is a variant *procès* which would give a better reading of 'in the documents'.

[2]*Saillinons*—Not identified.

[3]*Ptolon* = Either the land of Ptolomy, Egypt, or Acre, earlier called Ptolemais.

Even the proper names are obscure in this quatrain. France is clear and the Phocens, who were from Marseilles. The Barchinons may be from Barcelona. The Saillinons and Ptolons are unclear. Garencières suggests that Ptolons could be from Toulon. It is possible that the name could be contorted like this by Nostradamus.

4

Le duc de Langres assiegé dedans Dolle,	The Duke of Langres besieged at Dôle accompanied by people from Autun and Lyons. Geneva, Augsburg allied to those of Mirandola, to cross the mountains against the people of Ancona.
Accompaigné d'Ostun & Lyonnois:	
Geneve, Auspour, joinct ceux de Mirandole,	
Passer les monts contre les Anconnois.	

THE DUKE DE GUISE

This complicated verse describes the Duke de Guise (*Langres*) with soldiers from Autun and Lyons being besieged in Dôle during an attack on the Spanish. At the same time armies of the Empires from Geneva, Augsburg and Northern Italy will invade the Papal States (Ancona belonged to the Pope).

5

Vin sur la table en sera respandu,	Some of the wine on the table will be spilt, the third will not have that which he claimed. Twice descended from the black one of Parma, Perouse will do to Pisa that which he believed.
Le tiers n'aura celle qu'il pretendoit:	
Deux fois du noir[1] de Parme descendu,	
Perouse à Pize fera ce qu'il cuidoit.	

Pisa belonged to Tuscany, Perugia and Parma to the Vatican, the latter being given to his bastard son Pierluigi Farnese by Pope Paul III 1545. When the Farnese family died out Parma passed to the Bourbons. I cannot decipher this verse further.

[1]*noir*—The usual second meaning of *roi*, king, is possible here.

6

Naples, Palerme, & toute la Se- *cille,* *Par main barbare sera inhabitee,* *Corsicque, Salerne & de Sar-* *deigne l'isle,* *Faim, peste, guerre fin de maux* *intemptee.*	Naples, Palermo and all of Sicily will be uninhabited through Barbarian hands. Corsica, Salerno and the island of Sardinia, hunger, plague, war the end of extended evils.

This general verse predicts that Sicily and Southern Italy as well as Corsica and Sardinia will be ravaged by invasions of the Barbary pirates. There were many raids in the 16th Century both before and after Nostradamus wrote the Prophecies, so this may be a retroactive verse.

7

Sur le combat des grans cheveux *legiers,* *On criera le grand croissant con-* *fond.* *De nuict tuer monts, habits de* *bergiers,* *Abismes rouges dans le fossé pro-* *fond.*	Upon the struggle of the great, light horses, it will be claimed that the great crescent is destroyed. To kill by night, in the mountains, dressed in shepherds' clothing, red gulfs in the deep ditch.

POSSIBLE DEFEAT OF ISLAM

The crescent moon is the emblem of the Turks and Islam. Apparently Nostradamus sees them as suffering a great defeat. The third line suggests that some soldiers dress up as shepherds when attacking. The red gulfs almost certainly stand for rivers of blood.

8

Flora fuis, fuis le plus proche *Romain,* *Au fesulan² sera conflict donné:* *Sang espandu les plus grands* *prins à main,* *Temple ne sexe ne sera pardonné.*	Florence, flee, flee the nearest Roman, at Fiesole will be conflict given: blood shed, the greatest ones taken by the hand, neither temple nor sex will be pardoned.

¹*intemptee*—Latin, *intentatus* = extended, stretched.
²*fesulan*—Latin, *Faesulae* = Fiesole.

The quatrain seems to predict that Florence will suffer a severe attack by Vatican troops. Fiesole is only a few miles away and would naturally suffer the same fate.

9

Dame à l'absence de son grand capitaine,	The lady in the absence of her great master will be begged for love by the Viceroy. Feigned promise and misfortune in love, in the hands of the great Prince of Bar.
Sera priee d'amours du Viceroi,	
Faincte promesse & malheureuse estraine,[1]	
Entre les mains due grand Prince Barrois.	

DUKE DE GUISE AND DIANE DE POITIERS

France has never had a Viceroy, the only comparable offices are those of the Constable, or the Lieutenant-General, which de Guise held when Nostradamus wrote. The title Duke de Bar was that given to the eldest son of the Duke de Lorraine. As the Duke was a child there was no holder at that period. It is unlikely that Dame refers to the Queen, Catherine de' Medici, but it may well describe Henri II's influential mistress, Diane de Poitiers, who would have been in her late fifties.

10

Par le grand Prince limitrophe du Mans,	By the great Prince bordering le Mans, brave and valliant leader of the great army; by land and sea with Bretons and Normans, to pass Gibraltar and Barcelona to pillage the island.
Preux & vaillant chef de grand excercite:	
Par mer & terre de Gallotz & Normans,	
Caspre passer Barcelone pillé isle.	

DUKE D'AUMALE, 1526–1573

Le Mans used to be the main city of Maine in North Western France, whereas Mayenne the next most important city, belonged to de Guise. In Nostradamus' lifetime it was held by de Guise's brother Claude, whose titles were Marquess of May-

[1]estraine—O.F. = success in love, luck.

enne and Duke d'Aumale. The latter did fight at Metz in 1552 and later at Calais, St. Denis, Dreux and Montcontour, but he never invaded Spain or North Africa. Nostradamus seems to have foreseen a much greater future for him than that which actually happened.

11

L'enfant Royal contemnera la mere,	The royal child will scorn his mother, eye, feet wounded,
Ueil, piedz blessés, rude, inobeissant,	rude, disobedient; strange and very bitter news to the lady;
Nouvelle à dame estrange & bien amere,	more than five hundred of her people will be killed.
Seront tués des siens plus de cinq cens.	

This quatrain seems to refer to the quarrels of a Queen Regent with her son. Since Nostradamus' lifetime there has been one notable example between Louis XIII and his mother Marie de' Medici. In the ensuing battle Garencières states that more than five hundred of the Queen's supporters were killed.

12

Le grand puisné fera fin de la guerre,	The great younger son will make an end of the war, he
Aux dieux assemble les excusés:	assembles the pardoned before the gods; Ahors and
Cahors, Moissac iront long de la serre,	Moissac will go far from the prison, a refusal at Lectoure,
Reffus Lestore, les Agenois razés.	the people of Agen shaved.

A cadet or younger son was usually used to refer to the younger brother, or descendant of a younger brother of a king or ruler. This may refer to a son of the Guise family which were cadets of the Dukedom of Lorraine, all the towns being quite close together in Gienne, South-western France.

13

De la cité marine & tributaire,
La teste raze prendra la satrapie:
Chasser sordide qui puis sera con-
    traire
Par quatorze ans tiendra la tyr-
    annie.

From the marine tributary city, the shaven head will take up the satrapy; to chase the sordid man who will then be against him. For fourteen years he will hold the tyranny.

NAPOLEON I

Bonaparte (the shaven head) will retake Toulon the marine city in 1793 from the English, led by Sir Arthur Wellesley, who have made it a tributary. He will then overthrow the Directory (the sordid one) and put an end to the Republic. He will enjoy absolute power for fourteen years (9th November 1799–13th April 1814). This interpretation was made by le Pelletier who adds that 'the sordid one' may well mean the English!

14

Faux esposer viendra topogra-
    phie,
Seront les cruches des monuments
    ouvertes:
Palluler secte saincte philosophie,
Pour blanches, noirs, & pour
    antiques veres.

He will come to expose the false topography, the urns of the tombs will be opened. Sect and holy philosophy to thrive, black for white and the new for the old.

NATIONAL ASSEMBLY 1789

On 22nd December 1789, the National Assembly changed the ancient regional districts of France into Departments. At St Denis the tombs of the French kings will be violated and their ashes scattered. Anti-christian sects flourish and take the place of religion. People will accept that black is white and will accept new ideas for the old traditions.

15

Devant cité de l'Insubre¹ contree, *Sept ans sera le siege devant mis:* *Le tres grand Roi y fera son entree,* *Cité puis libre hors de ses ennemis.*	Before the city of the Insubrian lands, for seven years the siege will be laid; a very great king enters it, the city is then free, away from its enemies.

SIEGE OF MILAN

Nostradamus here predicts a very long drawn out siege of Milan lasting seven years. The liberating king is probably a French one freeing Milan from its Spanish masters.

16

Entrée profonde par la grand Roine faicte *Rendra le lieu puissant inaccessible:* *L'armee des trois lions sera deffaite,* *Faisant dedans cas hideux & terrible.*	The deep entry made by the great Queen will make the place powerful and inaccessible; the army of the three lions will be defeated causing within a thing hideous and terrible.

QUEEN MARY AND THE CAPTURE OF CALAIS, 1558

The great Queen, Mary Tudor, held Calais 'engraved upon her heart' until it was recaptured by the Duc de Guise in 1558. England was at that time an ally of Spain through Mary's marriage and the three lions form part of the English Standard. This is a comparatively successful quatrain.

17

Le prince rare de pitié & clemence, *Viendra changer par mort grand cognoissance:* *Par grand repos le regne travaillé,* *Lors que le grand tost sera estrillé.*	The prince who has little pity or mercy will come through death to change (and become) very knowledgeable. The kingdom will be attended with great tranquillity, when the great one will soon be fleeced.

¹*Insubre*—Latin, *Insubria* = the area around Milan.

18

Les assiegés couloureront leur
    paches,
Sept jours apres feront cruelle is-
    sue
Dans repoulsés feu, sang. Sept
    mis à l'hache
Dame captive qu'avoit la paix tis-
    sue.

The besieged will colour their
pacts, but seven days later
they will make a cruel exit:
thrown back inside, fire and
blood, seven put to the axe
the lady who had woven the
peace is a captive.

An obscure quatrain which apparently describes a treacherous
enemy who, while being besieged, pretends to sue for peace,
but seven days later makes a disastrous attack. Line 4 is quite
possible for that period. The peace of Cambrai, in 1529, was
known as the Ladies' Charter because it was negotiated by the
mother of Francis I and the aunt of Charles V.

19

Le fort Nicene ne sera combatu,
Vaincu sera par rutilant metal
Son faict sera un long temps de-
    batu,
Aux citadins estrange espouvan-
    tal.

The fort at Nice will not engage in combat, it will be overcome by shining metal. This
deed will be debated for a
long time, strange and fearful
for the citizens.

Nice has been captured twice since Nostradamus wrote the
Prophecies, in 1891 and 1705, both times by the French.

20

Ambassadeurs de la Toscane lan-
    gue,
Avil & Mai Alpes & mer passer:
Celui de veau[1] exposera
    l'harangue,
Vie Gauloise ne venant effacer.

Ambassadors of the Tuscan
language will cross the Alps
and the sea in April and May.
The man of the calf will deliver an oration, not coming
to wipe out the French way of
life.

[1]de veau—Some commentators think this should be de Vaud, a Swiss
Canton.

CAVOUR IN PARIS, 1856

The good relations which existed between Napoleon III and the Pope were spoiled when Cavour arrived in Paris in 1856 to plead the cause of Italian unity. The Congress at Paris took place in the months Nostradamus mentions, April and May. The reason for calling him man of the calf is obscure but fascinating, a typical Nostradamus contortion of facts. Cavour was the envoy of Turin, and Torino means the city of the bull. It was called Augusta Taurinorum by the Romans, and Cavour is thus the offspring of the calf.

21

Par pestilente inimitié Volsicque,	By the pestilential enmity of
Dissimulee chassera le tyran:	Languedoc, the tyrant dissi-
Au pont de Sorgues se fera la	mulated will be driven out.
traffique,	The bargain will be made on
De mettre à mort lui & son ad-	the bridge at Sorgues to put
herent.	to death both him and his fol-
	lower.

Probably a bridge at Sorgues, the main town on the river of the same name. It belonged to the Vatican States until 1791. Languedoc was a large province to the west of the Rhône.

22

Les citoyens de Mesopotamie,[1]	The citizens of Mesopotamia
Yrés encontre amis de Tarra-	angry with their friends from
conne,[2]	Tarraconne; games, rites,
Jeux, ritz, banquetz, toute gent	banquests, every person
endormie	asleep, the vicar at Rhône, the
Vicaire au Rosne, prins cité, ceux	city taken and those of Au-
d'Ausone.[3]	sonia.

POPE PIUS VI, 1799

Mesopotamia is used several times by Nostradamus but it is not wholly clear which town he meant. He does not seem

[1]*Mesopotamie*—Nostradamus means by this 'land between two rivers'. It could be modern Iraq or in France, Avignon, between the Rhône and the Durance, or Paris between the Seine and Marne.

[2]*Tarraconne*—Either from Latin, *Tarroca*, Tarragona in Catalonia, or from Tarraconensis, the north-eastern part of Roman Iberia.

[3]*Ausone*—Southern Italy, most probably Naples.

to refer to modern Iraq, and therefore it probably describes a European town. The Venaissin between the Rhône and the Durance and Avignon in particular seem to fit the prediction very well. The vicar in line 4 was the Pope Pius VI whom Nostradamus had captured and imprisoned at Valence in 1799. The second part of line 4 describes how a French army led by General Chaupionnet recaptured Rome and then went on to Naples in 1799.

23

Le Royal sceptre sera contrainct de prendre,	The Royal sceptre will be forced to take that which his predecessors had pledged. Because they do not understand about the ring when they come to sack the palace.
Ce que ses predecesseurs avoient engaigé:	
Puis que l'aneau on fera mal entendre,	
Lors qu'on viendra le palais saccager.	

Hugh Allen, an unreliable commentator on Nostradamus, wrote in 1943 that the scene of this pawnbroking of Royal Jewels would take place in Buckingham Palace! This is a very obscure quatrain.

24

L'enseveli sortira du tombeau,	He who was buried will come out of the tomb, he will make the strong one out of the bridge to be bound with chains. Poisoned with the roe of a barbel, the great one from Lorraine by the Marquis du Pont.
Fera de chaines lier le fort du pont:	
Empoisonné avec oeufz de Barbeau,	
Grand de Lorraine par le Marquis du Pont.[1]	

The barbel is a freshwater fish found throughout most of Europe. The Grand one of Lorraine is probably the Duke of that name, Charles III, who was taken to be reared in the French Court. The Marquis du Pont-à-Mousson was held by

[1]*Marquis du Pont*—The younger son of the house of Lorraine had the title of Marquis de Pont-à-Mousson.

the heir to the Duchy of Bar. After Bar passed to the house of Lorraine the title was given to the younger sons of the Duke of Lorraine. The quatrain predicts that among these families the Duke is to be poisoned by the Marquis, that is, by one of the younger sons.

25

Par guerre longue tout l'exercite expuiser,	Through long war all the army exhausted, so that they
Que pour souldartz ne trouveront pecune:	do not find money for the soldiers; instead of gold or sil-
Lieu d'or d'argent, cuir on viendra cuser,[1]	ver, they will come to coin leather, Gallic brass, and the
Gaulois aerain, signe croissant de Lune.	crescent sign of the Moon.

It is suggested that this quatrain refers to soldiers being paid with money made from leather after a severe war. Line 4 is very obscure.

26

Fustes & galees autour de sept navires,	Foists and galleys around seven ships, a mortal war will
Sera livree une mortelle guerre:	be let loose. The leader from
Chef de Madric recevra coup de vivres,[2]	Madrid will receive a wound from arrows, two escaped and
Deux eschapees & cinq menees à terre.	five brought to land.

NOVEMBER 1555

In November 1555 some privateers from Dieppe attacked a Spanish fleet in the Channel. *Vivres* is then translated as *viver*, a nautical verb to attack. Apparently the privateers concentrated upon the Admiral's flagship and they succeeded in capturing it and four other ships who came to its aid and towed them to Dieppe. Probably a retrospective quatrain.

[1]*cuser*—Latin, *cusare*. O.F. cudere = to coin money.
[2]*Vivres*—Alternative *vires* = arrows, seems better in context, or *viver* = to attack.

27

Au cainct¹ de Vast² le grand cav-
  alerie,
Proche à Ferrage empeschee au
  bagaige:
Pompt à Turin feront tel volerie,
Que dans le fort raviront leur
  hostaige.
	At the wall of Vasto the great
	cavalry are impeded by the
	baggage near Ferrara. At
	Turin they will speedily com-
	mit such robbery that in the
	fort they will ravish their hos-
	tage.

There are nine villages in France with the name of Vast plus
a monastery near Arras and a harbour near Cherbourg. The
reference may equally apply to Alphonso II, Marquis de Vasto
(1502–44) who from 1537 onwards was Governor of Milan.
He retired to Asti in 1554 and this may be what is meant by
Ferrara, as it was a duchy of the house of Este—and was seized
by the Papal States in 1597.

28

Le capitaine conduira grande
  proie,
Sur la montaigne des ennemis
  plus proche,
Environné, par feu fera tel voie,
Tous eschappex or³ trente mis en
  broche.
	The captain will lead a great
	herd on the mountain closest
	to the enemy. Surrounded by
	fire he makes such a way, all
	escape except for thirty put
	on the spit.

Most commentators understand 'put on a spit' as meaning to
be run through. I think it is Nostradamus' way of describing
them being burnt alive.

29

Le grand Duc d'Albe se viendra
  rebeller
A ses grans peres fera le tradi-
  ment:
Le grand de Guise le viendra de-
  beller,
Captif mené & dressé monument.
	The great one of Alba will
	come to rebel, he will betray
	his great forebears. The great
	man of Guise will come to
	vanquish him, led captive with
	a monument erected.

---

¹ *caint*—O.F., belt or waist. Possibly used here for encircling wall?
² *Vast*—Uncertain.
³ *or*—Misprint, in all editions for *hors* = without, except for.

DUKE OF ALBA, 1555–57

This is at first sight a very clear quatrain, but it is not very accurate. The Duke of Alba was the main Spanish general, and the Duke de Guise the main French one. Unfortunately de Guise never triumphed over Alba, yet alone take him captive. It is doubtful whether Nostradamus saw Alba crossing over to the French side, but he did fight with the French from 1555–7 against the Vatican states.

30

Le sac s'approche, feu, grand sang espandu
Po, grand fleuves, aux bouviers[1] l'entreprinse,
De Gennes, Nice, apres long attendu,
Foussan, Turin, à Savillon la prinse.

The sack approaches, fire and great bloodshed. Po the great rivers, the enterprise for the clowns; after a long wait from Genoa and Nice, Fossano, Turin the capture at Savigliano.

Nice, Fossano, Turin and Savigliano were all in Piedmont but all except Nice had been lost to the House of Savoy. Genoa was an independent state under Hapsburg domination.

31

De Languedoc, & Guienne plus de dix,
Mille voudront les Alpes repasser:
Grans Allobroges[2] marcher contre Brundis
Aquin & Bresse les viendront recasser.

From Languedoc and Guienne more than ten thousand will want to cross the Alps again. The great Savoyards march against Brindisi, Aquino and Bresse will come to drive them back.

These place names are obscure because they are all so separate; Languedoc and Guienne were in South-western France. Bresse belonged to Savoy until 1601. Brindisi is in South Italy and together with Aquino, belonged to the kingdom of the Two Sicilies. The action is totally unclear.

[1] *bouviers*—O.F. = either clowns or cowherdsmen.
[2] *Allobroges* = inhabitants of Savoy.

32

Du mont Royal naistra d'une cas-
    ane,[1]
Qui cave, & compte viendra tyr-
    anniser
Dresser copie de la marche Mil-
    lane,
Favene, Florence d'or & gens es-
    puiser.
	From the bank of Montereale
	will be born one who bores
	and calculates becoming a ty-
	rant. To raise a force in the
	marches of Milan, to drain
	Faenza and Florence of gold
	and men.

DE' MEDICI FAMILY

This may have been directed at one of the de' Medicis who came from an area of Florence called Montereale. Milan belonged to the Hapsburgs, Faenza was part of the Papal states and Florence, as above, belonged to the de' Medicis, but the action is again obscure.

33

Par fraude regne, forces expo-
    lier,[2]
La classe obsesse, passages à l'espie:
Deux fainctz amis se viendront
    rallier,
Esveiller haine de long temps as-
    soupie.
	The kingdom stripped of its
	forces by fraud, the fleet
	blockaded, passages for the
	spy; two false friends will come
	to rally to awaken hatred for
	a long time dormant.

FRANCE, 1940

This is one of Nostradamus' general prophecies which may have been fulfilled several times since it was written; mainly it is interpreted as the Fall of France in 1940, line 3 describing the Germans and the Russians, and the last line Anglo-French connections.

---

[1] *casane*—low Latin, *casana* = bank.
[2] *expolier*—O.F. = plunder, strip, despoil.

34

En grand regret sera la gent Gauloise	The French nation will be in great grief, vain and light-hearted, they will believe rash things. No bread, salt, wine nor water, venom nor ale, the greater one captured, hunger, cold and want.
Coeur vain, legier croirera temerité:	
Pain, sel, ne vin, eaue: venin ne cervoise	
Plus grand captif, faim, froit, necessité.	

FRANCE, 1940 *continued*

It is usually accepted that this quatrain carries on from the last, No. 33, and Nostradamus slipped up forgetting to change them about to muddle the reader as to their chronology. This is another general description of the Fall of France and its occupation under the Germans, which lasted until 1944.

35

La grand pesche viendra plaindre, plorer	The great fish will come to complain and weep for having chosen, deceived concerning his age: he will hardly want to remain with them, he will be deceived by those (speaking) his own tongue.
D'avoir esleu, trompés seront en l'aage:	
Guiere avec eux ne voudra demourer,	
Deçeu sera par ceux de son langaige.	

HENRI III

Henri III, the third son of Catherine de' Medici was elected King of Poland on the interpretation that Poland chose its kings in an unrestrained manner *'pesche'*. On the premature death of his brother Charles IX, he had to escape from Poland and resume his claim to the French throne. This upset the arrangements made by Poland and France to found dynasties. He was deceived (and also assassinated) by a fellow Frenchman, Jacques Clément. See II. 88.

36

Dieu, le ciel tout le divin verbe à l'unde,	God, the heavens, all the divine words in the waves, carried by seven red-shaven heads to Byzantium: against the anointed three hundred from Trebizond, will make two laws, first horror then trust.
Porté par rouges sept razes à Bisance:	
Contre les oingz trois cens de Trebisconde,	
Deux loix mettront, & horreur, puis credence.	

The seven red heads are almost certainly Cardinals, but what were they doing on their way to Constantinople? Perhaps they were trying to convert the Sultan? It seems very unlikely and there is no recorded incident that I can find to substantiate this.

37

Dix envoyés, chef de nef mettre à mort,	Ten sent to put the captain of the ship to death, are altered by one that there is open revolt in the fleet. Confusion, the leader and another stab and bite each other at Lerins and the Hyerès, ships, prow into the darkness.
D'un adverti, en classe guerre ouverte:	
Confusion, chef l'un se picque & mord,	
Lerin, stecades¹ nefz cap dedans la nerte.²	

This dramatic quatrain heralds the attempted assassination of a naval commander. The Lerin Islands are off Cannes and the Hyerès off Toulon.

38

L'aisné Royal sur coursier voltigeant,	The elder royal one on a frisky horse will spur so fiercely that it will bolt. Mouth, mouthful, foot complaining in the embrace; dragged, pulled, to die horribly.
Picquer viendra si rudement courir:	
Gueulle, lipee, pied dans l'estrein pleignant	
Trainé, tiré, horriblement mourir.	

¹*stecades*—Latin, *Stoechades* = the Islands of Hyères.
²*nerte*—O.F. = Black, or Greek, *nerthe* = underneath.

DEATH OF CROWN PRINCE FERDINAND, 1842
The heir of Louis Philippe was thrown and dragged by a frisky horse, and died on 13th July 1842.

39

Le conducteur de l'armeé Françoise,
Cuidant perdre le principal phalange:
Par sus pave de l'avaigne & d'ardoise,
Soi parfondra par Gennes gent estrange.

The leader of the French army will expect to lose the main phalanx. Upon the pavement of oats and slate the foreign nation will be undermined through Genoa.

40

Dedans tonneaux hors oingz d'huile & gresse,
Seront vingt un devant le port fermés,
Au second guet par mont feront prouesse:
Gaigner les portes & du guet assommés.

Within casks anointed outside with oil and grease twenty-one will be shut before the harbour, at the second watch; through death they will do great deeds; to win the gates and be killed by the watch.

It seems as though Nostradamus is describing a second Trojan horse which is trying to capture a seaport. They succeed in entering the town but are killed by the guards.

41

Les oz des piedz & des main enserrés,
Par bruit maison long temps inhabitee:
Seront par songes concavent deterrés,
Maison salubre & sans bruit habitee.

The bones of the feet and the hands locked up, because of the noise the house is uninhabited for a long time. Digging in dreams they will be unearthed, the house healthy and inhabited without noise.

Nostradamus seems to have believed in ghosts, because this is a description of a haunted house which is exorcized when the bones of the victim are removed. Perhaps an occupant of the house dreamt of the grave which led to the discovery of the skeleton?

42

Deux de poison saisiz nouveau venuz,	Two newly arrived have seized the poison, to pour it in the
Dans la cuisine du grand Prince verser:	kitchen of the great Prince. By the scullion both are caught
Par le souillard tous deux au faicts congneuz	in the act, taken he who thought to trouble the elder
Prins que cuidoit le mort l'aisné vexer.	with death.

This is a detailed, specific quatrain in which two conspirators on a Prince's kitchen staff try to poison him. They are caught red-handed by the kitchen boy but it appears that only one is captured so possibly his accomplice got away.

CENTURY VIII

1

PAU, NAY, LORON plus feu
    qu'à sang sera.
Laude nager, fuir grand au sur-
    rez.
Les agassas[1] entree refusera.
Pampon,[2] Durance les tiendra
    enserrez.

PAU, NAY, LORON will be
more of fire than blood, to
swim in praise, the great one
to flee to the confluence (of
rivers). He will refuse entry
to the magpies Pampon and
the Durance will keep them
confined.

NAPOLEON I

Although the names in the first line are all small towns in
Western France, Nostradamus does appear to be talking about
a man rather than places. The capital letters also indicate a
more fanciful reading by anagram, PAU, NAY, LORON becomes NAPAULON ROY—Napoleon the King. The spelling
of Napoleon's name with an 'au' instead of an 'o' was com-
monplace, and Nostradamus' orthography is not at all reliable.
The connection of the agassas or Pius would refer to Pius VI
and VII who were both imprisoned by Napoleon. The confluence of rivers refers to Valence where the Rhône and Isère
meet and where Pius VI was taken to die in 1798–9. Pius VII
was taken to Savona and then on to Fontainebleau in 1872,
therefore neither was imprisoned near the Durance of line 4.
But Durance did lie near Avignon which belonged to the Papacy until 1791, where the Rhône and the Durance meet.

2

Condon & Aux & autour de
    Mirande
Je voi du ciel feu qui les envi-
    ronne.
Sol Mars conjoint au Lion puis
    marmande
Fouldre, grand gresle, mur tombe
    dans Garonne.

Condom and Auch and
around Mirande, I see fire
from the sky which encom-
passes them. Sun and Mars
conjoined in Leo, then at
Marmande, lightning, great
hail, a wall falls into the Garonne.

All the towns mentioned are in the Department of Gers in the
south-west, except for Marmande which is about 50 miles

---

[1] agassas—Provençal, agassa = a magpie, known in French as pie,
which is also the French spelling of Pius. A typical Nostradamus con-
volution.

[2] Pampon—Doubtful, possibly Gk., Pamponeros = all depraved?

north. The wall may be falling here or in some other Garonne town such as Bordeaux, Agen or Toulouse?

3

Au fort chasteau de Viglanne[1] & Resviers
Sera serré le puisnay de Nancy:
Dedans Turin seront ards[2] les premiers,
Lors que de dueil Lyon sera transi.

Within the strong castle of Vigilance and Resviers the younger born of Nancy will be shut up. In Turin the first ones will be burned, when Lyons will be transported with grief.

THE DUKE DE MERCOEUR

The names in the first line of this quatrain are difficult to decipher, the best combinations are in Italy. There is a castle built by the Scaligers of Verona on the promontory at the south of Lake Garda. Another stands at Malescino. Also on the lake between San Vigilio and the Riviera is the monastery founded by St Francis. Thus we have three possible sites on the Garda. Nancy is the capital of Lorraine, and the cadet a younger brother or branch of the family. It is most likely to refer to Nicholas, Duke of Mercoeur, the father-in-law of Henri III, who did not die until 1577. So what Nostradamus is trying to say can be summarized thus. The Duke of Mercoeur will be confined in a castle on Lake Garda. Turin, in line 3, belonged to the French when Nostradamus wrote. 'Ards' is a difficult word for which to find a definite meaning.

4

Dedans Monech[3] le coq sera re-ceu,
Le Cardinal de France apparois-tra
Par Logarion[4] Romain sera de-ceu
Foiblesse à l'aigle, & force au coq naistra.

The cock will be received into Monaco, the Cardinal of France will appear; he will be deceived by the Roman lega-tion; weakness to the eagle, strength will be born to the cock.

[1]*Viglanne*—Most likely San Vigilio and the Riviera, but could be Rubbiera and Vignola.

[2]*ards*—Possibly from *ardere* = to burn, but uncertain.

[3]*Monech*—Latin, Monaceis = Monaco.

[4]*Logarion*—Other texts have legation, which reads much better in the context.

MISTAKEN QUATRAIN

This prediction did not come true, in fact just the opposite if one accepts that Logarion is a misreading for legation. It is concerned with the struggle for power in the Mediterranean between the French and Spanish. Monaco had nominal independence under the Grimaldis but was bound by treaty to help Spain. Nostradamus predicts that this protection will move to France, which occurred in 1614. The French Cardinal who intrigued so much during Nostradamus' time is probably a reference to Charles, second Cardinal of Lorraine (1524–74). Reading Logarion as legate, there were two in France, the Viceregal Legate at Avignon and another as Papal Ambassador. Nostradamus describes a legate deceiving the French, but in spite of this he foresees the Hapsburg power declining and that of France growing. In fact the exact opposite occurred. Monaco became a closer ally to the Spanish when a garrison took over from 1605–41, and the French were driven out of Italy in 1559.

5

Apparoistra temple luisant orné,
La lampe & cierge à Borne & Bretueil.
Pour la lucerne le canton destorné,
Quand on verra le grand coq au cercueil.

There will appear a shining ornate temple, the lamp and candle at Borne and Bretueil. For the canton of Lucerne turned aside, when one will see the great cock in his shroud.

This seems to predict that the Canton of Lucerne will be overcome, and that at the same period a great French king would die. This has not occurred.

6

Clarté fulgure à Lyon apparente
Luisant, print Malte subit sera estaine,
Sardon,[1] Mauris[2] traitera decepvante,
Geneve à Londes à coq trahison fainte.

Lightning and brightness are seen at Lyons shining, Malta is taken, suddenly it will be extinguished. Sardon, Maurice will act deceitfully, Geneva to London, feigning treason towards the cock.

[1]Sardon—Sardinia is the most likely interpretation for this word.
[2]Mauris—Probably St Maurice, patron Saint of much of French Alps and of Savoy.

FRANCE, SWITZERLAND, SAVOY AND ENGLAND
c. 1560

Malta was an independent state until the Revolution. The Turks attacked it in 1565. Maurice, according to legend, was a saint, leader of a Theban legion who were annihilated because they refused to murder Christians. His cult is strong in Switzerland and Savoy. Sardon may stand for Sardinia which belonged to the House of Savoy after 1720. Nostradamus thus indicates that the Savoy held both regions. The connection between Geneva and London probably describes Elizabeth I's involvement with Calvin in the Conspiracy of Amboise (1566).

7

Verceil, Milan donna intelligence,
Dedans Tycin[1] sera faite la paye.[2]
Courir par Siene eau, sang, feu par Florence.
Unique choir d'hault en bas faisant maye.[3]

Vercelli, Milan will give the news, the wound will be given at Pavia. To run in the Seine, water, blood and fire through Florence, the unique one falling from high to low calling for help.

Very obscure except for the fact that Vercelli and Pavia belonged to the Duchy of Milan and was finally taken over by the Hapsburgs until the 19th Century.

8

Pres de linterne[4] dans de tonnes fermez,
Chivaz[5] fera pour l'aigle la menee,
L'esleu cassé lui ses gens enfermez,
Dedans Turin rapt espouse emmenee.

Near Focia enclosed in some tuns Chivasso will plot for the eagle. The elected one driven out, he and his people shut up, rape with Turin, the bride led away.

---

[1]*Tycin* Latin, *Ticinum* – Pavia.
[2]*la paye*—Possible alternative is the plague.
[3]*maye* = (a) Kneading-trough. (b) *Ma aie,* help me!
[4]*linterne*—Now Focia near Naples.
[5]*Chivaz* = Chivasso.

The village of Focia which occupies the old site of Linternum is unlikely to be the subject of this. Chivasso, a few miles north-east of Turin was occupied by the French, and Nostradamus sees it plotting on behalf of the Emperor. Is the leader of the Chivasso plot exiled or sent to another town?

9

Pendant que l'aigle & le coq à Savone
Seront unis Mer Levant & Ongrie,
L'armee à Naples, Palerne, Marque d'Ancone
Rome, Venise par Barb'[1] horrible crie.

While the eagle is united with the cock at Savona, the Eastern Sea and Hungary. The army at Naples, Palermo, the marches of Ancona, Rome and Venice a great outcry by the Barbarian.

MUSLIM INVASION OF ITALY

At Savona Nostradamus foresees an alliance between the Emperor and the French. Both the Levant and Hungary belonged to the Turks except for the small area the Hapsburgs retained and paid for. Naples and Palermo were in the Hapsburg kingdom of the Two Sicilies, and Ancona belonged to the Papal States. Does Nostradamus envisage a Moslem invasion of Italy which will suddenly unify the Christian faces?

10

Puanteur grande sortira de Lausanne,
Qu'on ne saura l'origine du fait,
Lon mettra hors toute la gente loingtaine
Feu veu au ciel, peuple estranger deffait.

A great stench will come from Lausanne, but they will not know its origin, they will put out all the people from distant places, fire seen in the sky, a foreign nation defeated.

MARXISTS OR CALVINISTS

The stench from Lausanne probably refers to the Calvinist centre that it became in the 16th Century, and in particular while Calvin's second-in-command, de Bèze, was teaching there. A more modern meaning applies it to the very frequent meetings of early Marxists who also conspired there.

[1]Barb'—short for either barbarian, or the enigmatic Aenobarb = the red bearded one. See I. 74, II. 49, V. 45 etc.

11

Peuple infini paroistra à Vicence	A multitude of people will
Sans force feu brusler la Basi-	appear at Vicenza without
lique	force, fire to burn the Basil-
Pres de Lunage deffait grand de	ica. Near Lunage the great
Valence,	one of Valenza defeated: at
Lors que Venise par more prendra	a time when Venice takes up
pique.	the quarrel through custom.

SON OF PRINCE RAINIER OF MONACO

Vicenza was in the Republic of Venice, Valenza is Hapsburg Milan and Valence the town where the Rhône and Isère join. During the lifetime of Nostradamus the title of Valentinois belonged to Diane de Poitiers, Henri II's erstwhile mistress. It passed to the Grimaldis of Monaco and at the moment is held by the son of Grace Kelly and her husband, Prince Rainier.

12

Apparoistra aupres de Buffalorre	He will appear near to Buf-
L'hault & procere entré dedans	falora the highly born and tall
Milan	one entered into Milan. The
L'abbé de Foix avec ceux de saint	Abbe of Foix with those of
Morre	Saint-Meur will cause damage
Feront la forbe abillez en vilan.	dressed up as serfs.

Buffalora is a tiny village west of Milan, so small that it is unlikely that Nostradamus would know about it, unless he passed through it on his Italian wanderings. Those of St Mark mean the Benedictines, because St Maurus founded the order in France, while the Abbey at Foix belonged to the Augustinians. Quite what they hope to accomplish in line 4 is difficult to imagine.

13

Le croisé frere par amour effrenee	The crusader brother through
Fera par Praytus Bellerophon	impassioned love will cause
mourir,	Bellerophon to die through
Classe à mil ans la femme for-	Proetus; the fleet for a thou-
cenee,	sand years, the maddened
Beu le breuvage, tous deux apres	woman, the potion drunk,
perir.	both of them then die.

A story of poisoning based on the myth of Bellerophon and Proetus, king of Argos whose wife was furious when her advances to Bellerophon were refused. The Queen Anteia persuaded Proetus to send Bellerophon on a mortal mission in a sealed message to Lobates, king of Lycia. Lobates sent Bellerophon to kill the monster, Chimaera, and he succeeded with the help of his flying horse, Pegasus. In Nostradamus' situation the cuckold husband is poisoned as well as the wife.

14

Le grand credit d'or, d'argent l'abondance Fera aveugler par libide l'honneur Sera cogneu d'adultere l'offense, Qui parviendra à son grand deshonneur.	The great credit of gold and abundance of silver will cause honour to be blinded by lust; the offence of the adulterer will become known, which will occur to his great dishonour.

SPANISH MONEY IN 16th CENTURY

The first two lines appear to be a general condemnation of the great riches flowing from the Spanish-American mines into Europe, which caused great inflation throughout the 16th Century. Nostradamus apparently connects monetary lust very closely to sexual lust.

15

Vers Aquilon grans efforts par hommasse Presque l'Europe & l'univers vexer, Les deux eclipse mettra en tel chasse, Et aux Pannons vie & mort renforcer.	Great exertions towards the North by a man-woman to vex Europe and almost all the Universe. The two eclipses will be put into such a rout that they will reinforce life or death for the Hungarians.

GERMANY AND THE NAZIS

This quatrain almost certainly ties up with a prediction Nostradamus made in the preface as to the great German expansion. The mannish-woman may be understood as Germania. Many commentators apply this to the Nazi empire.

16

Au lieu que HIERON feit sa nef fabriquer,
Si grand deluge sera & si subite,
Qu'on n'aura lieu ne terres s'atacquer
L'onde monter Fesulan Olympique.

At the place where HIERON has his ship built, there will be such a great sudden flood, that one will not have a place nor land to fall upon, the waters mount to the Olympic Fesulan.

I cannot decipher HIERON although some commentators change it to JASON to fit the Greek atmosphere of the quatrain. It is hard to find any connection between that and *Fesulan* (Fiesole) in central Italy. As for the flooding Fiesole is 970 feet above sea level, whereas Mount Olympus is 9,570 feet above it.

17

Les bien aisez subit seront desmis
Par les trois freres le monde mis en trouble,
Cité marine saisiront ennemis,
Faim, feu, sang, peste & de tous maux le double.

Those at ease will suddenly be cast down, the world put into trouble by three brothers; their enemies will seize the marine city, hunger, fire, blood, plague, all evils doubled.

THE KENNEDY BROTHERS

It appears that when three brothers appear in positions of power during a century, those at ease, i.e. America will suddenly suffer trouble. The marine city seized by their enemies, whom I doubtfully connect with the Asian Antichrist, could be Formosa or even Singapore or Hong Kong. It will be fascinating to see what Edward Kennedy will achieve during the next few years. See VIII. 46, 77, II. 57, IX. 36, X. 26.

18

De Flora issue de sa mort sera cause,	The cause of her death will be issued from Florence, one time before drunk by young and old; by the three lilies they will give her a great pause. Save through her offspring as raw meat is dampened.
Un temps devant par jeune & vieille bueire,	
Par les trois lys lui feront telle pause,	
Par son fruit sauve comme chair crue mueire.	

Florence belonged to the de' Medicis and several daughters of that name, Catherine and Marie in particular, married into the Royal Family of France, as denoted by the fleur de lis. The last line probably means that poison was put into the meat—after all the Medicis were renowned for their mastery of poison.

19

A soubstenir la grand cappe¹ troublee,	To support the great troubled Cappe, the reds will march in order to clarify it; a family will be almost overcome by death. The red, red ones will knock down the red one.
Pour l'esclaircir les rouges marcheront,	
De mort famille sera presque accablee.	
Les rouges rouges le rouge assomeront.	

EXTREMISM IN THE FRENCH REVOLUTION

Cappe here probably is the shortened form of Capulet, the name of the French Royal family line. The French are described as not supporting the great Caputian family troubled by the Revolution. Republicans will march against them so that the family has to take enforced refuge in the Temple. The Royal Family will be almost completely destroyed except for the King's sister, Elizabeth, and possibly the eldest son, Louis XVII (see V. 1). Then the extremists, the red, red ones will guillotine the more moderate revolutionaries, the Girondins. Possibly the name of Robespierre (the red stone) is hinted at in the last line?

¹*cappe*—Here stands for Capulet instead of the more usual meaning of Pope.

20

Le faux messaige par election fainte	The false message about the rigged election to run through the city stopping the broken pact; voices bought, chapel stained with blood, the empire contracted to another one.
Courir par urban rompu pache arreste,	
Voix acheptees, de sang chappelle tainte,	
Et à un autre l'empire contraicte.	

This apparently describes the election of a Holy Roman Emperor who uses bribery—'voices bought'—to attain his ends. The false election will be followed by a short war, which ends when the Pretender is murdered.

21

Au port d'Agde trois fustes entreront	Three foists will enter the port of Agde carrying the infection and pestilence, not the faith. Passing the bridge they will carry off a million, the bridge is broken by the resistance of a third.
Portant l'infect non foi & pestilence	
Passant le pont mil milles embleront,	
Et le pont rompre à tierce resistance.	

The enormity of the figure of these victims of the plague make the quatrain somewhat suspect. The figures are more suitable for the 20th Century, as for instance Biafra and Pakistan. Agde is a seaport in the south-west of France, between Narbonne and Marseilles. Could it possibly be an indirect reference to the Second World War?

22

Gorsan, Narbonne, par le sel advertir	Coursan, Narbonne through the salt to warn Tuchan, the grace of Perpignan betrayed; the red town will not wish to consent to it, in a high flight, a copy flag and a life ended.
Tucham, la grace Parpignam trahie,	
La ville rouge n'y vouldra consentir.	
Par haulte vol drap gris vie faillie.	

COMMUNISM IN FRANCE?

A difficult quatrain. There are many Communist strong-holds in present-day France around Perpignan, the red town. The rest is obscure.

23

Lettres trouvees de la roine les coffres,	Letters are found in the queen's chests, no signature and no name of the author. The ruse will conceal the offers; so that they do not know who the lover is.
Point de subscrit sans aucun nom d'hauteur	
Par la police¹ seront caché les offres.	
Qu'on ne scaura qui sera l'amateur.	

THE CASKET LETTERS 1567

Unfortunately there is no proper noun to finally determine this quatrain but in that Nostradamus knew of Mary Queen of Scots and probably met her, while summoned to the Court in 1556, it may apply. The Casket Letters were documents relating to the murder of Darnley and the events of 1567. The Earl of Morton produced them before commissions in London and York. The originals disappeared after 1584 and their authenticity has always been held in doubt.

24

Le lieutenant à l'entree de l'huis,	The lieutenant at the door of the house, will knock down the great man of Perpignan. Thinking to save himself at Montpertuis, the bastard of Lusignan will be deceived.
Assommera le grand de Parpignan,	
En se cuidant saulver à Montpertuis.	
Sera deceu bastard de Luisgnan.	

The family of Lusignan died out before Nostradamus' time but ruled Jerusalem and Cyprus until 1489, its titles passing to the house of Savoy. Nostradamus' patron, the Count de Tende, Governor of Provence, was the son of the Grand Bastard of Savoy, as he was known. If this is so then Montpertuis is almost certainly the Perthus Pass in the Pyrenees, and Nos-

¹*police*—O.F. = (*a*) Ruse. (*b*) Government.

tradamus must have envisaged Tende defeating the Spanish around Rousillan (Perpignan) and then finding himself trapped in the Pyrenees with the Spanish blocking his return route to France.

25

Coeur de l'amant ouvert d'amour fertive
Dans le ruisseau fera ravir la Dame,
Le demi mal contrefera lassive,
Le pere à deux privera corps de l'ame.

The heart of the lover, awakened by furtive love will ravish the lady in the stream. She will pretend bashfully to be half injured, the father of each will deprive the body of its soul.

A possible history of incest and rape among Royalty? The plot is clear but the references too general to be of any use.

26

De Caton es[1] trouves en Barcel-lonne,
Mis descouvers lieu retrouvers & ruine,
Le grand qui tient ne tient vouldra Pamplonne.
Par l'abbaye de Montferrat bruine.

The bones of Cato found in Barcelona, placed, discovered, the site found again and ruined. The great one who holds, but does not hold, wants Pamplona, drizzle at the abbey of Montserrat.

None of Cato's famous family died at Barcelona, and only C. Pacius Cato died in Spain, at Tarragona.

27

La voye auxelle l'une sur l'autre forniz[2]
Du muy desert hor mis brave & genest
L'escript d'empereur le fenix[3]
Veu en celui ce qu'à nul autre n'est.

The auxiliary way, one arch upon the other, Le Muy deserted except for the brave one and his jennet. The writing of the Phoenix Emperor, seen by him which is (shown) to no other.

[1] es—Alternative reading, os = Bones. O.F., ez means planks or boards.
[2] forniz— = (a) Arch. (b) Brothel. In this case Nostradamus is describing an aqueduct.
[3] fenix = (a) The Phoenix. (b) The Phoenician.

This is set in Provence and the aqueduct is probably the one which ran from the River Saigne to Fréjus. A jennet is a small black horse. The commander with the Phoenix-like qualities is more of a problem.

28

Les simulacres d'or & d'argent enflez,	The copies of gold and silver inflated, which after the theft were thrown into the lake, at the discovery that all is exhausted and dissipated by the debt. All scrips and bonds will be wiped out.
Qu'apres le rapt au lac furent gettez	
Au desouvert estaincts tous & troublez.	
Au marbre script prescript intergetez.	

INFLATION AND PAPER MONEY

This quatrain may well be describing the monetary inflation which hit Europe during the nineteen twenties and again in the sixties and seventies. It is one of the few quatrains I have not translated literally, as it is too complex, and have used that of Dr Fontbrune (1939). It is an interesting idea for a man who lived long before paper money (the copies of gold and silver) was ever used. Another interesting suggestion is that the money 'thrown into the lake' was part of the vast plundered Nazi fortunes that have never been recovered.

29

Au quart pillier l'on sacre[1] à Saturne.	At the fourth pillar which they dedicate to Saturn split by earthquake and by flood; under Saturn's building an urn is found gold carried off by Caepio and then restored.
Par tremblant terre & deluge fendu	
Soubz l'edifice Saturnin trouvee urne,	
D'or Capion ravi & puis rendu.	

Saturn's building presumably means a temple dedicated to him, or the Church of Saint Saturnin (Sernin) in Toulouse. Under the fourth pillar an urn of gold will be found, stolen by Caepio who was a Roman consul who plundered Toulouse (106 BC). The treasure never reached Rome, for which Caepio was impeached and expelled from the Senate.

[1]*sacre = sacrere*—O.F. = to dedicate.

30

Dedans Tholoze non loing de Beluezer[1]	In Toulouse, not far from Beluezer making a deep pit
Faisant un puis long, palais d'espectacle,[2]	a palace of spectacle, the treasure found will come to vex
Tresor trouvé un chacun ira vexer,	everyone in two places and all near the Basacle.
Et en deux locz tout & pres del vasacle.[3]	

UNDISCOVERED TREASURE IN TOULOUSE

Beluezer is yet unidentified by all Nostradamus' commentators. VIII. 29 indicated that gold would be found when a pillar was struck by lightning, but here it seems more likely to be the result of men digging or a chance find, perhaps the two places referring to two different discoveries. This may be a quatrain yet to be fulfilled. See IX. 12.

31

Premier grand fruit le prince de Perquiere	The first great fruit of the prince of Pescheria, then will
Mais puis viendra bien & cruel malin,	come a cruel and wicked man. In Venice he will lose his
Dedans Venise perdra sa gloire fiere	proud glory, and is led into evil by the younger Selin.
Et mis à mal par plus joyne Celin.	

MUSSOLINI AND VICTOR EMMANUEL III

When Mussolini led the Fascists in revolt the first prize that fell to him was the Prince of Pescheria, i.e. Victor Emmanuel himself, who, at Pescheria did one of the noblest acts of his reign. He had gone to the front after Caporetto, and took command in person rejecting all proposals of surrender and determined to fight it out. The Council of War was also held at Pescheria. The cruel one is Mussolini, who will lose his glory in Venice and be delivered to the hands of the younger Selin. Since Selin means crescent or moon, Nostradamus foresaw

---

[1] *Beluezer*—Unidentified name, or anagram?

[2] Nostradamus presumably means a theatre.

[3] *vasacle* = The mill section of Toulouse, also of the castle protecting the main bridge and gate to the city.

some connection with Islam, which did not occur, at that time.
See III. 32, 68, IV. 68, VI. 31, 33.

32

Garde toi roi Gaulois de ton nepveu	French king, beware of your nephew who will do so much
Qui fera tant que ton unique filz	that your only son will be
Sera meutri à Venus faisant voeu,	murdered while making his
Accompaigné de nuit que trois & six.	vows to Venus; accompanied at night by three and six.

A clear prophecy which does not seem to have taken place.
See III. 32, 68, IV. 68, VI. 31, VIII. 33.

33

Le grand naistra de Veronne & Vincence,	The great one who will be born of Verona and Vincenza
Qui portera un surnom bien indigne.	who carries a very unworthy surname; he who at Venice
Qui à Venise vouldra faire vengeance,	will wish to take vengeance, himself taken by a man of the
Lui mesme prins homme du guet & signe.	watch and sign.

MUSSOLINI

The great one born in the North of Italy, where both towns
mentioned are situated, bearing an unworthy name, is Mussolini which literally means muslin maker. The vengeance he
desires was against those powers who frustrated his dream of
Mare Nostrum. The last line, more difficult, implies that he
is taken in a snare by a man who watches and ambushes—
presumably Hitler, who became Mussolini's inspiration, and
finally the cause of his downfall. See III. 32, 68, IV. 68, VI.
31.

34

Apres victoire du Lyon au Lyon	After the victory of the Lion
Sur la montaigne de JURA Se-catombe[1]	over the Lion, there will be great slaughter on the moun-tain of JURA; floods and dark-coloured people the seventh of a million, Lyons, Ulm at the mausoleum death and the tomb.
Delues[2] *& brodes*[3] *septieme mil-lion*	
Lyon, Ulme à Mausol mort & tombe.	

The Jura mountains run through Franche-Comté which be-longed to the Hapsburgs until 1674. If '*brodes*' is normally used as and refers to dark skinned people this suggests another quatrain where the vast amount of population implies the 20th Century. See IV. 3, VI. 8.

35

Dedans l'entree de Garonne & Baise	At the entrance to Garonne and Baise and the forest not far from Damazan, discover-ies of the frozen sea, then hail and north winds. Frost in the Dardonnais through the mis-take of the month.
Et la forest non loing de Dama-zan	
Du marsaves[4] *gelees, puis gresle & bize*	
Dordonnois gelle[5] *par erreur de mezan.*[6]	

This seems to be a general summary of unseasonable weather which will occur in all the above mentioned places.

[1]*Secatombe*—An obvious misprint for hecatombe.

[2]*Delues*—Uncertain, possibly from Latin, *diluvies* = flood/destruc-tion.

[3]*brodes*—Yet again these strange people derived from the O.F., *brode* = black, brown and decadent.

[4]*marsaves*—Compound word made up from O.F., *mar* = sea and O.F., *save* = discovery.

[5]*gelle*—O.F., without extra syllable for scansion = frost.

[6]*mezan*—From Latin, *mensa* = a month by metathesis.

36

Sera commis conte oingdre ad-uché[1]	It will be committed against the anointed brought from Lons le Saulnier, Saint Aubin and Bell'oeuvre. To pave with marble taken from distant towers, not to resist Bletteram and his masterpiece.
De Saulne & sainct Aulbin & Bell'oeuvre[2]	
Paver de marbre de tours loing espluché	
Non Bleteram resister & chef d'oeuvre.	

A difficult quatrain with an enigma, see footnote. Bletteram is in Franche Comté which used to belong to the Hapsburgs until 1647.

37

La forteresse aupres de la Tamise	The fortress near the Thames will fall when the king is locked up inside. He will be seen in his shirt near the bridge, one facing death then barred inside the fortress.
Cherra par lors le Roi dedans serré,	
Aupres du pont sera veu en chemise	
Un devant mort, puis dans le fort barré.	

CHARLES I

One of Nostradamus' more exciting quatrains, and reasonably exact too. After his defeat and captivity Charles I was taken to Windsor Castle overlooking the Thames, in December 1648. He remained there until 9th January 1649. In a sense the castle did fall because it was in the hands of the Parliamentarians. On 30th January after a trial, Charles was beheaded dressed in a white shirt. The nearest bridge would be London Bridge, for Westminster Bridge was not built at this time. This quatrain is definitely connected with IX. 49. See III. 80, IX. 11, 49.

[1] *aduché*—Provençal, *aducha* = brought.
[2] *Bell'oeuvre*—Most probably an enigmatic place-name or it may translate literally 'beautiful work'.

38

Le Roi de Blois dans Avignon regner	The King of Blois will reign in Avignon, once again the
Une autre fois le peuple emono-pole[1]	people covered in blood. In the Rhône he will make swim
Dedans le Rhosne par murs fera baigner	near the walls up to five, the last one near Nolle.
Jusques à cinq le dernier pres de Nolle.[2]	

39

Qu'aura esté par prince Bizantin,	He who will have been for the
Sera tollu par prince de Tholoze.	Byzantine prince will be taken
La foi de Foix par le chief Tho-lentin,	away by the prince of Tou-louse. The faith of Foix
Lui faillira ne refusant l'espouse.	through the leader of Tolen-tino will fail him, not refusing the bride.

The identity of the characters here is completely unclear. A Byzantine prince is either a Sultan or a Moslem leader; the prince of Toulouse may be its Archbishop or any one of the hereditary Montmorency family. Tolentino is part of the Papal States so presumably its leader is the Pope. Foix belonged to the House of Navarre.

[1]*emonopole*—A difficult compound Nostradamus word. Probably the nearest is the Greek, *aimapnoos* meaning bloodthirsty, or *aimatopotes*, blood drinker.

[2]*Nolle*—Probably an enigmatic proper name; possible Nola in Italy, but it does not fit the context.

40

Le sang du Juste par Taurer la daurade,[1]	The blood of the Just for Taur and La Duarade in order to avenge itself against the Saturnines. They will immerse the band in the new lake, then they will march against Alba.
Pour se venger contre les Saturnins[2]	
Au nouveau lac plongeront la maynade.[3]	
Puis marcheront contre les Albanins.[4]	

If one accepts that the two churches stand for Toulouse, the quatrain seems to imply that the inhabitants are fighting both Calvinism, or the Huguenots, as well as a Spanish attack led by the Duke of Alba.

41

Esleu sera Renad ne sonnant mot,	A fox will be elected without speaking one word, appearing saintly in public living on barley bread, afterwards he will suddenly become a tyrant putting his foot on the throats of the greatest men.
Faisant le faint public vivant pain d'orge,[5]	
Tyranniser apres tant à un cop,[6]	
Mettant à pied des plus grans sus la gorge.	

NAPOLEON III

Napoleon III was indeed as cunning as a fox and when elected President was known as '*le Taciturne*'. The prediction of line 3 was fulfilled by the *coup d'état* he exerted to make way for the Second Empire, 2nd December 1851. He certainly used his newly acquired power to fulfil line 4.

[1]*Taurer la daurade* = Two Churches in Toulouse. (*a*) St Saturnin du Taur. (*b*) Ste Marie de la Daurade.

[2]*Saturnins*—Either those of Saturn or of St Saturnin.

[3]*maynade*—Provençal, *marinada* = (*a*) Band, (*b*) Servants, household.

[4]*Albanins*—Probably the troops of the Duke of Alba, the Hapsburg general for Emperors Charles V and Philip II. Just possibly Albanian mercenaries.

[5]*vivant pain d'orge*—Has a secondary meaning—to feather one's nest, which is singularly appropriate.

[6]*cop*—Alternative spelling of coup, for the rhyme.

42

Par avarice, par force & violence	Through avarice, through
Viendra vexer les siens chiefz	force and violence the chief
d'Orléans,	of Orléans will come to vex
Pres saint Memire[1] assault & re-	his supporters. Near St Merri,
sistance.	assault and resistance. Dead
Mort dans sa tante diront qu'il	in his tent they will say he is
dort leans.	asleep inside.

LOUIS PHILIPPE D'ORLÉANS

Louis Philippe will upset his supporters and will engage in combat around St Merri (not *Memire*). That Nostradamus got the title of Orléans is astonishing because the founder of the House was the brother of Louis XIII, born long after Nostradamus' death. After his victory Orléans is unable to cope and sleeps like a dead man within his tent.

43

Par le decide[2] de deux choses bas-	Through the fall of two bas-
tars	tard creatures the nephew of
Nepveu du sang occupera le regne	the blood will occupy the
Dedans lectoyre seront les coups	throne. Within Lectoure there
de dars	will be blows of lances, the
Nepveu par peur plaira l'enseigne.	nephew through fear will fold
	up his standard.

THE DEFEAT OF LOUIS NAPOLEON, 1870

The only important nephew in French history occurred over 300 years after Nostradamus' death; Louis Napoleon, son of King Louis of Holland who was the brother of Napoleon I. The two bastards that fall are presumably the government of Louis Philippe, for whom Nostradamus has little liking, and that of the Second Republic. Lectoyre is an anagram of Le Torcey, a suburb of Sedan, the scene of Louis Napoleon's defeat by the Germans and Prussians. He ordered a flag of surrender to be hung on Sedan's church and then on its citadel, after which the Emperor formally surrendered to the Germans at Douchery two miles away from Le Torcey, in 1870.

[1] *St Memire*—An unidentified place name.

[2] *decide*—From Latin, *decidere* = to fall.

44

Le proceé naturel dogmion,[1]
 De sept à neuf du chemin destor-
    ner
 A roi de longue & ami aumi hom,
 Doit à Navarre fort de PAU pros-
    terner.
	The natural offspring of Ogmios will turn off the road from seven to nine. To the king long friend of the half man, Navarre must destroy the fort at Pau.

Ogmios turns up in several quatrains; he was the Celtic equivalent of Hercules or Mercury. Apart from this, the only clear fact seems to be the destruction of the fortress at Pau where Henri IV of Navarre was born.

45

La main escharpe & la jambe
    bandee,
 Longs puis nay de Calais portera.
 Au mot du guet la mort sera tar-
    dee
 Puis dans le temple à Pasques
    saignera.
	With his hand in a sling and his leg bandaged, the younger brother of Calais will reach far. At the word of the watch, the death will be delayed, then he will bleed at Easter in the Temple.

46

Pol mensolee mourra trois lieus
    du Rosne[2]
 Fuis les deux prochains tarasc
    destrois:
 Car Mars fera le plus horrible
    trosne,
 De coq & d'aigle de France, freres
    trois.
	Paul the celibate will die three leagues from Rome, the two nearest flee the oppressed monster. When Mars will take up his horrible throne, the Cock and the Eagle, France and the three brothers.

WAR LINKED WITH A POPE PAUL, AND A KENNEDY BROTHER

There have been four Pope Pauls since Nostradamus' time: Paul VI–1621, Paul VI–1978, John Paul I–1978, and John

[1]*Ogmion* = the Celtic Hercules.

[2]Possible misspelling for Rome or Rhône.

Paul II, 1978–? The linking of the present Pope with one of
the Kennedy brothers helps us to date the quatrain in the
near future. A contemporary Pope will die either just outside
of Rome, or in France if the river Rhône is intended. At this
point the two great allies (see V. 78) are troubled, threatened
by a great war. The Cock stands for France which appears to
have an important role to play through the Ayatollah and the
Eagle stands for the USA, the home of the Kennedys. See I.
26, VIII. 46, 77, IX. 36, X. 26.

47

Lac Trasmenien portera tesmoig-
    nage,
Des conjurez serez dedans Per-
    ouse,
Un despolle contrefera le sage,
Truant Tedesque de sterne &
    minuse.
	Lake Trasimene will bear wit-
	ness of the conspirators locked
	up inside Perugia. A fool will
	imitate the wise one, killing
	the Teutons, destroying and
	cutting to pieces.

48

Saturne en Cancer, Jupiter avec
    Mars,
Dedans Feurier Chaldondon[1] sal-
    vaterre.
Sault Castallon[2] affailli de trois
    pars,
Pres de Verbiesque[3] conflit mor-
    telle guerre.
	Saturn in Cancer, Jupiter with
	Mars in February 'Chaldon-
	don' salva tierra. Sierra Mor-
	ena besieged on three sides
	near Verbiesque, war and
	mortal conflict.

[1]*Chaldondon*—Possibly from Latin, *Chaldens* = a soothsayer, otherwise incomprehensible.
  [2]*Sault Castallon*—Probably Latin, *Saltus Castulonensis* = Sierra Mor-
ena.
  [3]*Verbiesque*—An unsolved place name, probably near to Sierra Mor-
ena.

49

Saturn: au beuf joue en l'eau, Mars en fleiche,	Saturn in Taurus, Jupiter in Aquarius. Mars in Sagittarius,
Six de Fevrier mortalité donra,	the sixth of February brings
Ceux de Tardaigne[1] à Briges si grand breche,	death. Those of Tardaigne so great a breach at Bruges, that
Qu'à Ponteroso[2] chef Barbarin mourra.	the barbarian chief will die at Ponteroso.

According to Wöllner again, this conjunction occurred in 1736 and not again in the foreseeable future. However McCann (1942) says that it occurred on 6th February 1971 so Nostradamus seems to have been wrong on both counts, unless it refers to those Mafia chiefs who were put on an island off Sardinia in enforced exile in 1971?

50

La pestilence l'entour de Capadille,	The plague around Capellades, another famine is near
Un autre faim pres de Sagont s'appreste:	to Sagunto; the knightly bastard of the good old man will
Le chevalier bastard de bon senille,	cause the great one of Tunis to lose his head.
Au grand de Thunes fera trancher la teste.	

CAPTURE OF TUNIS, 1573

This quatrain is a very successful hit for Nostradamus. In 1573 (after Nostradamus' death in 1566), Don John of Austria, the bastard son of Charles V, the old man, recaptured Tunis for his half-brother, Philip of Spain. Although there is no record of a famine, Spain was suffering from sporadic outbursts of plague between 1570–4.

[1]*Tardaigne*—Almost definitely misreading for Sardaigne = Sardinia.

[2]*Ponteroso*—Unidentified, may mean the red bridge.

51

Le Bizantin faisant oblation,
Apres avoir Cordube à soi re-
    prinse:
Son chemin long repos pampla-
    tion,¹
Mer passant proi par la Co-
    longna² prinse.

The Byzantine makes an oblation after having taken back
Cordoba. A long rest on his
road, the vines cut down, at
sea the passing prey captured
by the Pillar.

In this, Nostradamus seems to predict that the leader of Constantinople, whatever nation it might be, will invade Spain near
Cordoba, having first made an offering to the Gods. Cordoba
had belonged to the Arabs until 1031, and then to the Moslems
until 1236. Line 4 may suggest that this Turkish leader, or
whatever, is likely to be caught when returning through the
Pillars of Hercules, i.e. Gibraltar.

52

Le roi de Blois dans Avignon reg-
    ner,
D'amboise & seme³ viendra le
    long de Lyndre
Ongle à Poitiers sainctes aesles
    ruiner
Devant Boni.⁴

The king of Blois to reign in
Avignon, from Amboise and
'Seme' the length of the Indre:
claws at Poitiers holy wings
ruined before Boni....

Line 1 is identical to the first line of VIII. 38. The various
rivers are in France. Either the final line was not completed
or was cut by the Catholic censor because it was dangerous or
heretical. It is a pity because, with it, one might have gleaned
some meaning from this quatrain.

¹pamplation—Dubious, probably from Latin, pampinatio = to cut
vines.
²Colongna—From Collonnes d'Hercule = Gibraltar.
³seme—Possibly the Seine, otherwise not identified.
⁴Boni—Incomplete line.

53

Dedans Bolongne vouldra laver ses fautes,	Within Boulogne he will want to wash away his misdeeds, he
Il ne pourra au temple du soleil,	cannot at the temple of the
Il volera faisant choses si haultes	Sun. He will fly away, doing
En hierarchie n'en fut oncq un pareil.	very great things: In the hierarchy he had never an equal.

NAPOLEON'S FAILURE TO INVADE ENGLAND

Many commentators apply this to Napoleon by reading Bolongne as Boulogne, but there is just a possibility that it may mean Bologna in the Papal States. Westminster Abbey, which Napoleon could not enter by conquest, was traditionally built on the Temple of Apollo, which was destroyed by an earthquake in AD 154. Napoleon flew so high as to think of taking Russia as well as England. Certainly he had no equal during his lifetime.

54

Soubz la colleur du traicte mariage,	Under the colour of the marriage treaty, a magnanimous
Fait magnamine par grand Chyren selin,	act by the 'Chyren selin': St Quintin and Arras recovered
Quintin, Arras recouvrez au voyage	on the journey; By the Spanish a second butcher's bench
D'espaignolz fait second banc macelin.	is made.

See II. 29, VI. 27, 70, IX. 41.

55

Entre deux fleuves se verra enserré,	He will find himself shut in between two rivers, casks and
Tonneaux & caques unis à passer outre,	barrels joined to cross beyond: eight bridges broken,
Huict pontz rompus chef à tant enferré,	their chief run through so many times, perfect chil-
Enfans parfaictz sont jugetez en coultre.[1]	dren's throats slit by the knife.

[1]*coultre*—O.F. = knife.

Specific details of an unknown battle.

56

La bande foible le terre occupera
Ceux de hault lieux feront hor-
ribles cris,
Le gros troppeau d'estre coin
troublera
Toute pres D.nebro descouvers les
escris.

The weak band will occupy the land, those of high places will make dreadful cries. The large herd of the outer corner troubled, near Edinburgh it falls discovered by the writings.

SCOTLAND AND CHARLES II

D.nebro is taken as meaning Edinburgh, through a phonetic pun, 'Edinbro'. This quatrain then describes very clearly the battle of Dunbar which took place 25 miles east of the city. Charles II landed in Scotland in 1650. The highlanders (line 1) were more numerous than the Cromwellians but their position was weak. (The phrase *estre en coin* is interesting because before the battle the Scots boasted they had Cromwell cornered 'in a pound'.) Therefore the weaker band, the Cromwellians, routed the Scots on 3rd September. Perhaps line 4 can be explained by the fact that Cromwell took possession of all the papers in the Scottish War Office?

57

De soldat simple parviendra en
empire,
De robe courte parviendra à la
longue
Vaillant aux armes en eglise ou
plus pire
Vexer les prestres comme l'eau fait
l'esponge.

From simple soldier he will attain to Empire, from the short robe he will grow into the long. Brave in arms, much worse towards the Church, he vexes the priests as water fills a sponge.

NAPOLEON I

From a simple lieutenant Napoleon attained to the government of the French Empire. He exchanged his short consular robe for the long robe of Imperial Majesty. Although brave in battle he mishandles the Clergy, and troubles the priests by the abolition of the Clergy just as much as water fills a sponge. An explicit quatrain to describe Napoleon's progress. Note that the word Empire definitely refers the quatrain to Napoleon and not to Cromwell who ran a Protectorate.

58

Regne en querelle aux freres divisé,
Prendre les armes & le nom Britannique
Tiltre Anglican sera guard advisé,
Surprins de nuict mener à l'air Gallique.

A kingdom divided by two quarrelling brothers to take the arms and the name of Britain. The Anglican title will be advised to watch out, surprised by night (the other is), led to the French air.

JAMES II AND WILLIAM OF ORANGE, 1688

Since Nostradamus' death there have been no brothers fighting for the English throne, the loser fleeing to France. The nearest this came to fulfilment was when James II and his son-in-law, the Anglican William of Orange, came to open disagreement in 1688. The Anglican Church may well have exerted influence on the Catholic James II, but nevertheless he fled to France 'to take the Gallic air'.

59

Par deux fois hault, par deux fois mis à bas
L'orient aussi l'occident foiblira
Son adversaire apres plusieurs combats,
Par mer chassé au besoign faillira.

Twice put up and twice cast down, the East will also weaken the West. Its adversary after several battles chased by sea will fail at time of need.

EAST AND WEST, 20th CENTURY

This seems again to describe the geopolitical state of the 20th Century better than any other. From this quatrain it appears that Asia will make two violent attacks upon the Western Powers which will affect them somewhat. But finally the East will lose at sea. See reference to 'Victor born on American soil.' IV. 95. Also I. 16, 91, II. 89.

60

Premier en Gaule, premier en Romanie	First in Gaul, first in Roumania, over land and sea against the English and Paris. Marvellous deeds by that great troop, violent, the wild beast will lose LORRAINE.
Par mer & terre aux Anglois & Paris	
Mervilleux faitz par celle grand mesnie	
Violent terax perdra le NOR-LARIS.	

NAPOLEON II?

Napoleon II is the only French leader to lose the Lorraine, but the rest of the quatrain does not fit him well. James Laver applies it to Napoleon I, saying he can be described as first in France and in Rome. This may be a split quatrain describing father and son, or maybe Nostradamus was confused, and saw the two men as one.

61

Jamais par le descouvrement[1] du jour	Never by the revelation of daylight will he attain the mark of the sceptre bearer. Until all his sieges are at rest, bringing to the Cock the gift of the armed LEGION.
Ne parviendra au signe sceptri-fere[2]	
Que tous ses sieges ne soient en sejour,	
Portant du coq don du TAG[3] amifere.	

The Cock bearing the gift of arms is the Cock symbolizing France, which was an obscure symbol until the Revolutionaries adopted it. The rest most commentators apply to Napoleon III; although I am not happy with this interpretation I cannot find a better.

[1]*descouvrement*—O.F. = discovery.
[2]*sceptrifere*—Latin = sceptre bearing, i.e. royal.
[3]*TAG*—Variant in editions, *tagma* = body of soldiers or legion.

62

Lors qu'on verra expiler[1] le saint temple,	When one sees the holy temple plundered, the greatest of the Rhône profaning their sacred things; because of them a very great pestilence will appear, the king, unjust, will not condemn them.
Plus grand du rosne leurs sacrez profaner:	
Par eux naistra pestilence si ample.	
Roi fuit injuste ne fera condamner.	

A very general quatrain in which an unjust king commits sacrilege which results in a plague.

63

Quand l'adultere blessé sans coup aura	When the adulterer wounded without a blow will have murdered his wife and son out of spite; his wife knocked down, he will strangle the child; eight captives taken, choked beyond help.
Merdri la femme & le filz par despit,	
Femme assoumee l'enfant estranglera:	
Huit captifz prins, s'estouffer sans respit.	

Too general to identify.

64

Dedans les Isles les enfans transportez,	The infants transported into the islands, two out of seven will be in despair. Those of the soil will be supported by it, the name 'shovel' taken, the hope of the leagues fails.
Les deux de sept seront en desepoir,	
Ceux du terrouer[2] en seront supportez,	
Nom pelle[3] prins, des ligues fui l'espoir.	

---

[1] *expiler*—Latin, *expilare* = to rob, plunder.

[2] *terrouer*—O.F. = soil, land, ground.

[3] *pelle*—This has never been deciphered. Garencières got nearest with his suggestion of Montpellier. Alternative = shovel.

NAZIS AND BRITAIN

This quatrain is applied by most modern commentators to Britain, besieged by the Nazis in the Second World War. But even with this, *pelle* is not satisfactorily deciphered.

65

Le vieux frustré du principal es-
  poir,
Il parviendra au chef de son em-
  pire:
Vingt mois tiendra le regne à
  grand pouvoir,
Tiran, cruel en delaissant un
  pire.

The old man disappointed in his main hope, will attain to the leadership of his Empire. Twenty months he will hold rule with great force, a tyrant, cruel, giving way to one worse.

MARSHAL PÉTAIN, 1940–2

If one accepts that most general quatrains are assumed to occur in France, as I do, this may well refer to that country in 1940. In that year on 10th July, a rump session of the French Assembly invested Pétain with plenary powers until a new constitution could be formed. After increasing pressure from the Germans to collaborate he handed most of his powers over to Laval on April 1942.

66

Quand l'escriture, D.M.[1] *trou-*
  vee,
En cave antique à lampe descou-
  verte,
Loi, Roi, & Prince Ulpian[2] *es-*
  prouvee
Pavillon rouge & Duc sous la
  couvert.

When the inscription D.M. is found in the ancient cave, revealed by a lamp. Law, the King and Prince Ulpian tried, the Queen and Duke in the pavilion under the cover.

Many commentators have suggested very ingenious solutions for D.M., but as I say in the footnote, it is just the equivalent of There Lies...in English. James Laver takes it to mean *du*

[1]*D.M.*—Probably stands for Latin inscription, *Diis Manibus* which was put on many Roman tombstones.
[2]*Ulpian*—Ulpius a Roman name, e.g. Trajan's was Marcus Ulpius Trajanus.

manuscrit, of the manuscript. It probably ties in with the puzzling quatrain of IX. 84.

67

PAR. CAR. NERSAF, à ruine grand discorde, *Ne l'un ne l'autre n'aura election,* *Nersaf du peuple aura amour & concorde.* *Ferrare, Callonne grande protection.*	PARIS, CARCASSONE, FRANCE to ruin in great disharmony, neither one nor the other will be elected. France will have the love and good will of the people, Ferara, Colonna great protection.

PAR, and *CAR* probably stand for Paris and Carcasonne, but *NERSAF* is not a very good anagram for France, although by the rules one is allowed to change one letter. Although Ferara was joined with the Franco-Papal troops fighting Spain in 1557, Colonna was always firmly pro-Spanish. The key to this quatrain lies in the word *Nersaf.*

68

Vieux Cardinal par le jeune deceu, *Hors de sa change se verra desarmé,* *Arles ne monstres double soit aperceu,* *Et Liqueduct & le Prince embausmé.*	The old Cardinal is deceived by the young one, he will find himself disarmed, out of his position: Do not show, Arles, that the double is perceived, both Liqueduct and the Prince embalmed.

DEATHS OF CARDINAL RICHELIEU AND LOUIS XIII, 1642–3

Cardinal Richelieu is supplanted by the younger Cinq Mars and loses the favours of Louis XIII and has to resign. But at Arles he will receive a copy of a treaty with Spain, signed by Cinq Mars and the king's brother, in 1642. He tells the king of this treachery, and although very ill, travels to Paris on a barge. *Liqueduct* means literally 'led by the water', an excellent description of the Cardinal's voyage. But the Cardinal died at the end of 1642 and the king five months later, and as Nostradamus says, both bodies were embalmed.

69

Aupres du jeune le vieux ange baisser	Beside the young one the old angel falls, and will come to
Et le viendra surmonter à la fin:	rise above him at the end; ten
Dix ans esgaux au plus vieux rabaisser,	years equal to most the old one falls again, of three two
De trois deux l'un huitiesme seraphin.	and one, the eighth seraphin.

This quatrain seems to describe the rivalry of favourites; apart from this it is very obscure.

70

Il entrera vilain, mechant, infame	He will enter, wicked, unpleasant, infamous, tyranniz-
Tyrannisant la Mesopotamie,	ing over Mesopotamia. All
Tous amis fait d'adulterine d'ame,	friends made by the adulter-
Terre horrible, noir de phisonomie.	ous lady, the land dreadful and black of aspect.

Usually Mesopotamia has described Avignon, at the joining of the Rhône and the Durance. If this is so, the villain is the Cardinal Legate governing it in place of the Pope.

71

Croistra le nombre si grand des astronomes	The number of astrologers will grow so great, that they
Chassez, bannis & livres censurez,	will be driven out, banned, and their books censored. In
L'an mil six cents & sept par sacre glomes	the year 1607 by sacred assemblies so that none will be
Que nul aux sacres ne seront asseurez.	safe from the holy ones.

URBAN VIII AND DEKKERS' ALMANACH 1607

In 1607 Pope Urban VIII banned Dekkers' Almanach under pain of expulsion which caused great controversy. A good quatrain. However, the Almanach had exercised great influence on English astrology. See X. 91.

72

Champ Perusin d'enorme deffaite
Et le conflit tout au pres de Rav-
  enne,
Passage sacre lors qu'on fera la
  feste,
Vainqueur vaincu cheval manger
  la venne.

Oh what a huge defeat on the
Perugian battlefield and the
conflict very close to Ravenna. A holy passage when
they will celebrate the feast,
the conqueror banished to eat
horse meat.

RAVENNA, 1512

This is probably a retrospective quatrain which had already
occurred when Nostradamus wrote the Prophecies. Both Perugia and Ravenna were Papal States and this quatrain describes accurately enough the victory of Gaston de Foix at
Ravenna in 1512.

73

Soldat barbare le grand Roi frap-
  pera,
Injustement non esloigné de mort,
L'avare mere du fait cause fera
Conjurateur & regne en grand
  remort.

The king is struck by a barbarian soldier, unjustly, not
far from death. The greedy
will be the cause of the deed,
conspirator and realm in great
remorse.

If used correctly the word '*barbare*' refers to the pirates from
Barbary (Algeria), but it is used widely for Moslems and others
not of the Christian faith. This could possibly refer in a general
way to 20th Century Middle East.

74

En terre neufue bien avant Roi
  entré
Pendant subges lui viendront
  faire acueil,
Sa perfidie aura tel reconntré
Qu'aux citadins lieu de feste &
  receuil.

A king entered very far into
the new land while the subjects will come to bid him welcome; his treachery will have
such a result that to the citizens it is a reception instead
of a festival.

USA

The new land is an interesting phrase because it was one of the names for America in Nostradamus' day. If the USA is meant, the verse implies that a world leader comes to that country and is given an excellent welcome whereas the whole time the guest is planning treachery. Since I first wrote this book there have been several visits between China and the USA.

75

Le pere & filz seront meurdris ensemble	The father and son will be murdered together, the leader
Le prefecteur dedans son pavillon	within his pavilion. The
La mere à Tours du filz ventre aura enfle.	mother at Tours will have her belly swollen with a son. A
Criche verdure de failles papillon.	verdure chest with little pieces of paper.

ASSASSINATION IN PORTUGAL, 1908?

The first line of this quatrain is very clear, the murder of a father and son. It cannot apply to France as no French kings and Dauphins were assassinated together. In the case of Louis XVI and his son there were over two years between the king's and his son's presumed death. There was no pregnant widow at Tours involved with the family. The most important father and son assassination outside France was in 1908, when Carlos I and Louis Philippe of Portugal were murdered at Lisbon. But still no explanation of the widow at Tours or the puzzling last line.

76

Plus Macelin[1] que roi en Angleterre	More of a butcher than a king in England, born of obscure
Lieu obscure nay par force aura l'empire:	rank will gain empire through force. Coward without faith,
Lasche sans foi, sans loi saignera terre,	without law he will bleed the land; His time approaches so
Son temps approche si presque que je soupire.	close that I sigh.

[1]*Macelin*—Latin, *macellum* = a meat basket. Used elsewhere with the above meaning by Nostradamus.

OLIVER CROMWELL

Apparently Nostradamus had little sense of time because Oliver Cromwell did not appear until over 30 years after his death (1599–1658). He is described as more of a butcher than a king because of the bloodshed of the Civil War. He was of the Protestant faith and Nostradamus regards him as a heretic. He was of comparatively humble origins and attained his position through military force. The reference to his being a coward is interesting as Cromwell was supposed to wear a corselet of some kind, because he was afraid of assassination.

77

L'antechrist trois bien tost annichilez,	The antichrist very soon annihilates the three, twenty-seven years his war will last. The unbelievers are dead, captive, exiled; with blood, human bodies, water and red hail covering the earth.
Vingt & sept ans sang durera sa guerre.	
Les heretiques mortz, captifs, exilez.	
Sang corps humain eau rougi gresler terre.	

ANTICHRIST, THE THREE BROTHERS AND WAR

Three separate Antichrists appear in Nostradamus' Epistle. It is usually accepted that Napoleon was the first and Hitler the Second, so the Third is still to come. Line 1 can be read either as 'the third Antichrist will soon be annihilated' or 'the Antichrist will soon annihilate the three', implying by this the three Kennedy brothers, two of whom are already dead. It makes more sense in this context to assume that the Antichrist is a way of life, i.e. Russian Communism or Chinese Communism, since obviously one man did not kill both brothers. It seems as though Edward Kennedy must be a psychological assassinee since even Nostradamus foresaw his death four hundred years ago! The war is a long one of attrition; it may refer to the length of time needed before the cities would be safe from harmful radioactive fallout. After the atomic bombing of Nagasaki and Hiroshima large black raindrops fell, full of dust. This was recorded by survivors so perhaps Nostradamus is not so far out when he speaks of red rain. See I. 16, 26, IV. 14, VIII. 46, 77, IX. 36. NB. occult no: of quatrain.

78

Un Bragamas[1] avec la langue torte	A soldier of fortune with twisted tongue will come to the sanctuary of the gods. He will open the door to heretics and raise up the Church militant.
Viendra des dieux le sanctuaire,	
Aux heretiques il ouvrira la porte	
En suscitant l'eglise militaire.	

This is a general quatrain that can be applied either to France during the Wars of Religion (1562–98) or to Germany during the Thirty Years War (1618–48).

79

Qui par fer pere perdra nay de Nonnaire,[2]	He who loses his father by the sword, born in a Nunnery, upon this Gorgon's blood will conceive anew; in a strange land he will do everything to be silent, he who will burn both himself and his child.
De Gorgon sur la sera sang perfetant[3]	
En terre estrange fera si tout de taire,	
Qui bruslera lui mesme & son enfant.	

The legendary Gorgon was a hateful monster, who turned everyone who looked at her into stone. Nostradamus is therefore describing an appalling woman who causes a man to kill himself and the child he has had by her. An interesting footnote is that Hugh Allen in his book on Nostradamus in 1943, applies this quatrain to himself, on page xii!

80

Des innocens le sang de vefue & vierge.	The blood of innocents, widow and virgin, so many evils committed by means of the Great Red One, holy images placed over burning candles, terrified by fear, none will be seen to move.
Tant de maulx faitz par moyen se grand Roge	
Saintz simulacres trempez en ardent cierge	
De frayeur crainte ne verra nul que boge.	

[1]*Bragamas*—O.F. = broadsword, or Provençal, *Briamanso* = a soldier of fortune.
[2]*Nonnaire*—Low Latin, *nonneria* = nunnery.
[3]*perfetant*—Latin, *superfetens* = to conceive while pregnant.

THE RUSSIAN REVOLUTION

The great Red One of line 2 is a revolution, but it is difficult to decide if the French or Russian Revolution is meant. I am inclined to accept the latter as the Communist Party is described as Red, and Nostradamus describes the French Revolutionary tricolour elsewhere. The first line would then refer to the deaths of the Czar and Czarina and their 'virgin' children. Line 3 smacks faintly of the influence of the Church through the priest Rasputin. The last line would then imply that Anastasia did not escape assassination, and that those who claim to be her are pretenders.

81

Le neuf empire en desolation
Sera changé du pole aquilonaire.
De la Sicile viendra l'esmotion
Troubler l'emprise à Philip tributaire.

The new empire in desolation will be changed from the Northern Pole. From Sicily will come such trouble that it will bother the enterprise tributary to Philip.

CHANGE OF WORLD POWER CENTRES

The first two lines make this quatrain sound very modern by the sheer scope of their concept. A ravaged empire moves itself and its civilization southwards. This might well occur after an atomic war. But the last two lines bring us back to 16th Century Europe where Nostradamus seems to see a Hapsburg civil war between Philip and Ferdinand over the division of Charles V's empire. The uprising against Philip is predicted as starting in Sicily.

82

Ronge long, sec faisant du bon valet,
A la parfin n'aura que son congie[1]
Poignant poison & lettres au collet
Sera saisi eschappé en dangie.[1]

Thin tall and dry, playing the good valet in the end will have nothing but his dismissal; sharp poison and letters in his collar, he will be seized escaping into danger.

[1]*congie* and *dangie*—The latter word shortened to keep the rhyme.

ANTHONY BLUNT

A valet who tries to poison his master is caught and dismissed. This is somewhat fanciful but is a very good description of the situation of the traitor Anthony Blunt, ex-keeper of the Queen's pictures.

83

Le plus grand voile hors de port de Zara,	The largest sail set out of the port of Zara, near Byzantium
Pros de Bisance fera son entreprinse,	will carry out its enterprise.
D'ennemi parte & l'ami ne sera,	Loss of enemy and friend will not be, a third will turn on
Le tiers à deux fera grand pille & prinse.	both with great pillage and capture.

FOURTH CRUSADE, 1202

Another retroactive prophecy describing the atrocities of the Fourth Crusade, 1202. Venice agreed to cross to Egypt with the Crusaders for a large sum of money and half the plunder. The Crusaders could not raise the money and so they captured Zara (then Hungarian, now in Yugoslavia). The Pope excommunicated the whole Crusade, whereupon they sacked Constantinople (Byzantium) and set up Romania, the Roman Empire of the East.

84

Paterne orra de la Sicile crie,	Paterno will hear the cry from Sicily, all the preparations in
Tous les aprests du goulphre de Trieste,	the Gulf of Trieste; it will be heard as far as Sicily flee oh
Qui s'entendra jusque à la trinacrie[1]	flee, so many sails, the dreaded pestilence!
Tant de voiles, fui, fui, l'horrible peste.	

The Spanish empire of the two Sicilies owned Catonia and Paterno, whereas Trieste belonged to Venice of the Hapsburg branch. So this is probably a continuation of VIII. 81.

[1] *Trinacrie*—Trinicia, poetic name for Italy.

85

Entre Bayonne & à Saint Jean de Lux
Sera posé de Mars la promottoire[1]
Aux Hanix[2] d'Aquilon Nanar[3] hostera lux,[4]
Puis suffocqué au lict sans adjutoire.[5]

Between Bayonne and St Jean de Luz will be placed the promontory of Mars. To the Hanix of the North, Nanar will remove the light, then suffocate in bed without assistance.

NAPOLEON III'S DEATH?

Nostradamus foresees a war zone (Mars) between Bayonne and St Jean de Luz in South-west France. The difficulty of interpretation lies in Hanix and Nanar, see below. Another suggestion is that the promontory is Biarritz, where Napoleon III, like Mars the God of War, retired into the arms of loving women when the North wind ceases to blow. *Hanix* would then come from the Greek, *ansiscus*, without force. Napoleon died from an operation for the stone, but his bad physical condition, because of his debauchery, may have made him much weaker.

86

Par Arami Tholoser ville franque,
Bande infini par le mont Adrian,
Passe riviere, Hutin[6] par pont la planque
Bayonne entrera tous Bihoro[7] criant.

Through Emani, Tolosa and Villefranche, an infinite band through the mountains of Adrian. Passes the river, Combat over the plank for a bridge, Bayonne will be entered all crying Bigore.

NAVARRE

The three towns of line 1 and the mountain of Adrian in line 2 are all close together on the south-western tip of the Spanish Pyrenees. The only river to the north between them

[1] *promottoire*—Variant spelling of *promontoire*.
[2] *Hanix*—Possibly from Gk., *anikatos* = unconquerable, or Latin, *Hamaxaeci* = the nomads of Northern Europe.
[3] *Nanar*—Possibly Latin, *nonaria* = prostitute?
[4] *lux*—Latin = light.
[5] *adjutoire*—O.F. = assistance, aid.
[6] *Hutin*—O.F. = dispute, combat, hostility.
[7] *Bihoro*—Bigorre was the battle cry of the Huguenots of Navarre.

and Bayonne is the Bidassoa. As I have said before, Bigorre was the battle cry of the Huguenots of Navarre, and the original Navarre covered the area south of the Pyrenees and north into France. It became a separate state in 1515 until it was reunified with France by the accession of Henri IV of Navarre to the French throne after Nostradamus' death.

87

Mort conspiree viendra en plein effect,	A death conspired will come to its full effect, the charge
Charge donnee & voiage de mort,	given and the voyage of death.
Esleu, crée, receu par siens deffait.	Elected, created, received (then) defeated by his followers, in remorse the blood of
Sang d'innocence devant foi par remort.	innocence in front of him.

LOUIS XVI

The conspiracy to rob Louis XVI of both his crown and life is successfully carried off. The change to the position of constitutional king and his flight to Varennes (voyage of death) will be the final cause of his death. He will be defeated by his own nation who earlier elected him. His innocent blood will be a source of remorse to the French.

88

Dans la Sardaigne un noble Roi viendra	A noble king will come to Sardinia, who will only rule for
Que ne tiendra que trois ans le royaume,	three years in the kingdom. He will join with himself sev-
Plusieurs coulleurs avec soi conjoindra,	eral colours; he himself, after taunts, care spoils slumber.
Lui mesmes apres soin someil marrit[1] scome.[2]	

KING OF SARDINIA, 1798–1802

King Charles Emmanuel IV, when the French Republic took most of his lands retired to Sardinia where he reigned for three years (1798–1802). He abdicated in favour of his brother, Victor Emmanuel I. He then went to Rome humili-

---

[1] marrit—O.F. = to afflict, spoil.
[2] scome—Latin, scomma = scoff, taunt, jeer.

ated and unhappy and joined the Jesuit Order with whom he stayed until his death in 1819. This is one of the few times in modern history that Sardinia had its own king and not a titular one.

89

Pour ne tumber entre mains de son oncle,	In order not to fall into the hands of his uncle who
Qui ses enfans par regner trucidez.[1]	slaughtered his children in order to reign. Pleasing with
Orant au peuple mettant pied sur Peloncle[3]	the people, putting his foot on 'Peloncle', dead and
Mort & traisné entre chevaulx bardez.	dragged between armoured horses.

I have not been able to decipher *Peloncle* and therefore the quatrain remains unbroken.

90

Quand des croisez un trouvé de sens trouble	When those of the cross are found their senses troubled,
En lieu du sacre verra un boeuf cornu	in place of sacred things he will see a horned bull, through
Par vierge porc son lieu lors sera comble	the virgin the pig's place will then be filled, order will no
Par roi plus ordre ne sera soustenu.	longer be maintained by the king.

The men of the cross are either Crusaders, or Nazis. The bull may mean in Taurus, and the Virgin, Virgo, but it doesn't get us much further.

---

[1] *trucidez*—Latin, *trucidare* = to slaughter, massacre.
[2] *Orant*—Latin, *orans* = pleading, arguing.
[3] *Peloncle*—Doubtful, possibly Pellonia, the goddess who put enemies to flight?

91

Frymy[1] les champs des Rodanes[2]
entrees
Ou les croisez seront presque unis,
Les deux brassieres[3] en pisces ren-
contrees
Et un grand nombre par deluge
punis.

Entered among the fields of the Rhône (dwellers) where those of the cross are almost united, the two lands meeting in Pisces and a great number punished by the flood.

The conjunction of Pisces with Venus is the time clue for this quatrain, linked with flooding above the Rhône.

92

Loin hors du regne mis en hazard
voyage
Grand ost[4] duira[5] pour soi
l'occupera,
Le roi tiendra les siens captif os-
trage
A son retour tout pays pillera.

Far distant from his kingdom, sent on a dangerous journey, he will lead a great army and keep it for himself. The king will hold his people captive and hostage, he will plunder the whole country on his return.

A very clear and dramatic quatrain which does not seem to have been fulfilled.

93

Sept mois sans plus obtiendra pre-
lature
Par son deces grand scisme fera
naistre:
Sept mois tiendra un autre la pre-
ture
Pres de Venise paix union re-
naistre.

For seven months, no longer, will he hold the office of prelate, through his death a great schism will arise; for seven months another acts as prelate near Venice, peace and union are reborn.

[1]*Frymy*—Misprint in some editions for *Parmi* = among.
[2]*Rodans*—Latin, *Rhodanus* = the Rhône, or possibly its people.
[3]*brassieres*—lead strings, probably standing for Venus who was bound to Mars by an unbreakable thread forged by Vulcan.
[4]*ost*—O.F. = army.
[5]*duira*—O.F., *duire* = to lead.

UNTIMELY DEATHS OF POPES

The only popes to live for less than seven months after election were Sixtus V, Urban VII, who died after two weeks, followed by Gregory XIV, who died after ten months, and Pope John Paul I (1978) who reigned for less than a month. Unfortunately, there is no definite record of a schism although the death of John Paul I caused a great deal of contemporary scandal that was quickly hushed up by the Vatican.

94

Devant le lac ou plus cher fut getté	In front of the lake where the dearest one was destroyed for
De sept mois, & son host desconfit	seven months and his army
Seront Hispans par Albanois gastez	routed; Spaniards will be devastating by means of Alba,
Par delai perte en donnant le conflict.	through delay in giving battle, loss.

BAY OF CADIZ, 1596

Ward applies this quatrain to the English attack on Cadiz by Essex, Howard and Raleigh in June 1596. In line 1 the word *cher* becomes treasure or valuables, because the ships were heavy with booty having come in from a seven months' voyage. Cadiz bay is called a lake because the word Gaddir, from which Cadiz comes, means 'an enclosed space'. Forty galleons and thirteen warships were destroyed. What makes this quatrain so interesting is that Nostradamus must have foreseen the war between Spain and England, whereas when he wrote England's queen was the wife of Spain's king (Mary Tudor).

95

Le seducteur sera mis en la fosse	The seducer will be placed in
Et estaché jusques à quelque temps,	a ditch and will be tied up for
Le clerc uni le chef avec sa crosse[1]	some time. The scholar joins the chief with his cross. The
Picante droite attraira[2] *les contens.*	sharp right will draw the contented ones.

[1] *crosse*—O.F. = possibly abbey; or cross.
[2] *attraira*—O.F. = to draw, attract.

96

La synagogue sterile sans nul fruit	The sterile synagogue without any fruit, will be received by the infidels, the daughter of the persecuted (man) of Babylon, miserable and sad, they will clip her wings.
Sera receu entre les infideles	
De Babylon la fille du porsuit	
Misere & triste lui trenchera les aisles.	

FLIGHT OF JEWS TO MOSLEMS, *c.* 1550–1566
This prophecy was already partly fulfilled in Nostradamus' lifetime. After the wave of persecution that they were suffering in Christian countries, the Sultan of Turkey, Suleiman the Magnificent, offered hospitality to Jews who came and settled in Constantinople, and Salonika in particular. One of them became very powerful and in 1566, the year of Nostradamus' death, Don Joseph Nassi was created Duke of Naxos and became the principal adviser to Selim II.

97

Aux fins du VAR changer le pompotans,	At the ends of the VAR the great powers change; near the bank three beautiful children are born. Ruin to the people when they are of age; in the country the kingdom is seen to grow and change more.
Pres du rivage les trois beaux enfants naistre.	
Ruine au peuple par aage competans.	
Regne ay pays changer plus voir croistre.	

In X. 100 '*pempotan*' stands for England. The problem is to decide whether it does so in this case, probably not. The river Var flows into the Mediterranean between Cannes and Nice and it was the approximate border of Savoy in Nostradamus' time. The three beautiful brothers who bring trouble to the nation may link up with the Kennedy theme. Certainly the USA is changing during their lifetimes and presumably growing in influence to become a world power.

98

Des gens d'eglise sang fera espandu,	Of the church men the blood will be poured forth as abundant as water in (amount); for a long time it will not be restrained, woe, woe, for the clergy ruin and grief.
Comme de l'eau en si grand abondance:	
Et d'un long temps ne sera restranché	
Ve, ve[1] au clerc ruine & doleance.	

Another quatrain about the Persecution of the Clergy *c.* 1792 in France.

99

Par la puissance des trois rois temporelz	Through the powers of three temporal kings, the sacred seat will be put in another place, where the substance of the body and the spirit will be restored and received as the true seat.
En autre lieu sera mis le saint siege:	
Où la substance & de l'esprit corporel,	
Sera remis & receu pour vrai siege.	

The only time that the Pope's seat has been moved from the Vatican to date is when Pope Pius VI was moved to Valence and died there. Pius VII managed to return to Rome. Maybe one of the future Popes will move out of the Vatican. Lines 3 and 4 imply a revival of religious fervour.

[1]*Ve, ve*—Latin, *vae* = alas, woe.

100

Pour l'abondance de larme res-
pandue
Du hault en bas par le bas au
plus hault
Trop grande foi par jeu vie per-
due
De soif mourir par habondant
deffault.[1]

By the great number of tears
shed, from top to bottom and
from the bottom to the very
top, a life is lost through a
game with too much faith, to
die of thirst through a great
deficiency.

A nonsensical quatrain to present-day readers.

[1]The whole of this line is difficult. It probably means drowned, or
even to drink oneself to death.

CENTURY IX

1
2
3
4
5   National Assembly, 1848
6
7
8
9   Nîmes, 1557
10
11   Death of Charles I, 1649 followed by Great Plague
      of 1655
12
13
14
15
16   General Franco and de Rivera
17   French Revolution
18   Louis XIII
19   Mistaken Quatrain
20   Louis XVII Flight to Varennes 1791
21
22
23   Louis XVI and his Son
24
25
26
27   Louis VII?
28
29   Capture of Calais, 1558
30
31
32
33

391

77	Fates of Marie Antoinette and Mme. du Barry
78	
79	
80	
81	
82	
83	Earthquake after 10th May. San Andreas Fault?
84	Tomb of St Peter?
85	
86	3 July 1851
87	
88	Calais, 1557
89	Louis Philippe, 1830–48
90	Hitler
91	
92	New York?
93	Louis XIV
94	
95	
96	
97	
98	
99	Napoleon's Retreat from Moscow
100	Pearl Harbor, 1941

1

Dans la maison du traducteur de Bourc[1]	In the house of the translator from Bourc letters will be
Seront les lettres trouvees sur la table	found on the table. One-eyed, red-and-white-haired will hold
Bourgne, roux, blanc chanu tiendra de cours,	the course, which will change for the new constable.
Qui changera au nouveau connestable.	

This is a fascinating quatrain. One of the best known 16th-Century French scholars was a man called Etienne de la Boétie. If *'Bourc'* stands for Boétie then the prophecy makes some sort of sense, in that the latter had a famous quarrel with the then Constable of France, Anne de Montmorency over the publication of a book, 'La Servitude Voluntaire'. Nostradamus seems to predict that Boétie would have even more trouble with the Constable's successor, Henri de Montmorency. This did not occur as Boétie died four years before Anne de Montmorency, in 1563. See also IX. 81.

2

Du hault du mont Aventin voix ouie,	A voice is heard from the top of Aventine Hill. Go, go, all
Vuidez, vuidez de tous les deux costez,	on both sides! The anger will be appeased by the blood of
Du sang des rouges sera l'ire assomie,[2]	the red ones. From Rimini and Prato, Colonna expelled.
D'Arimin Prate, Columna[3] *debotez.*[4]	

Another quatrain centered around the feuds of the Vatican states with the great Italian families, the Colonnas and the Orsinis etc. In Nostradamus' time they were allied to the Spanish and thus got deeply involved with the Vatican's anti-Spanish policies of Pope Paul IV.

[1]*Bourc* = Bourg, north of Bordeaux; the inhabitants were called Bourcais.
[2]*assomie*—O.F. = to appease.
[3]*Columna*—Original spelling of the Colonnas of Rome.
[4]*desbotez*—O.F., *debouter* = expel, drive out.

3

La magna vaqua[1] *à Ravenne grand trouble,* *Conduictz par quinze enserrez à Fornase* *A Rome naistre deux monstres à teste double* *Sang, feu, deluges, les plus grands à l'espase.*	The magna vaqua near Ravenna in great trouble, led by fifteen shut up at Fornese; at Rome two monsters with double heads are born, blood, fire, floods, the greatest in the air.[2]

This is similar to the last quatrain with the added enigma of *magna vaqua*, literally 'the great cow'. It seems to be involved with the Papal states and the Vatican, together with hanging and two-headed monsters, two of which were shown to Nostradamus in his capacity of prophet in the early 1560s near Salon, when he declared them to predict a disunited France to come. I saw a stuffed two-headed lamb this year.

4

L'an ensuivant descouvertz par deluge, *Deux chefs esluez le premier ne tiendra* *De fuir ombre à l'un d'eux le refuge,* *Saccagee case*[3] *qui premier maintiendra.*	The following year revealed by a flood, two leaders elected, the first will not hold on; for one of them refuge in fleeing shadows, the victim plundered who maintained the first.

Another quatrain describing a discovery, or treasure, combined with vague threats.

5

Tiers doit du pied au premier semblera. *A un nouveau monarque de bas hault* *Qui Pise & Lucques Tyran occupera* *Du precedant corriger le deffaut.*	The third toe will look like the first one of a new king, of low height, he who will occupy as a tyrant Pisa and Lucca, to correct the fault of his predecessor.

[1]*magna vaqua*—Either the valley and port named Magnavalca between Ravenna and Ferrara, or an unsolved name?
[2]i.e., hanged.
[3]*case*—Provençal *casa* = victim of hunt or the hunt.

NATIONAL ASSEMBLY OF 1848

The third estate, established for a second time in 1848, will seem no more than a toe of the first, i.e. very insignificant. Louis-Napoleon found it easier to deal with than did Napoleon I. In 1831 Louis Napoleon was involved with Italian revolutionaries and helped to try to seize Civila Castellana which is in Tuscany as are Pisa and Lucca. The fault of Napoleon's predecessor was Napoleon II's failure to obtain real power.

6

Par la Guienne infinité d'Anglois
Occuperont par nom d'Angla-
quitaine
Du Languedoc Ispalme[1] Bour-
delois.
Qu'ilz nommeront apres Barbox-
itaine.[2]

A great number of English in Guienne will occupy it, calling it Anglaquitain. In Languedoc, Ispalme, Bordelais which they will name after Barboxitaine.

The English occupied Gienne, the Languedoc and Bordelais steadily between the 12th and 15th Centuries, but not since Nostradamus' lifetime. Bordelais was one of the centres of English dominance in southern France. Perhaps Ispalme is a misprint for Lapalme near Narbonne? Barboxitaine seems to mean 'the Beard's' south-western France, the Beard being the man variously referred to as Bronze Beard or Aenobarbe (see V. 59). Not a successful quatrain on the whole.

7

Qui ouvrira le monument trouvé
Et ne viendra le serrer prompte-
ment.
Mal lui viendra & ne pourra
prouvé,
Si mieux doit estre roi Breton ou
Normand.

The man who opens the tomb when it is found, and who does not come and shut it immediately; evil will come to him, no one will be able to prove it. It might have been better were he a Breton or a Norman King.

[1]*Ispalme*—Unidentified place name.
[2]*Barboxitaine*—Probably derived from Barbe-Occitanie, Barbe referring to the enigmatic Bronze Beard and Occitanie, the medieval name for the Mediterranean coast.

Another quatrain about the discovery of a tomb, and it may
be linked with I. 27. The last line is suitably enigmatic: I. 27
is regarded by some as being a threat against the opening of
Nostradamus' tomb which was desecrated by Republican soldiers in 1813. He was reburied in the wall of the Church of
St Laurent where his bones remain to this day. See II. 27.

8

Puisnay Roi fait son pere mettra à mort,	The younger son will put his father, the king to death, after
Apres conflit de mort tres inhoneste:	the quarrel, to a death very dishonest. Writings found,
Escrit trouvé soubson donra remort,	suspicion will bring remorse,
Quand loup chassé pose sus la couchette.	when the chased wolf lies on the bedcover.

Although the statement of a younger son taking over his
father's throne, in a way that involves murder, sounds quite
reasonable, it is hard to find any possible fulfilment since Nostradamus' lifetime, and also of the strange details of the last
two lines.

9

Quand lampe ardente de feu inextinguible,	When the lamp burning with eternal fire, will be found in
Sera trouvé au temple des Vestales,	the temple of the Vestals. A
Enfant trouvé feu, eau passant par trible:[1]	child found (in the) fire water passing through the sieve,
Perir eau Nîmes, Tholose cheoir les halles.	Nîmes to perish in water, the markets will fall in Toulouse.

1557

Nostradamus may have cheated on this verse because in
1557 the most enormous cloudburst occurred over Nîmes
(popularly held to be the site of a Temple of Diana, tended

---

[1]*trible*—Mod. French, *crible* = a sieve.

by the Vestal Virgins). The water was over six feet deep in some places and many of the beautiful monuments were uncovered. But nothing remarkable occurred in Toulouse around that time.

10

Moine moinesse d'enfant mort exposé,	The child of a monk and a nun will be exposed to die, to die by a she bear, and carried off by a boar; the army will be camped near Foix and Parmiers, Carcassonne will raise the pillage against Toulouse.
Mourrir par ourse & ravi par verrier.[1]	
Par Foix & Pamyes le camp sera posé	
Contre Tholose Carcas, dresser forrier.	

A quatrain set in South-west France, the first part describing the tragic circumstances and death of a baby, the second part great military events.

11

Le juste à tort à mort l'on viendra mettre	They will come to put the just man wrongfully to death, publicly in the midst he is extinguished. So great a plague will be born in this place that the judges will be forced to flee.
Publiquement & du millieu estaint:	
Si grande peste en ce lieu viendra naistre,	
Que les jugeans[2] fouir seront constraint.	

DEATH OF CHARLES I, 1649 FOLLOWED BY GREAT PLAGUE OF 1655

This quatrain is usually applied to England. It states that after someone is unjustly executed, a great plague occurs in that place causing the people who caused the death to flee. It is understood to describe Charles I who was beheaded in 1649, his death to be followed by the great plague of London 1655–6. See III. 80, VIII. 37, IX. 11, 49.

[1] *verrier*—Probably made up by Nostradamus from Latin, *verez* = a boar.

[2] *jugeans* = judges, again invented by Nostradamus.

12

Le tant d'argent de Diane & Mercure	The great amount of silver of Diana & Mercury, the images
Les simulacres au lac seront trouvez,	will be found in the lake. The sculptor looking for new clay,
Le figulier cherchant argille neufve	both he and his followers will be soaked in gold.
Lui & les siens d'or seront abbrevez.	

Another treasure quatrain relating in particular to that in Toulouse of VIII. 28–30.

13

Les exilez autour de la Soulonge	The exiles around Sologne,
Condus de nuit pour marcher à Lauxois,	led by night to march into Auxas, two from Modena
Deux de Modene truculent¹ de Bologne,	for the cruel one of Bologna; put, discovered, by the fire of
Mis descouvers par feu de Burançois.	the Buzançais.

14

Mis en planure chaulderons d'infecteurs,²	The dyers' cauldrons put in a flat place, wine, honey and
Vin, miel & l'huile, & bastis sur forneaulx	oil and built over furnaces. They will be drowned, with-
Seront plongez sans mal dit mal facteurs	out saying or doing an evil thing, seven of Borneaux, the
Sept. fum extaint au canon des borneaux.	snake extinguished from the cannon.

A typical, unintelligible Nostradamus quatrain at its worst.

---

¹*truculent*—From Latin, *truculentus* = ferocious, hard, cruel.
²*infecteur*—Latin, *infector* = dyer.

15

Pres de Parpan les rouges de-tenus	The red ones detained near Perpignan, those in the middle, ruined, led far away.
Ceux du milieu parfondrez menez loing:	Three cut into pieces and five badly supported for the Lord and Prelate of Burgundy.
Trois mis en pieces, & cinq mal soustenus,	
Pour le Seigneur & Prelat de Bourgoing.	

Perpignan belonged to Spain until 1659, and red was the colour of the Spanish. Nostradamus seems to foresee a Franco-Spanish struggle around the Pyrenees. The Governor of Burgundy, in Nostradamus' time the Duke of Aumale, died in 1573, the country had four (not five) bishops under him.

16

De castel¹ Franco sortira l'assemblee	From Castille Franco will bring out the assembly, the ambassadors will not agree and cause a schism. The people of Riviera will be in the crowd, and the great man will be denied entry to the Gulf.
L'ambassadeur non plaisant fera scisme:	
Ceux de Ribiere seront en la mes-lee	
Et au grand goulphre desnier ont l'entree.	

FRANCO AND DE RIVERA
This is an extraordinary verse with the names of two personages in it. The Dictator Primo de Rivera and also Francisco Franco, who helped depose him, and was exiled to Morocco, returning triumphantly when his party came to power. The last line is held to describe Franco's exile when he was not allowed to cross the Mediterranean (*goulphre*) to his native Spain. Castel should be read as Castille. See III. 8, 54.

¹*castel* = Castille.

17

Le tiers premier pis que ne fait Neron,
Vuidex vaillant que sang humain respandre:
R'edifier sera le forneron,
Siecle d'or, mort, nouveau roi grand esclandre.

The third one firstly does worse than Nero, go, flow, brave human blood. The furnace will be rebuilt, a golden century; (then) death, a new king and great scandal.

THE FRENCH REVOLUTION

The third first is the National Convention of the Tiers État in Revolutionary France. Nostradamus describes it as being far crueller than Nero's reign with blood flowing freely from the guillotines. The machine will be put at the Place de la Révolution opposite the Tuileries, where formerly tile kilns were built. The golden century of the Kings Louis XIV-XVI is over! The great scandal is possibly a reference to the killing of the Royal Family. See also III. 59.

18

Le lis Dauffois portera dans Nancy
Jusques en Flandres electeur de l'empire,
Neufve obturee au grand Mont-morency,
Hors lieux provez delivre à clere peyne.

The lily of the Dauphin will be taken as far as Nancy, the elector of the empire as far as Flanders. A new prison for the great Montmorency, to the usual place delivered up to Clerepeyne.

LOUIS XIII

Louis XIII was the first bearer of the lilies of France and the title of Dauphin since Nostradamus' death. He entered Nancy in September 1633. The city of Trèves had been recovered the year before by the Maréchal d'Estrées who re-established the authority of the Elector. However in 1633 the Elector was carried off by the Spanish and taken as a prisoner to Brussels (*Flandres*). At the same time 1632, a revolt was led in southern France by the great Montmorency. His family pleaded for his release in vain, but did obtain the doubtful privilege of execution by a private, rather than public, executioner. He was beheaded in the court of the prison Hôtel de Ville, quite recently built, i.e. 'not in the usual place'. *'Delivre à clere peyne'* has two meanings. It means delivered to clear punishment, but also *clere peyne* is declared by some commentators to be the name of the executioner. A typical Nostradamus pun. I have not been able to verify the name. It first appears in a commentary by Jaubert, 1656.

19

Dans le millieu de la forest Myenne,
Sol au lyon la fouldre tombera.
Le grand bastard issu du gran du Maine,
Ce jour fougeres pointe en sang entrera.

In the middle of the Mayenne forest, the Sun in Leo, the lightning will fall. The great bastard born of the great man of Maine, on that day a point will enter the blood of Fougères.

MISTAKEN QUATRAIN

Mayenne in North-western France has a large forest west of the city. Fougères is about twenty miles further west, the seat of a great family bearing the name which died out in the 13th Century. It was used in the 15th Century by Diane de Poitiers, Henri II's mistress, and also by Henri III when he was still Duke of Anjou. No other great families are connected with the house, and the Fougères line was long dead, unfortunately for Nostradamus.

20

De nuict viendra par la forest de Reines,
Deux pars vaultort Herne[1] la pierre blanche,
Le moine noir[2] en gris dedans Varennes
Esleu cap. cause tempeste feu sang tranche.

By night will come through the forest of Reins two partners, by a roundabout way; the Queen, the white stone. The monk-King dressed in grey at Varennes the Elected Capet causes tempest, fire and bloody slicing.

LOUIS XVI's FLIGHT TO VARENNES, 1791

The royal couple, Louis XVI and his wife, Marie Antoinette, escaped by night through the forest of Reins, having fled from

[1]*Herne*—Anagram for *Reine*.
[2]*noir*—Usual anagram for king.

the Tuileries through a secret door in the Queen's apartment. They lost their way and chose an extremely bad route (*vaultort*). The pierre blanche probably refers to the affair of the diamond necklace which demolished Marie Antoinette's fragile popularity with the French people. It may also refer to the fact that her lady in waiting said that the Queen's hair turned white overnight, and that she always wore white dresses. The King was wearing a simple grey suit (perhaps the word monk refers to his earlier impotence), when they entered Varennes. He was a Capet, an elected king, the first France had ever had, and as Nostradamus declares, was the cause of a revolution and the shedding of blood. *Tranche* is the verb meaning to slice, and the sound is particularly apposite in this context of the guillotine. See IX. 34. Saulce.

21

Au temple hault de Blois sacre Solonne,	At night, the high temple of Blois at Sacré Solonne a priest
Nuict pont de Loire, prelat, roi pernicant[1]	on the Loire bridge, a king dying; a messenger, victory
Curseur[2] *victoire aux marestz de la lone*[3]	for the marshes on the water. Destruction for a priestly gift
Dou prelature de blancs à borméant.[4]	from the whites.

Sacré Solonne is the church of Saint Solenne, the Cathedral at Blois. Nostradamus repeats in several quatrains his conviction that France would gain a king from Blois.

22

Roi & sa court au lieu de langue halbe,[5]	The king and his court in the place of the clever tongue, in
Dedans temple vis à vis du palais.	the temple, facing the palace.
Dans le jardin Duc de Mantor & d'Albe,	In the garden the Duke of Mantua and Alba, Alba and
Albe & Mantor poignard langue & palais.	Mantua dagger, tongue and the palace.

[1] *pernicant*—From either Latin, *pernecare* = to kill, or *pernix* = swift.
[2] *curseur*—O.F. = runner, messenger.
[3] *lone*—Provençal, *lona* = a pool, still water.
[4] *borméant*—Latin, *aboriri* = to miscarry. Provençal, *abouriment* = destruction.
[5] *halbe*—O.F., *habler* = to talk a lot.

The key to this quatrain lies in the identities of Mantor and Alba. In 1536 the places of Alba and Mantua had been joined together by Charles V. The ruler from 1550–87 was Gonzaga who did suffer an assassination attempt at Casale, but not at Blois. Also the famous Château de Blois does not face the Cathedral.

23

Puisnay jouant au fresch dessouz la tonne,	The younger son playing outdoors under the arbour, the
Le hault du toict du milieu sur la teste,	top of the roof on the middle of his head. The father king
Le pere roi au temple fait Solonne,	in the Temple is solemn, sacrificing, he will consecrate the
Sacrifiant sacrera fum de feste.	smoke of the feast.

LOUIS XVI AND HIS SON

The younger child is the second son of Louis XVI and his wife who was allowed out to play in the Temple gardens while Louis was imprisoned in a tower away from the rest of his family. Line 3 actually repeats this fact, and we continue on to the King's gloomy future when he will be sacrificed to the Festival of the French Revolution.

24

Sur le palais au rochier¹ des fenestres	At the palace from the balcony of the windows, the two
Seront ravis les deux petits royaux,	little royal ones will be carried off. To pass Orléans, Paris
Passer aurelle² Luthece³ Denis cloistres	and the cloisters of Saint Denis, a nun, the flies devouring the
Nonain, mallods⁴ avaller verts noyaulx.	green pits.

¹rochier—Derived from roche, and in the context of windows probably means a balcony.

²aurelle—Latin, *Aurelianum*, Orléans.

³Luthece—Latin, *Lutetia*, Paris.

⁴mallods?—O.F., *malots* = flies? *malois* = wicked? or Latin, *malum* = an apple?

St Denis was about ten miles from Paris in Nostradamus' age.
All that is clear in this verse is the fact that two young royal
children are kidnapped.

25

Passant les ponts venir pres des rosiers,[1]	Crossing the bridges to come near the Roisiers, sooner than
Tard arrivé plustot qu'il cuidera,[2]	he thought, he arrived late.
Viendront les noves[3] *espaingnolz à Beziers,*	The new Spaniards will come to Béziers, so that this chase
Qui icelle chasse emprinse[4] *cassera.*	will break the enterprise.

Nostradamus' new Spaniards are the interesting point in this
quatrain. Béziers was on the Spanish invasion route about fifty
miles north-east of the pre-1659 border. The river is probably
the one which became the Canal du Midi.

26

Nice sortie sur nom[5] *des letres aspres,*	Departed by the bitter letters the surname of Nice, the great
La grande cappe[6] *fera present non sien,*	Cappe will present something, not his own; Near Vol-
Proche de vultry aux murs de vertes capres	tai at the wall of the green columns, after Piombino the
Apres plombin[7] *le vent à bon essien.*	wind in good earnest.

[1] *rosiers*—Either the place or rosebushes.
[2] *cuiderer*—O.F. = to think.
[3] *noves*—O.F. = new.
[4] *emprinse*—O.F. = enterprise.
[5] *sur nom*—Either surname or 'under the name of'.
[6] *cappe*—Referring to Pope as a Cope, modern French, cape.
[7] *plombin*—Either of Piombino, or leaden, from lead.

27

De bois la garde vent cloz rond pont sera, *Hault le receu frappera le Daulphin,* *Le vieux teccon¹ bois unis passera,* *Passant plus oultre du duc le droit confin.*	The forester, the wind will be close around the bridge, received highly, he will strike the Dauphin. The old craftsman will pass through the woods in a company, going far beyond the right borders of the Duke.

LOUIS XVII

This quatrain may be another confirming the escape of the Dauphin who was reported dead in June 1795. It implies that he is taken out of France, but the method is very obscure. The possible reference to a ball game would be in context with amusing a ten-year-old child. See V. 1.

28

Voille Simacle² port Massiliolique,³ *Dans Venice port marcher aux Panons:* *Partir du goulfre & sinus⁴ Illirique,* *Vast⁵ à Socile, Ligures coups de canons.*	The Allied fleet from the port of Marseilles, in Venice harbour to march against Hungary. To leave from the gulf and the bay of Illyria, devastation in Sicily, for the Ligurians, cannon shot.

This quatrain covers a lot of ground, geographically. We have Panonia, Hungary, Marseilles, and the gulf of Illyria which is the Adriatic sea, but despite so many place names I cannot decipher it.

¹*teccon*—O.F. = a game played with a ball. Possibly from Gk., *tekton*, a craftsman?
²*Simacle*—Gk., *symmachos* = allied with, auxiliary.
³*Massiliolique*—Latin, *Masilioticus* = of Marseilles.
⁴*sinus*—Latin = a bay.
⁵*Vast*—Latin, *vastum* = destruction, devastation.

29

Lors que celui qu'à nul ne donne lieu,	When the man will give away to none, will wish to abandon
Abandonner vouldra lieu prins non prins:	a place taken, yet not taken; Ship afire through the
Feu nef par saignes, bitument¹ à Charlieu,	swamps, bitumen at Charlieu, St Quintin and Calais will be
Seront Quintin Balez² reprins.	recaptured.

CAPTURE OF CALAIS, 1558

The last line of this quatrain is interesting. The fall of Calais to the French was unexpected when the Duke de Guise recaptured it on 6th January 1558. St Quentin was given back to the French in the general settlement of 1559.

30

Au port de P.U.O.L.A. & de saint Nicolas,	At the port of POLA and Saint Nicolo, a Normand will
Perir Normande au goulfre Phanatique,³	punish in the Gulf of Quarnero: Capet to cry alas in the
Cap.⁴ de Bizance raues crier he-las,	streets of Byzantium, help from Cadiz and the great
Secours de Gaddez⁵ & du grand Philipique.	Philip.

All the places mentioned, except Cadiz, are in Yugoslavia. If Philip is intended to be Philip II, Nostradamus was predicting a Franco-Turkish attack on the Hapsburgs in the south, with the Spaniards helping against the French.

¹*bitument*—O.F. = bitumen—a mineral pitch, asphalt.
²*Balez*—Probably anagram for Calais.
³*Phanatique?*—Latin, *Sinus Flanaticus* = the Gulf of Quaerno?
⁴*Cap*—Possible apocope of Capet, the French Royal line?
⁵*Gaddez*—Latin, *Gades* = Cadiz.

31

Le tremblement de terra à Mortara,	The trembling of the earth at Mortara the tin island of St George half sunk; drowsy with peace, war will arise, at Easter in the temple abysses opened.
Cassich[1] saint George[2] à demi perfondrez,	
Paix assoupie, la guerre esveillera,	
Dans temple à Pasques abismes enfondrez.	

The St George islands here seem unlikely to be Great Britain because it is unusual to suffer earthquakes so far outside the earthquake zone, and secondly that an earthquake in Mortara would incur a disturbance of over 1,000 miles from Britain. This one is left for the reader. However, there have been slight earthquakes in Britain in 1978–1980. Possibly the sunken island refers to II. 22?

32

De fin porphire profond collon trouvee	A deep column of fine porphyry is found, inscriptions of the Capitol under the base; bones, twisted hair, the Roman strength tried, the fleet is stirred at the harbour of Mitylene.
Dessoubz la laze[3] escriptz capitolin:[4]	
Os poil retors Romain force prouvee,	
Classe[5] agiter au port de Methelin.	

See also I. 43.

[1]Cassich—probably from Greek Cassiterides, the tin islands, a name given to Cornwall and the Scilly Isles.
[2]saint George—Possibly England, as he was adopted as patron saint in the 14th Century.
[3]laze—Greek = foot or base.
[4]capitolin—Belonging to the Capital of Rome—i.e. Latin.
[5]Classe—Latin, classis = fleet.

33

Hercules Roi de Romme &	Hercules, king of Rome and
d'Annemarc[1]	of 'Annemarc' three times the
De Gaule trois Guion[2] *surnommé*	leader of France to be sur-
Trembler l'Italie & l'unde de	named (de Gaule). Italy will
sainct Marc[3]	tremble and the waters round
Premier sur tous monarque re-	St Mark, the first to be re-
nommé.	nowned over all (the) kings.

Perhaps a reference to General de Gaulle? For Annemarc see also IV. 27. etc: Princess Anne and Mark Phillips?

34

Le part solus mari sera mitré,	The partner, solitary but
Retour conflict passera sur le	married, will be mitred, the
thuille:	return, fighting will cross over
Par cinq cens un trahir sera tiltré,	the Tuileries. By five hundred
Narbon & Saulce par couteaux	one traitor will be ennobled,
avons d'huile.	Narbonne & Saulce, we will
	have oil for knives.

LOUIS XVI AND SAULCE

This is one of the most extraordinary of the quatrains. When Louis XVI and Marie Antoinette were stopped at Varennes (IX. 20) they passed the night at the house of a man named Saulce (line 4). The Sauces (modern spelling) have been chandlers and *marchands-épiciers* there since the 16th Century. The fact that the king alone is mitred refers to Louis' return to the Tuileries on 20th June 1792 when the mob invaded the palace, and the king was forced to wear the revolutionary cap of liberty, which looks very like a mitre. It is thought that *couteaux* in line 4 should be read as *quartants*, which means oil sold in retail, which was exactly what Saulce did. In Thiers' History of France, he states that the mob when they returned (*retour*) to the Tuileries (*thuile*), for a second time, numbered exactly five hundred. A very convincing quatrain. See IX. 20.

---

[1] *Annemarc?* Hungary and Bohemia, Moravia.
[2] *Guion*—O.F. guide, chief, leader.
[3] *Saint Marc*—Venice, of whom he is the patron.

35

Et Ferdinand blonde sera des- *corte,*[1]	And the fair-haired Ferdi- nand will be detached to
Quitter la fleur suivre le Mace- *don.*[2]	abandon the flower and to follow the Macedonian. In
Au grand besoing defaillira sa *routte,*	great need his course will fail him and he will march against
Et marchera contre le Myrmi- *don.*[3]	the Myrmidons.

FERDINAND OF BULGARIA, 20th CENTURY

This may well describe King Ferdinand of Bulgaria with
the Macedonians, Germans and Greeks during the Second
World War.

36

Un grand Roi prins entre les *mains d'un Joine,*	A great king captured by the hands of a young man, not far
Non loing de Pasque confusion *coup cultre:*[4]	from Easter, confusion, a state of the knife. Everlasting cap-
Perpet.[5] *captifs temps que fouldre* *en la husne,*	tives, times when the light- ning is on the top, when three
Lorsque trois freres se blesseront *& meutre.*	brothers will be wounded and murdered.

KENNEDYS?

If this refers to the Kennedys, the theme of three brothers
from America, which runs through the Prophecies, this verse
indicates that the brothers are murdered and that this may
happen around Easter. Since J. F. Kennedy died on 22nd
November 1963 and Robert Kennedy on 6th June 1968, perhaps another assassination may occur around April, with perhaps a storm thrown in, 'the lightning on the top'. Equally the
lightning may refer to a gun on the top of a tall building, as
happened at Dallas in 1963. See I. 26, IV. 14, VIII. 46, 77,
X. 26.

[1]*descorte*—O.F. = detached, in disagreement.
[2]*Macedon*—Nostradamus probably means the Spanish.
[3]*Myrmidon*—Achilles' tribe, renowned for their obedience to all
commands.
[4]*cultre*—Latin, *culter* = a knife.
[5]*Perpet*—Probably apocope. Latin, *Perpetualis* = everlasting.

37

Pont & molins en Decembre ver-
  sez,
En si haut lieu montera la Garonne:
Murs, edifices, Tholose renversez,
Qu'on ne scaura son lieu avant
  matronne.[1]

Bridges and milk overturned
in December, the Garonne
will rise to a very high place.
Walls, buildings, Toulouse
overthrown, so that none will
know his place before Ma-
tronne.

38

L'entree de Blaye par Rochelle
  & l'Anglois,
Passera outre le grand Aemath-
  ein[2]
Non loing d'Agen attendra le
  Gaulois,
Secours Narbonne deceu par en-
  tretien.

The entry at Blaye for la Rochelle and the English, the
great Macedonia will pass beyond; not far from Agen the
Gaul will wait,[3] help from
Narbonne misled by a con-
versation.

39

En Arbissel à Veront[4] & Carcari,
De nuict conduitz pour Savonne
  attraper,
Le vifz Gascon Turbi, & la
  Scerry
Derrier mur vieux & neuf palais
  gripper.

In Albisobla to Veront & Car-
cara, led by night to seize Savona, the swift Gascon, La
Turbie and l'Escarene, to seize
the old and new palace behind the wall.

¹matronne—May well be disguised place name.
²Aemathein—Latin, Emathia = poetic name for Macedonia and
Thessaly.
³will wait—Alternatively, he will wait for the Frenchman...
⁴Veront—Not Verona as other places close to Albisobla; unsolved
place name?

40

Pres de Quintin dans la forest bourlis[1]	Near St Quentin, deceived in the forest, in the Abbey the Flemish will be cut up. The two youngest half-stunned by blows, their followers crushed, and the guard all cut to pieces.
Dans l'abbaye seront Flamens ranches,[2]	
Les deux puisnays de coups mi estourdis	
Suitte oppressee & garde tous aches.	

BATTLE OF ST QUENTIN, 1557

Before the battle of St Quentin in 1557 the Spaniards seized the Abbey of Vermandois: this was followed by the battle on 10th August 1557.

41

Le grand Chyren[3] *soi saisir d'Avignon,*	The great 'Chyren' will be seized from Avignon, from Rome will come honeyed letters full of bitterness. The letter and embassy to leave from Chanignon, Carpentras taken by the Black Duke with the red feather.
De Romme letres en miel plein d'amertume	
Letre ambassade partir de Chanignon,[4]	
Carpentras pris par duc noir rouge plume.	

Henri II is here seen to capture Avignon, which belonged to the Papacy, but unfortunately it did not come into French hands until 1791, although it was twice occupied in 1663–4 and 1768–74. The letters are doubtless from an irate Vatican. Chanignon is still undeciphered. Carpentras is near Avignon and was part of the Pope's lands. See II. 29, VI. 27, 70.

---

[1] *bourlis*—Possibly a proper name or derivative of *boucle* = deceived?
[2] *ranches*—Error for *tranches* in all editions.
[3] *Chyren*—Anagram for Henryc?
[4] *Chanignon*—Unsolved place or proper name.

42

De Barcellonne, de Gennes &
Venise,
De la Secille peste Monet[1] unis,
Contre Barbare classe[2] prendront
la vise
Barbare, pulse bien loing jusqu'à
Thunis.

From Barcelona, from Genoa
and Venice, from Sicily a pestilence allied with Monaco;
they will take aim against the
barbarian fleet, the barbarian
driven as far back as Tunis.

BATTLE OF LEPANTO, 7th OCTOBER 1571

This prophecy was well fulfilled in 1571 when the allied
fleets of the Papacy, Venice and Spain crushed the Turks at
Lepanto. By 1573 Don John of Austria the leader of the expedition went on to recapture Tunis. Much of the Turkish
fleet was composed of ships from their ally the Algerian Bar-
bari, or pirates.

43

Proche à descendre l'armee Cru-
cigere[3]
Sera guettez par les Ismaëlites[4]
De tous cottez batus par nef Ra-
viere[5]
Prompt assaillis de dix galeres
eslites.

Ready to land, the army of the
Cross will be watched for by
the Ishmaelites; struck from
all sides by the ship Raviere,
quickly attacked by ten chosen galleys.

This is probably a continuation of the last quatrain.

[1]*Monet*—Unusual spelling for Monech, Monaco from Latin, *Herculi
Monoeciis.*
[2]*classe*—Latin = fleet.
[3]*Crucigere*—Bearing a cross, a Crusader.
[4]*Ismaëlites*—Biblical name for the Arabs.
[5]*Raviere*—O.F., *raviere* = impetuosity. Nostradamus must be hinting at an unsolved name here.

44

Migres migre de Genesvue trestous,	Leave, leave Geneva everyone, Saturn will change from gold into iron. Those against RAYPOZ will all be exterminated. Before the rush the sky will show signs.
Saturne d'or en fer se changera,	
Le contre RAYPOZ[1] exterminera tous,	
Avant l'a ruent de ciel signes fera.	

Geneva was famous in Nostradamus' time as being the Protestant equivalent of the Vatican because Calvin made it his centre. Nostradamus is either warning the victims of a Calvinist purge, or warning them that they will be attacked by Philip II. Raypoz is another unsolved personal name.

45

Ne sera soul jamais de demander,	There will never be a single person to ask, great Mendosus will attain his Empire. Far from the court he will have countermanded Piedmont, Picardy, Paris, Tuscany the worst.
Grand Mendosus[2] obtiendra son Empire	
Loing de la cour fera contremander	
Pimond, Picard, Paris, Tyrron[3] le pire.	

Mendosus is an anagram for the family of Vendôme, earlier spelt Vendosme, in which case the quatrain should describe either Henri IV, or his father Anthony de Navarre, Duke de Vendosme. Unfortunately despite this excellent lead the rest of the quatrain is very obscure. Piedmont was Italian and belonged to Savoy, Picardy is a Normandy province of France.

---

[1] *RAYPOZ*—An anagram, but not solved except for one suggestion. Zopyre who betrayed Babylon to Darius.

[2] *Mendosus*—Erroneous, or an anagram for Vendosme, the Bourbon branch who won the French throne in 1594.

[3] *Tyrron*—Probably from Latin, *Tyrrheni* = the Etruscans.

46

Vuidez, fuyez de Tholose les rouges	Be gone, flee from Toulouse
Du sacrifice faire expiation,	the red ones, make expiation
Le chef du mal dessouz l'ombre des courges	for the sacrifice. The main cause of evil in the shadow of the gourds, dead, to strangle
Mort estranger carne omination.[1]	the prognostication of flesh.

47

Les soulz signez d'indigne delivrance,	The undersigned to an infamous delivery, and receiving
Et de la multe auront contre advis,	contrary advice from the crowds; a monarch changes,
Change monarque mis en perille pence,[2]	thoughts are put in danger, shut in a cage they will see
Serrez en caige se verront vis à vis.	each other face to face.

Possibly this quatrain can be applied to Francis II, 1559–60?

48

La grand cité d'occean maritime,	The great city of the maritime
Environnee de maretz en cristal:	ocean, surrounded by a swamp
Dans le solstice hyemal[3] *& la prime*[4]	of crystal; in the winter solstice and the spring will be
Sera tempté de vent espouvantal.	tried by a dreadful wind.

This is described by Allen (1943) as the destruction of Central Park, and by Boswell (1941) as the destruction of Tokyo, but by Russian chemical bombs. The latter was almost correct in his own prediction i.e. Nagasaki and Hiroshima 1945.

[1]*carne omination*—Prognostic of flesh.

[2]*pence*—This may either be from *penser*, to think, or if Nostradamus knew some English, pence.

[3]*hyemal*—Latin = *hiemalis*, of winter.

[4]*prime*—O.F., springtime.

49

Gand & Bruceles marcheront contre Envers	Ghent and Brussels march against Antwerp; the Parliament of London will put their king to death; the salt and wine will oppose him; because of them he will have the kingdom in trouble.
Senat du Londres mettront à mort leur Roi	
Le sel & vin lui seront à l'envers,	
Pour eux avoir le regne en dessarroi.	

EXECUTION OF CHARLES I, 1649

This quatrain implies that lines 1 and 2 are simultaneous. Charles I was executed in 1649 new style, or 1648, old style, when New Year's day was held on 25th March. Philip IV made great attempts to reconquer the Netherlands but by 1648 they were anxious to get the Dutch out of the war, and ceded to them several key towns. By doing this, they closed the Scheldt which ruined Antwerp. Note that the quatrain is also numbered 49, the date of King Charles' death, a very fortunate coincidence. See III. 80, VIII. 37, IX. 11.

50

Mandosus tost viendra à son hault regne	Mendosus will soon come to his great reign putting behind somewhat the Nolaris; the pale red one, the man in the interregnum, the frightened young man and the fear of the Barbaric ones.
Mettant arriere un peu de Nolaris:	
Le rouge blaisme, le masle à l'interregne	
Le jeune crainte & frayeur Barbaris.	

HENRI IV

Mendosus as we saw in IX. 45 and X. 18, is an anagram of Vendosme, and Nolaris one of the Lorraine, the home of the Guise family. The quatrain says that Vendosme, Henri IV, will soon come to the throne and relegate the house of Guise to the wings. The '*rouge blesme*' is probably the old Cardinal of Bourbon, pallid from age and red in his Cardinal's robes. He was proclaimed King Charles X in 1589 but died the next year. The '*masle*' is the Duke de Mayenne who was Lieutenant-General during the interregnum. The young man is the Duke de Guise, and Barbaris is Philip II of Spain who claimed the throne of France through his daughter Isabella.

51

Contre les rouges sectes se banderont,	Against the red ones will unite, fire, water, iron, the rope will weaken through peace. Those who plot are at the point of dying except one who above all will ruin the world.
Feu, eau, fer, corde par paix se minera,[1]	
Au point mourir, ceux qui macheront,	
Fors un que monde sur tout ruinera.	

RUSSIAN AND MOSLEM CONFLICT

This quatrain must have a 20th century interpretation. The Reds fit better here in a modern politico-social setting than anywhere else. The one who will eventually rule the world is yet again a reference to the third Antichrist. It is unclear as to which side is victorious, but see the reference to victory on the American side. IV. 95.

52

La paix s'approche d'un costé, & la guerre	Peace approaches from one side; and war never was the pursuit of it so great. Men and women moan, innocent blood on the land, and this will be throughout the whole of France.
Oncques ne feut la poursuitte si grande,	
Plaindre homme, femme, sang innocent par terre	
Et ce fera de France à toute bande.	

PEACE OF CATEAU CHAMBRESIS, 1559

On 13th April 1559, the King of France declared that he would stop fighting the Spanish and turn his attention to liquidating the heretics in France. The peace is between France and Spain, the war the civil war between Catholics and Huguenots, declaring a time of bloodshed for all of France.

[1]*se miner*—O.F. = to ruin, destroy, spoil.

53

Le Neron jeune dans les trois cheminées
Fera de paiges vifs pour ardoir[1] getter,[2]
Hereux qui loing sera de telz menees,
Trois de son sang le feront mort guetter.

In three chimneys the young Nero will make the living pages thrown out to burn. He is happy who will be far from such happenings; three of his family will ambush him to death.

There is one record of a young man being thrown into a fireplace by his prince in the historical novels of Rafael Sabatini; otherwise I can offer no clue.

54

Arrivera au port de Corsibonne,[3]
Pres de Ravenne qui pillera la dame,
En mer profonde legat de la Ullisbonne
Souz roc cachez raviront septante ames.

There will arrive at Porto Corsini, near Ravenna, one who will plunder the lady. The legate from Lisbon in the deep sea; hidden under a rock they will carry off seventy souls.

The Dame here may well be the Catholic Church that is plundered at Porto Corsini, eight miles north of Ravenna.

55

L'horrible guerre qu'en l'occident s'apreste
L'an ensuivant viendra la pestilence,
Si fort horrible que jeune, vieux, ne beste,
Sang, feu, Mercure, Mars, Jupiter en France.

The dreadful war which is prepared in the West, the following year the pestilence will come, so very horrible that young, nor old, nor animal (will survive) blood, fire, Mercury, Mars, Jupiter in France.

[1]*ardoir*—O.F. = to burn.
[2]*getter*—O.F. spelling of *jeter* = to throw.
[3]*Corsibonne* = Porto Corsino, the port of Ravenna.

INFLUENZA EPIDEMIC, 1918

This quatrain is usually applied to the First World War which was followed by the dreadful influenza epidemic of 1917–18, governed by the conjunction of Mercury, Mars and Jupiter.

56

Camp pres de Noudam passera Goussan ville,
Et à Maiotes¹ laissera son en-signe,
Convertira en instant plus de mille,
Cherchant les deux remettre en chaine & legne.²

The army near Noudan will pass Goussainville, and will leave its mark at Maiotes; in an instant more than a thousand will be converted, looking for the two to put back chain and firewood(?).

Houdan and Goussainville are both to the west of Paris. But Maiotes is still unsolved and I cannot find a clear meaning for *legne*.

57

Au lieu de DRUX³ un Roi re-posera,
Et cherchera loi changeant d'Anatheme,
Pendant le ciel si tres fort ton-nera,
Porter neufve Roi tuera soy-mesme.

In the place of DRUX a king will rest, and will look for a law to change Anathema. While the sky thunders so loudly the king will kill himself at the new gate.

58

Au costé gauche à l'endroit de Vitry
Seront guettez les trois rouges de France:
Tous assoumez rouge, noir non murdri
Par les Bretons remis en asseur-ence.

To the left side of the place of Vitry the three red ones of France will be watched. All those killed, red, the black not murdered, in safety reassured by the Bretons.

¹*Maiotes*—Either a place name, Mantes? or from the Greek, *memaotes* = keen soldiers.
²*legne*—Possibly Provençal, *legna* = firewood.
³*DRUX*—Possibly anagram for Dreux?

59

A la Ferté prendra la Vidame
Nicol tenu rouge qu'avoit produit
la vie.
La grand Loisne naistra que fera
clame.[1]
Donnant Bourgongne à Bretons
par envie.

At the Ferté Vidame he will take, Nicol the red who had produced life; to the great Louise who acts secretly one will be born, who gives Burgundy to the Bretons through envy.

60

Conflict Barbar en la Cornere
noire.
Sang espandu trembler la
d'Almatie,
Grand Ismaël[2] mettra son promontoire,
Ranes[3] trembler secours Lusi-
tanie.

In a black head-dress the Barbarian fights, blood shed, Dalmatia trembles. The great Ishmaël will make his promontory, frogs tremble under aid from Portugal.

61

La pille faite à la coste marine,
In cita nova & parents amenez
Plusieurs de Malte par le fait de
Messine,
Estroit serrez seront mal guar-
donnez.

The plunder taken on the sea coast, in the new city and relations brought forward; Several of Malta through the deeds of Messina, will be closely shut up, poorly rewarded.

62

Au grand de Cheramon agora
Seront croisez par ranc tous at-
tachez,
Le pertinax[4] Oppie,[5] & Mandra-
gora,[6]
Rougon[7] d'Octobre le tiers seront
laschez.

To the great one of Cheramon agora will all the crosses by rank be attached, the long lasting Opium and Mandrake, the Rougon will be released on October the third.

[1]clame—Latin, clam = secretly.
[2]Ismaël = An ancestor of the Arab nation, therefore Arabs.
[3]Ranes—Latin, rama = a frog.
[4]pertinax—Latin = long lasting.
[5]Oppie—Greek = opium.
[6]Mandragora—Greek = mandrake.
[7]Rougon—Unsolved place name.

MAGIC PRACTICES?

A very odd verse. Ceramon-agora was actually the name of a town in Asia Minor which is believed to be present-day Usak. Both the herbs of opium and mandrake had mysterious virtues and were used in occult practices.

63

Plainctes & pleurs cris & grands urlemens
Pres de Narbon à Bayonne & en Foix
O quel horrible calamitz changemens,
Avant que Mars revolu quelques fois.

Complaints and tears, cries and great howls, near Narbonne and Bayonne and in Foix; oh what dreadful calamities and changes, before Mars has revolved a few times.

Each revolution of Mars lasts 687 days, which may be relevant if the quatrain is to be taken literally. The rest is obscure.

64

L'Aemathion[1] passer montz Pyrenees,
En Mars Narbon ne fera resistance,
Par mer & terre fera si grand menee
Cap.[2] n'ayant terre seure pour demeurance.

The Aemathian will cross the Pyrenees in March, Narbonne will not make any resistance. He will carry on a very great intrigue by land and sea, Cap. having no land in which to stay safely.

65

Dedans le coing de luna[3] viendra rendre,
Ou sera prins & mis en terre estrange,
Les fruitz immeurs seront à la grand esclandre
Grand vitupere à l'un grande louange.

He will come to take himself to the corner of Luna, where he will be taken and placed on foreign land. The unripe fruit will be the subject of great scandal, great blame, to the other great praise.

[1]*Aemathian*—Either Macedonian or Thessaly as before IX. 38.
[2]*Cap.*—Nostradamus' usual shortening of the Capetian name of the French royal line.
[3]*luna*—Possibly Lunigiana, or even the Moon?

ABORTIVE MISSION OF APOLLO 13

If Luna is to be taken literally as the Moon, this quatrain makes surprising sense. The first astronaut to land on the moon will most certainly be taken and placed on a foreign land, 'taken' in his space capsule. The unripe fruit probably indicates the great trouble, as America had with Apollo 13— the rockets were not functioning properly, and the efforts to return the astronauts to earth were certainly the cause of scandal, blame and praise. It was admitted that the odds of their returning safely were extremely low.

66

Paix, union sera & changement,	There will be peace, union and change, estates and offices (that were) low, (are) high, those high, very low. To prepare for a journey torments the first child; war to cease, legal processes, debates.
Estatz, offices bas hault, & hault bien bas.	
Dresser voyage le fruict premier torment,	
Guerre cesser, civil proces debatz.	

This could apply to any post-war period.

67

Du hault des montz à l'entour de Lizer	From the top of the mountains around Isàere, a hundred assembled at the gate to the Valencian rock; from Châteauneuf, Pierrelatte, in Douzære; against the Crest, Romans assembled in faith.
Port à la roche Valen. cent assemblez	
De chasteau neuf pierre late en donzere	
Contre le crest Romans foi assemblez.	

Crest is probably a shortening of *Chrestiens,* Christians, which makes this obscure verse imply some sort of religious strife.

68

Du mont Aymar[1] sera noble ob- *scurcie,* *Le mal viendra au joinct de sonne* *& rosne.[2]* *Dans bois caichez soldatz jour de* *Lucie,[3]* *Qui ne fut onc un si horrible* *throsne.*	The noble of Mount Aymar will become obscure, the evil will come at the junction of the Saone and the Rhône, soldiers hidden in the woods on Lucy's day, there never was so horrible a throne.

SACK OF LYONS, 13th DECEMBER 1793

Two facts are obvious in this quatrain, Lyons and December the 13th. This is probably describing the sack of Lyons in 1793 which was performed by the Revolutionary soldiers and was a great scandal at the time. Mount Aymar is still unclear.

69

Sur le mont de Bailly & la Bresle[4] *Seront caichez de Grenoble les* *fiers,* *Oultre Lyon, Vien. eulx si grande* *gresle,* *Langoult[5] en terre n'en restera un* *tiers.*	On the mountain of Sain Bel and l'Arbresle will be hidden the proud people of Grenoble. Beyond Lyons, at Vienne there will be such great hail, locust on the land, not a third of it will remain.

70

Harnois trenchant dans les flam- *beaux cachez* *Dedans Lyon le jour du Sacre-* *ment,[6]* *Ceux de Vienne seront trestous* *hachez* *Par les cantons Latins[7] Mascon* *ne ment.*	Sharp armour hidden in the torches at Lyons, on the day of the sacrament; all those of Vienne will be cut to pieces by the Latin cantons, Mâcon does not lie.

[1]*Mont Aymar*—Possibly Montelimart? or by the mountain of slaughter.

[2]Junction of the rivers is at Lyons.

[3]*jour de Lucie*—St Lucy's day, 13th December.

[4]The most likely two combinations.

[5]*Langoult*—O.F., *langouste* = a locust, not a lobster as in modern French.

[6]*jour du Sacrament*—Understood as Corpus Christi, the first Thursday after Trinity Sunday.

[7]*Latins*—Possibly the Grisone where most of the Italian-speaking Swiss live.

71

Au lieux sacrez animaux veu à trixe,[1]	Animals with hair seen at the holy places with one who does not dare (to face) the day; Carcassonne is suitable for the disgrace, and will be left for a longer stay.
Avec celui qui n'osera le jour:	
A Carcassonne pour disgrace propice,	
Sera posé pour plus ample sejour.	

72

Encor seront les saincts temples pollus,	Again the holy temples will be polluted and plundered by the Senate of Toulouse; Saturn having completed two or three cycles in April and May there will be people of a new leaven.
Et expillez par Senat Tholossain,	
Saturne deux trois cicles revollus,	
Dans Avril, Mai, gens de nouveau levain.[2]	

The cycle of Saturn is 29.5 years, so two or three cycles can be added presumably to the date of the sack of Toulouse. Nostradamus appears to think that the Calvinists will take over and despoil the churches. It is possible that line 3 means two × three cycles of Saturn, i.e. six, which would be 177 years, a figure Nostradamus mentions also in the Preface.

73

Dans Foix entrez Roi ceiulee[3] Turbao,	The king enters Foix wearing a blue turban, he will reign for less than a revolution of Saturn; the king with the white turban, his heart banished to Byzantium, Sun, Mars and Mercury near Aquarius.
Et regnera moins revolu Saturne,	
Roi Turban blanc Bisance coeur ban,	
Sol, Mars, Mercure pres la hurne.[4]	

[1] trixe—Greek, thrix = hair or wool, possibly sheep in this context?
[2] levain—i.e. Protestants disputing the Eucharist.
[3] ceiulee—Latin, caeruleus = blue.
[4] hurne—Variant spelling of l'urne, Aquarius.

18 FEBRUARY 1981. POSSIBLE DOWNFALL
OF AYATOLLAH KHOMEINI?

This verse apparently describes a Moslem or Eastern invasion, because of the turbans. Foix is understood to belong to a blue-turbaned man, a king who reigns for less than 29.5 years. He appears to defeat the Ayatollah. See references: II. 2, V. 27, VI. 80. The white figures presumably refer to the white turbans of Islam. However, where this man in the blue turban comes from at the moment remains a mystery. He may be in some way connected with Constantinople (Byzantium). According to McCann (1942) this quatrain is dated by the planets as 18 February 1981. See X. 75.

74

Dans la cité de Fersod[1] homicide,
Fait & fait multe beuf arant ne macter,[2]
Retour encores aux honneurs d'Artemide,
Et à Vulcan corps morts sepulturer.[3]

In the homicidal city of Fertsod, again and again many oxen plough, not sacrificed; again a return to the honours of Artemis, and to Vulcan the corpses of the dead to bury.

75

De l'Ambraxie & du pays de Thrace
Peuple par mer mal & secours Gaulois,
Perpetuelle en Provence la trace,
Avec vestiges de leur coustume & loix.

From Arta & the country of Thrace, people ill by sea, help from the Gauls; in Provence their perpetual trace and remnants of their customs and laws.

This seems to describe the Greeks returning to ask aid from Southern France, and particularly Provence, of which their early colonial settlers were particularly fond.

[1]*Fersod—La Ferté*—Sodom?
[2]*macter*—Latin, *mactare* = to slaughter.
[3]*sepulturer*—O.F., *sepultrer* = to bury.

76

Avec le noir[1] Rapax & sangui-
naire,
Issu du peaultre[2] de l'inhumain
Neron
Emmi[3] deux fleuves main gauche
militaire,
Sera murtri par Joine chaul-
veron.[4]

With the rapacious and bloody king, sprung from the pallet of inhuman Nero; between two rivers, the military on the left hand, he will be murdered by a bald young man.

77

Le regne prins le Roi conujera,[5]
La dame prinse à mort jurez à
sort,
La vie à Roine fils on desniera,
Et la pellix[6] au sort de la consort.

The kingdom taken, the King will plot, the lady taken to death by these sworn by lot; they will refuse life to the Queen's son, and the mistress suffers the same fate as the wife.

FATE OF MARIE ANTOINETTE AND MME. DU BARRY

After the Royal Family's imprisonment, Louis XVI was executed in January 1793. He was condemned by the Convention who elected these powers to itself. However, the Queen, who was not executed until the following October, had a newly created revolutionary tribunal to judge her which was served by a jury selected by lot. This was an institution unknown to France in Nostradamus' day. The third line tells the fate of Louis XVII, whether he died or lived abroad is irrelevant, his kingdom was denied to him. Finally the most interesting line of all. While the Queen was imprisoned in the Conciergerie, the old mistress of Louis XV, Mme. du Barry, was taken for a while to the prison of Sainte Pelagie. An impressive quatrain.

[1] Anagram for *roi*, king, or the black one?
[2] *peaultre* = pallet, brothel, rudder (Laver).
[3] *Emmi*—O.F., = between.
[4] *chaulveron*—Diminutive of *chauve* = bald.
[5] *conujera*—Alternative, will make advances?
[6] *pellix*—Latin = mistress or concubine.

78

La dame Greque de beauté lay-
     dique,[1]
Hereuse faicte de procs innumer-
     able,
Hors translater au regne Hispa-
     nique,
Captive prinse mourir mort mis-
     erable.

The Greek lady of the beauty
of Lais is made happy by in-
numerable suitors; trans-
ferred out to the Spanish
kingdom she is captive taken
to die a wretched death.

It has been suggested that the incomparable lady is in fact
democracy, which was founded in Greece, and which starts to
die out in Europe beginning with Spain in 1936.

79

Le chef de la classe[2] par fraude
     stratageme,
Fera timides sortir de leurs gall-
     eres,
Sortis meutris chef renieur de
     cresme,
Puis par l'embusche lui rendront
     les saleres.

The leader of the fleet through
deceitful trickery will make
the scared ones come out of
their galleys. Come out, murdered, the leader to renounce
the holy oil. Then through an
ambush they give him his de-
serts.

80

Le Duc voudra les siens exter-
     miner
Envoyera les plus forts lieux es-
     tranges,
Par tyrannie Pize & Luc rui-
     nera,
Puis les Barbares sans vin feront
     vendanges.

The Duke will wish to kill his
followers, he will send the
strongest to the strangest
places; through tyranny he
ruins both Pisa and Lucca,
then the Barbarians will harvest grapes without wine.

[1] laydique—Lais was the most beautiful woman in Corinth. Possibly
means ugly from laid?
[2] classe—Latin, classis = fleet.

81

Le Roi rusé entendra ses embusches	The crafty king will understand his ambushes, from three sides the enemies threaten; a large amount of strange tears from the hooded (ones), the splendour of the translator will fail.
De trois quartiers ennemis affaillir,	
Un nombre estranges larmes de coqueluches[1]	
Viendra Lemprin[2] du traducteur faillir.	

Perhaps the translator in this quatrain is the same as in IX. 1, in trouble with the church and the state?

82

Par le deluge & pestilence forte	By the flood and the great plague the great city is assailed for a long time. The sentry and guard killed by hand, suddenly captured, but none wronged.
La cité grande de long temps assiegee,	
La sentinelle & garde de main morte,	
Subite prinse, mais de nul oultragee.	

Another vague, general quatrain; a great city which is suffering from the plague and flooding, is seized by a surprise attack at night.

83

Sol vingt de taurus si fort terre trembler.	The sun in twenty degrees of Taurus, there will be a great earthquake; the great theatre full up will be ruined. Darkness and trouble in the air, on sky and land, when the infidel calls upon God and the Saints.
Le grand theatre rempli ruinera,	
L'air ciel & terre obscurcir & troubler	
Lors l'infidelle Dieu & sainctz voguera.	

[1] *coqueluches* = hooded men, i.e. monks.
[2] *Lemprin*—Greek, *lampros* = splendour.

EARTHQUAKE AFTER 10th MAY,
SAN ANDREAS FAULT?

The day but not the year of this great earthquake is given; such an apocalyptic verse makes one think of the San Andreas Fault. *'Sol vingt de Taurus'* means twenty days after the sun moves into Taurus which is May 10th.

84

Roi exposé parfaira l'hecatombe,
Apres avoir trouvé son origine,
Torrent ouvrir de marbre & plomb
*   la tombe*
D'un grand Romain d'enseigne
*   Medusine.*[1]

The king discovered will complete the slaughter once he has found his origin; a torrent to open the tomb of marble and lead, of a great Roman with the Medusine device.

TOMB OF ST PETER

Yet another verse about the discovery of a tomb. The key lies in the word Medusine. If it is an anagram of "Deus in me," this would mean it was the real tomb of St Peter, as that was his emblem, and that the one which was declared to be found some years ago is of another early Pope.

85

Passer Guienne, Languedoc &
*   le Rosne,*
D'Agen tenans de Marmande &
*   la Roole,*
D'ouvrir par foi parroi[2] *Phocen*[3]
*   tiendra son trosne*
Conflit aupres saint Pol de Mau-
*   seole.*[4]

To pass Guienne, Languedoc and the Rhône from Agen, holding Marmande and La Réole; to open the wall through the king, Marseilles will hold its throne a battle near St Paul-de-Mausole.

---

[1]*Medusine*—Device of Medusa? Device of Pegasus? Device of 'Deus in me'?
[2]*parroi*—Possibly *parroi* = wall?
[3]*Phocen* = Marseilles.
[4]*St Paul de Mausole*—A convent, then an asylum (where Van Gogh stayed) just outside St Rémy.

86

Du bourg Lareyne ne parvien-dront droit à Chartres *Et feront pres du pont Anthoni panse,*[1] *Sept pour la paix cautelleux comme martres.* *Feront entree d'armee à Paris clause.*	From Bourge-la-Reine they will not come straight to Chartres, they will pause near the Pont d'Anthony; seven as crafty as martens for peace they will enter with weapons into a closed Paris.

3rd JULY 1815

The seven allied nations who joined against Napoleon were Austria, England, Prussia, Portugal, Sweden, Spain and Russia, they entered Paris on 3rd July 1815. The city was stripped of its troops when the French army was evacuated to Chartres taking up positions on the way to the Loire, passing Bourge-la-Reine and the Pont d'Anthony under which it is reputed to have camped.

87

Par la forest du Touphon[2] *essar-tee,* *Par hermitage sera posé le temple,* *Le duc d'Estampes par sa ruse inventee,* *Du mont Lehori prelat donra ex-emple.*	In the cleared forest of Touphon the temple will be placed near the hermitage. The Duke of Étampes through the ruse he invented will give an example to the priest of Montlhery.

The clue to this verse probably lies in the title in line 3. Three of the kings of France's greatest mistresses held the title, first Anne de Pisseleu, then Diane de Poitiers, and later Henri IV's Gabrielle d'Estrées. I cannot get any further with this.

---

[1]*panse*—Should be *pause* to rhyme with line 4.
[2]*Touphon*—Doubtful. There is a place called Forfou but it has no forest. Possibly from the Gk., *tophion* = a plaster quarry, or French, *touffe* = a clump.

88

Calais, Arras secours à Ther-
oanne,
Paix & semblant simulera les-
coutte,[1]
Soulde[2] *d'Alabrox*[3] *descendre par*
Roane
Destornay peuple qui deffera le
routte.[4]

Calais & Arras help to Thérou-
anne, the spy will simulate
peace and semblance; the soldiers of Savoy go down by
Roanne; those people who
would stop the rout turned
away.

1557

This quatrain must be dated 1557 since Calais fell to the French in 1558. Both Arras and Théronanne belonged to Spain. When Calais fell, Philip II, husband of the English Queen, lost all rights to Calais. On 5th February 1556 the Treaty of Vaucelles was declared between France and Spain. Therefore this quatrain was probably written between the Truce and the Spanish attack of 1557. Savoy (Allobrox) was almost completely French occupied at this period, so it is possible that a garrison of soldiers was sent up after St Quentin. The borders of Savoy were only thirty-five miles from Rouanne.

89

Sept ans sera Philip. fortune
prospere,
Rabaissera des Arabes l'effaict,
Puis son midi[5] *perplex rebours*
affaire
Jeune ognion[6] *abismera son fort.*

Fortune will favour Philip for
seven years, he will cut down
again the exertions of the Arabs. Then, in the middle a
perplexing, contrary affair,
young Ogmios will destroy his
stronghold.

LOUIS PHILIPPE, 1830–48

The first seven years of Louis Philip's reign, 1830–8 were extremely fortunate. He managed to subdue the Arabs and

[1]*l'escoute*—O.F. = a spy.
[2]*soulde*—O.F. = pay or mercenaries.
[3]*Allobrox* = classical inhabitants of Savoy.
[4]*routte*—Either O.F., *route* = rout; or route—road?
[5]*son midi*—Either in middle age, or to the South?
[6]*ogmios*—The Celtic Hercules.

consolidate the French occupation of Algeria. In the middle
of his reign, 1838–40, he will be troubled by the Eastern question and the result will be shameful for him. Finally the French
proclaiming the new republic, 24th February 1848, will de-
throne him and keep him under guard.

90

Un capitaine de la grand Ger-
manie
Se viendra rendre par simulé se-
cours
Un roi des rois aide de Pan-
nonie,[1]
Que sa revolte fera de sang grand
cours.

A captain of the greater Germany will come to deliver
false help, king of kings; to
support Hungary; His war
will cause a great shedding of
blood.

HITLER

The Greater Germany sounds uncannily like the Grossen-
deutschland of Hitler's Third Reich. The second line is brilliant. Hitler invaded Poland under the pretence of giving help,
as Nostradamus says elsewhere. Hitler for a time was a king
of kings, lord of all he surveyed. He also captured Hungary
and the war he started killed about 14 million people among
the soldiers of both sides, and according to some estimates as
many again among the civilian population, and quite probably
more. See I. 34, II. 24, III. 35, 53, 58, 61, IV. 40, 68, V. 29,
94, VI. 7, 49, 51.

91

L'horrible peste Perynte[2] *& Ni-*
copolle,[3]
Le Chersonnez[4] *tiendra & Mar-*
celoyne,[5]
La Thessalie vastera l'Amphipolle,[6]
Mal incogneu & le refus
d'Anthoine.

The dreadful plague at Perinthus and Nicopolis will take
the Peninsula and Mace-
donia; it will lay waste Thessaly and Amphipolis, an unknown evil, and refused by
Anthony.

[1]*Panonie*—Classical Hungary.
[2]*Perinthe*—Modern Eski Eregli.
[3]*Nicopolle*—Modern Prevesa.
[4]*Chersonnez*—Either the Gallipoli peninsular (Chersonese) or the
Poloponnesus.
[5]*Marceloyne*—Probably error for Macedoine.
[6]*Amphipolle*—Near modern Salonika.

The Anthony here may be Anthony of Navarre, father of Henri IV, but the setting of the quatrain in Greece makes this unlikely.

92

Le roi vouldra dans cité neuf entrer
Par ennemis expugner[1] lon viendra
Captif libere faulx dire & perpetrer
Roi dehors estre, loin d'ennemis tiendra.

The king will want to enter the new city, they come to subdue it through its enemies; a captive falsely freed to speak and act; the king to be outside, he will stay far from the enemy.

NEW YORK?

This may refer to New York, as in I. 87, VI. 97 and X. 89, and continue the three quatrains describing the city being attacked during the next war. This is a logical possibility which must be futuristic as it has not occurred to date. The king far from the enemy is probably the President in some secret underground shelter from which he will continue to direct the war. See X. 49.

93

Les ennemis du fort bien eslongnez,
Par chariots conduict le bastion,
Par sur les murs de Bourges esgrongnez,
Quand Hercules battra l'Haemathion.[2]

The enemies are very far from the strong man, the bastion is brought by wagons. Above the crumbled walls of Bourges when Hercules strikes the Macedonian.

LOUIS XIV

This quatrain tells that when Aemathion, who can here stand for Louis XIV, has pushed back his enemies and consequently enlarged the borders of France, bastions of earth were constructed in the fortification system of Vauban. At this time Bourges falls into decay when its Grosse Tour (great tower) fell into ruin during Louis' reign. The final line refers

[1]expugner—Latin, expugnare = to subdue, capture, storm, violate etc.

[2]Haemathion—As Aemathion, Macedonian or from Thessaly.

to a labour of Hercules, which was in this case the lengthy Languedoc canal. Started in 1666 and finished in 1681 at a cost of 34,000,000 francs it was the wonder of the times. It also freed the French from dependency on the Western area of the Mediterranean and became their equivalent of the Pillars of Hercules, i.e. Gibraltar.

94

Foibles galleres seront unies ensemble,
Ennemis faux le plus fort en rampart:
Faible assaillies Vratislaue tremble,
Lubecq & Mysne tiendront barbare part.

Weak galleys will be joined together, the false enemy is strongest on the ramparts. Bratislava trembles, the weak attacked, Lubeck & Meissen will take the Barbarian's side.

95

Le nouveau faict[1] conduira l'exercite,[2]
Proche apamé[3] jusques au pres du rivage,
Tendant secour de Milannoile[4] eslite,
Duc yeux privé à Milan fer de cage.

The new fact will lead the army, almost cut off as far as to the river bank, holding for help from the Milanese élite; the Duke loses his eyes in an iron cage in Milan.

Milan belonged to the Hapsburgs until 1859. A lot of commentators equate the last line with Mussolini but the quatrain is really too general.

[1]Or the newly made one?
[2]*exercitus*—Latin = army.
[3]*apamé*—Greek, *apamao* = to cut off.
[4]Almost certainly means Milanese.

96

Dans cité entrer excercit[1] desniee,
Duc entrera par persuasion,
Aux foibles portes clam[2] armee
*   amenee,*
Mettront feu, mort de sang ef-
*   fusion.*

The army denied entry to the city, the Duke will enter through persuasion; secretly the army led to the weak gates, they put it to fire, death and flowing of blood.

97

De mer copies[3] en trois parts div-
*   isees,*
A la seconde les vivres failliront,
Desesperez cherchant champs
*   Helisees,*
Premier en breche entrez victoire
*   auront.*

The forces at sea divided into three parts, the second one will run out of supplies; in despair looking for the Elysian Fields, the first entering the breach will have victory.

Here are two battles; we start with a naval one and end up on land. Apart from the fact that the Elysian Fields were the Greek heaven, I cannot decipher this muddled quatrain.

98

Les affligez par faute d'un seul
*   taint,*
Contremenant[4] à partie opposite,
Au Lygonnois mandera que con-
*   traint*
Seront de rendre le grand chef de
*   Molite.[5]*

Those afflicted through the fault of a single infected one, the transgressor will be in the opposite party. He will send to the Lyonnais and compel that they should be given up to the great leader of Molite.

---

[1] *exercite*—Latin, *exercitus* = army.
[2] *clam*—Latin = secretly.
[3] *copies*—Latin, *copia* = troops, army.
[4] *Contremenant*—Error for *contrevenant*.
[5] *Molite?*—either from Melita, Malta, or Greek, *molos* = war?

99

Vent Aquilon fera partir le siege, *Par murs gerer cendres, chauls,* * & pousiere,* *Par pluie apres qui leur fera bien* * piege,*[1] *Dernier secours encontre leur* * frontiere.*	The north wind will cause the siege to be raised, to throw over the walls cinders, lime and dust; afterwards through rain which does them much harm, the last help is met at their frontier.

RETREAT FROM MOSCOW?

If Aquilon is a synonym for North, most commentators take this as describing Napoleon's retreat from Moscow. He finds help only at the frontiers of his empire having lost so many men on the expedition (the rain and snow which does them much harm).

100

Navalle pugne[2] *nuit sera su-* * peree,*[3] *Le feu aux naves*[4] *à l'Occident* * ruine:* *Rubriche neufue la grand nef* * coloree,* *Ire à vaincu, & victoire en bruine.*	A naval battle will be overcome at night. Fire in the ruined ships of the West, a new coding the great coloured ship, anger to the vanquished and victory in a mist.

PEARL HARBOR, 1941

Pearl Harbor was attacked in the very early morning by the Japanese planes. The great tankers were set alight to the ruin of America, the West. I think 'the new coding' of line 3 is the formula for this new type of attack which finally brings anger to a defeated Japan and hazy glimpses of victory to a stunned America. The 'colour' of the ship probably refers to camouflage.

---

[1] *piege*—Provençal, *piegi* = worse, harmful.
[2] *pugne*—Latin, *pugna* = battle.
[3] *superee*—Latin, *superatus* = overcome.
[4] *naves*—Latin = ships.

CENTURY X

1	France. Vichy Régime
2	
3	
4	Battle of Worcester, 1651
5	
6	9th September 1557
7	
8	15th June 1856
9	
10	Napoleon
11	
12	Sudden Death of Pope
13	
14	
15	
16	Louis XVIII
17	Madame Royale, 1787–99
18	Henri of Navarre
19	Elizabeth of England?
20	Italy and Common Market
21	
22	Abdication of Edward VIII, 1936
23	Louis XVIII
24	The Hundred Days, 1815
25	
26	Death of Robert Kennedy. Britain and Common Market
27	
28	
29	
30	
31	
32	
33	

437

1

A l'ennemy l'ennemy foi promise
Ne se tiendra les captifs retenus:
Prins preme[1] mort & le reste en
chemise,
Damné le reste pour estre sous-
tenus.

To the enemy, the enemy faith promised will not be kept, the captives retained; one is taken near to death and the rest in their shirts, the rest damned for being support-ers.

FRANCE—VICHY RÉGIME

This is usually read as a general quatrain about the Vichy régime, when the Germans failed to make collaboration a two-way proposition to the French people.

2

Voille gallere voil de nef cachera,
La grande classe[2] viendra sortir
la moindre.
Dix naves[3] proches le tourneront
poulser,
Grande vaincue unis à foi joindre.

The ships sail will hide the sailing galley, the great fleet will cause the lesser one to go out. Nearby ten ships will turn to drive it back, the great one conquered united to join in faith.

There seems possibly to be a connection between this quatrain and IX. 100. It describes a naval battle with ships either camouflaged or hidden by a smoke screen. The great one who is conquered may then refer to the USA who joins the Allies after Pearl Harbor. Alternatively it may apply to one of the many actions in the Mediterranean 1940–1943.

3

En apres cinq troupeau ne mettra
hors un
Fuytif pour Penelon[4] l'aschera,
Faulx murmurer secours venir
par lors,
Le chief le siege lois habandon-
nera.

After the fifth will not put out a flock, a fugitive will be turned loose for Penelon. Falsely to murmur, then to come in aid then the chief will abandon the siege.

[1] *preme*—O.F. = next, close near.
[2] *classe*—Latin, *classis* = fleet.
[3] *naves*—Latin, *navis* = ship.
[4] *Penelon?*—Possibly an anagram for Polone, Poland?

The key word in this quatrain is Penelon which is not definitely deciphered, see footnote, page 440.

4

Sus la minuict conducteur de l'armee
Se saulvera, subit evanoui,
Sept ans apres la fame non blasmee
A son retour ne dira oncq oui.

At midnight the leader of the army will run away, suddenly disappeared. Seven years later, his reputation unblemished, to his return 'yes' will not once be said (i.e. many times).

BATTLE OF WORCESTER, 1651

After his defeat at the Battle of Worcester, Charles II fled to France via Scotland, in disguise. His usurper Cromwell actually reigned for seven years, and Charles was restored in 1560. It is a general quatrain but can be applied to these events quite accurately.

5

Albi & Castres feront nouvelle ligue,
Neuf Arriens[1] Lisbons & Portugues,
Carcas, Tholosse consumeront leur brigue
Quand chef neuf monstre de Lauragues.

Albi & Castres will make a new alliance, nine Arians Lisbon and the Portuguese; Carcassonne, Toulouse will join their intrigue when a new chief is the monster from the Lauragues.

The new Arians are the interesting subject here. Unfortunately it is most likely that Nostradamus was reverting to the Crusade (1208–13) of the Albigensians. Alternatively could the New Arians be the Russians who have invaded Afghanistan?

[1]*Arriens* = (*a*) The 13th Century heretics. (*b*) People now dwelling in Afghanistan.

6

Sardon¹ Nemans si hault desbor-
  deront,
Qu'on cuidera² Ducalion re-
  naistre,
Dans le collosse la plus part fui-
  ront,
Vesta sepulchre feu estaint ap-
  paroistre.

The Gardon will flood Nîmes
so high that they will think
Ducalion has been reborn. In
the colossus the greater part
will flee, Vesta's fire appears
extinguished in the tomb.

9th SEPTEMBER 1557

According to Jaubert a storm broke out at Nîmes in 1557
which lasted from 5 a.m. to 9 p.m., and this combined with a
flood from the Gardon. Apparently many antiquities were revealed when the flood waters withdrew. Menard's History of
Lyons confirms the flood as 1 p.m. to 9 p.m. but does not
mention the Gardon.

7

Le grand conflit qu'on appreste
  à Nancy,
L'aemathien dira tout je soub-
  metz,
L'isle Britanne par vin, sel, en
  solci,
Hem. mi deux Phi. long temps ne
  tiendra Metz.

The great fight that they prepare at Nancy, Aemathien
will say I subjugate all; the
British Isles through wine and
salt are in trouble, Hem. mi
Philip two, Metz will not hold
for long.

The reference to wine and salt connects this quatrain in some
manner to England, see IX. 49. But I am not happy with any
of the ingenious comments to date. It seems more probable
that '*deux Phi.*' refers to Philip II attacking French-occupied
Lorraine. Metz was finally ceded in 1648 but was in French
control from 1552, in which case Nostradamus is only stating
a known fact. Nancy was handed back to its Duke in 1661
having been occupied for twenty-seven years.

¹*Sardon*—Error for Gardon.
²*cuidera*—O.F. = To think, believe.

8

Index & poulse parfondera[1] le
  front
De Senegalia le Conte à son filz
  propre
Les Myrnarmee[2] par plusieurs de
  prinfront
Trois dans sept jours blesses mors.

With index finger and thumb
he will wet the forehead, the
Count of Senigallia to his own
son, through several, Venus
in short order, three are
wounded to death in seven
days.

15th JUNE 1856

On this date the Prince Imperial, son of Napoleon III, was
baptized. His godfather was Pope Pius IX who was the son of
Count Mastoi Ferretti of Senigallia. Venus is interpreted as
the Empress Eugenie but line 4 is still unexplained.

9

De Castillion figuires jour de
  brune,
De fame infame naistra souver-
  ain prince.
Surnon de chausses perhume lui
  posthume,
Onc Roi ne faut si pire en sa
  province.

In the Castle of Figueras on
a misty day a sovereign prince
will be born of an unworthy
woman. The surname of
Chausses on the ground will
make him posthumous, never
was a king so bad in his province.

See X. 11 for this verse. Loomis suggests this verse describes
one of Nostradamus' Antichrists.

10

Tasche de murdre enormes ad-
  ulteres,
Grand ennemi de tout le genre
  humain
Que sera pire qu'ayeulx, oncles ne
  peres
En, fer, feu, eau, sanguin & inhumain.

Stained with murder and
enormous adulteries, great
enemy of all mankind, he will
be worse than his ancestors,
uncles and fathers, in steel,
fire and water, bloody and inhuman.

[1]perfundere   Latin = to sprinkle, moisten.
[2]Mimnermia—A surname of Venus.

NAPOLEON

The epithet of line 2 was applied to Napoleon Bonaparte by the Venetian ambassador, Morenigo.

11

Dessouz lonchere du dangereux passage
Fera passer le posthume sa bande,
Les monts Pyrens passer hors son bagaige
De Perpignam courira duc à tende.

In the dangerous passage underneath Junquera, the posthumous one will cross his men. To cross the Pyrenean mountains without his baggage the duke will hasten to Perpignan from Tende.

This obscure verse seems to be related to X. 9, particularly the reference to the posthumous child.

12

Esleu en Pape, d'esleu sera mocqué,
Subit soudain esmeu prompt & timide,
Par trop bon doulz à mourir provocqué,
Crainte estainte la nuit de sa mort guide.

Elected as Pope, he will be mocked when elected, suddenly and unexpectedly moved, prompt and timid: caused to die through too much goodness and kindness he will fear for the guide killed on the night of his death.

SUDDEN DEATH OF POPE

This is normally applied to the Cardinal Santa Severina who was elected Pope Gregory XIV, but died two months later in 1591, the election being declared illegal. However his successor Innocent IX also died in under two months, and John Paul I died within less than a month from suspected poisoning in 1979.

13

Soulz pa pasture d'animaux rum-
  inant[1]
Par eux conduicts au ventre her-
  bipolique[2]
Soldatz caichez les armes bruit
  menant,
Non loing temptez de cité Anti-
  polique.

Beneath the food of ruminat-
ing animals, led by them into
the centre of the food place;
soldiers hidden, their weapons being noise, tried not far
from the city of Antibes.

14

Urnel Vaucile[3] sans conseil de soi
  mesmes
Hardit timide par crainte prins
  vaincu,
Accompaigné de plusieurs pu-
  tains blesmes
A Barcellonne aux chartreux
  convaincu.

'Urnel Vaucile' without a plan
of his own, bold, timid for
fear of being taken and captured; accompanied by several pale whores converted in
the Carthusian convent at
Barcelona.

The interpretation here depends on the *Urnel Vaucile* line,
which has no connections to date with the monastery at de
Urgel, near Llanos to the town of the same name. The Carthusian monastery mentioned is that of Mont Allegro.

15

Pere duc vieux d'ans & de soif
  chargé,
Au jour extreme filz desniant les
  guiere[4]
Dedans le puis vif mort viendra
  plongé,
Senat au fil[5] la mort longue &
  legiere.

The father duke old in years
and troubled with thirst, on
the last day his son denying
him the jug: into the well
plunged alive he will become
dead: the Senate to the son a
death long and light.

[1]i.e. under a load of hay.
[2]Into the market place?
[3]*Urnel Vaucile?*—Llanos de Urgel? Plain of Urgel?
[4]*guiere*—Mod. French, *aiguiere* = jug.
[5]*fil*—Probably should read *filz* = son.

A son is hanged for giving his thirsty father an excess of water, by putting him down the well. Impossible to place this quatrain.

16

Heureux au regne de France, heureux de vie	Happy in the kingdom of France, happy in life, igno-
Ignorant sang mort fureur & rapine,	rant of blood, death, anger and rage. By a flattering name
Par nom flateurs seras mis en envie,	he will be envied, a king robbed, too much faith in the
Roi desrobé trop de foi en cuisine.[1]	kitchen.

LOUIS XVIII

When he is happily re-established on the French throne, Louis XVIII will not die a violent death but lives happily. He was given the name of Louis le Desiré (line 3). His guilt will lie in the fact that he does not sufficiently occupy himself with the public good, and that he is a renowned glutton.

17

La roine Ergaste[2] voiant sa fille blesme,	The barren queen, seeing her pale daughter because of un-
Par un regret dans l'estomac encloz,	happiness locked up in her stomach. Lamentable cries will
Cris lamentables seront lors d'Angoulesme,	then come from Angoulême and the marriage to the cousin
Et au germain mariage fort clos.	greatly impeded.

MADAME ROYALE, 1787–99

The *Roine Ergaste* is a queen confined to the manual labour found in any penitentiary. When imprisoned in the Temple Marie Antoinette was compelled to sew her own clothes. The adjective can also mean captive, which indeed the Queen was

[1] i.e. in his servants.
[2] *Ergaste*—Latin, *Ergastulus* = penitentiary?

She sees her daughter, Madame Royale, pale with the family misfortunes. Madame Royal was betrothed to the Duke of Angoulême in 1787, and married him in 1799. It is suggested that her childless marriage '*l'estomac enclos*' was due to her sufferings with her family in the Temple.

18

Le ranc Lorrain fera place à Vendosme,	The house of Lorraine will make way for Vendôme, the high put low and the low exalted. The son of Hamon will be elected in Rome, and the two great ones will be put at a loss.
Le huult mis bas & le bas mis en hault,	
Le filz d'Hamon[1] sera esleu dans Rome,	
Et les deux grands seront mis en deffault.	

HENRI DE NAVARRE

This is a very successful prophecy for Nostradamus. Henri IV, Duke of Vendôme, will eclipse the house of Lorraine, and earlier known as '*le petit Béarnais*' will be elevated to the high rank of king of France. This son of Hamon, i.e. heretic, will be accepted as King in Rome. The two great ones who lose out on this are the two Pretenders, the Duke de Guise and the Duke de Mayenne.

19

Jour que sera par roine saluee	The day she will be saluted as queen, the prayer the day after the blessing. The account is right and valid, once humble, there was never a woman so proud.
Le jour apres le salut, la priere,	
Le compte fait raison & valbuee,[2]	
Par avant humbles oncques ne feut si fiere.	

Suggested as applying to Elizabeth I of England when she succeeded to her sister, the childless Mary Tudor.

[1]*Hamon*—Mamon in some editions.
[2]*valbuee*—Unsolved word. *Valable* is suggested as an alternative?

20

Tous les amis qu'auront tenu parti,	All of the friends who have belonged to the party, put to
Pour rude en lettres mis mort & saccagé,	death and looked for the uncouth letters. The public possessions, the great one anni-
Biens publiez par sixe grand neanti,[1]	hilated by six, never were the
Onc Romain peuple ne feut tant outragé.	Roman people so wronged.

ITALY AND COMMON MARKET

This quatrain probably applies to the troubles caused to the Italians by the Common Market Policy when it consisted only of the seven original members.

21

Par le despit du Roi soustenant moindre,	Through the king's spite in supporting the lesser one, he
Sera meurdri lui presentant les bagues,	will be murdered presenting the jewels to him. The father
Le pere au filz voulant noblesse poindre	wishing to impress his son with nobility did what the
Fait comme à Perse jadis feirent les Mague.	Magi once used to do in Persia.

22

Pour ne vouloir consentir au divorce,	For not wanting to consent to the divorce, which then after-
Qui puis apres sera cogneu indigne,	wards will be recognized as unworthy, the King of the is-
Le Roi des Isles sera chassé par force	lands will be forced to flee, and one put in his place who
Mis à son lieu que de roi n'aura signe.	has no sign of kingship.

ABDICATION OF EDWARD VIII, 1936.
10th DECEMBER
Edward VIII's abdication was not popular among the Brit-

[1] *neantir*—to annihilate. *Neanti,* adj.—annihilated.

ish people, who had little love for Mrs. Simpson. Edward was therefore forced to leave Britain because of her social standing, 'cogneu indigne'. Finally George VI, who was not in line for the kingship is forced to accede to the throne. See also X. 40.

23

Au peuple ingrat faictes les remonstrances,
Par lors l'armee se saisira d'Antibe,
Dans l'arc Monech feront les
  doleances
Et à Frejus l'un l'autre prendra
  ribe.[1]

Remonstrances are made to the ungrateful people, then the army will seize Antibes. In the arch of Monaco the complaints will occur, and at Fréjus the shore will be taken by one from the other.

LOUIS XVIII

When Louis XVIII issued a proclamation urging fidelity to the new régime the only place that remained loyal to Napoleon was Antibes. Both Louis and Napoleon used Fréjus; the former to embark for England, the latter when embarking for Elba.

24

Le captif prince aux Italles vaincu
Passera Gennes par mer jusqu'à
  Marseille,
Par grand effort des forens[2] sur-
  vaincu
Sauf coup de feu barril liqueur
  d'abeille.

The captive prince conquered in Italy will cross from Genoa to Marseilles by sea; by a great effort the foreigners will be overcome except for a gun shot, a barrel of bees' honey.

THE HUNDRED DAYS, 1815

This quatrain must be linked with IV. 26 in which Napoleon's emblem of bees also appears. Napoleon, a closely guarded prisoner on Elba, escapes by sea in March and lands at Cannes, near Marseilles. He is overcome again at Waterloo, where he seeks death in vain, and the bees of his emblem spill all their sweetness.

[1]ribe—Provençal riba = bank, shore.
[2]forens—O.F. = foreigner, stranger.

25

Par Nebro ouvrir de Brisanne¹ passage,	Through the Ebro will be opened a passage to Brissane far away the Tago will make a demonstration. The outrage will be committed in Pelligoux, of the great lady sitting in the orchestra.
Bien eslongnez el tago fara muestra,	
Dans Pelligouxe² sera commis l'outrage	
De la grand dame assise sur l'orchestra.	

26

Le successeur vengera son beau frere,	The successor will avenge his handsome brother and occupy the realm under the shadow of vengeance, he, killed, the obstacle of the blameworthy dead, his blood; for a long time Britain will hold with France.
Occupera regne souz umbre de vengeance,	
Occis ostacle son sang mort vitupere,	
Long temps Bretaigne tiendra avec la France.	

DEATH OF SECOND KENNEDY BROTHER. BRITAIN AND COMMON MARKET

The quatrain seems to indicate that Robert Kennedy will die following the death of his handsome brother, J. F. Kennedy. It is interesting to note that Nostradamus foresees two brothers killed within a short period of time. Robert Kennedy's stand in the name of his dead brother does him no good. One wonders what it will bring to Edward Kennedy. See I. 26, VIII. 46, 77, IX. 36.

27

Par le cinquieme & un grand Hercules,	Through the fifth and a great Hercules they will come to open the temple with the hand of war; one Clement, Julius and Ascans put back, the sword, the key, the eagle never once felt so great a dislike.
Viendront le temple ouvrir de main bellique,	
Un Clement, Iule & Ascans recules,	
Lespe, clef, aigle n'eurent onc si grand picque.	

¹*Brisanne*—Unsolved place name.
²*Pelligouxe*—Unsolved place name.

28

Second & tiers qui font prime musicque	Second and third make first class music they will be sub-
Sera par Roi en honneur subli-mee,	limely honoured by the king: Through fat and thin, even
Par grasse & maigre presque demi eticque	half emaciated, to be made debased by the false report of
Raport de Venus faulx rendra deprimee.	Venus.

29

De Pol MANSOL dans caverne caprine[1]	In the great cave of Saint Paul de MAUSOLE, hidden and
Caché & prins extrait hors par la barbe,	seized, pulled out by the beard, the captive led like a mastiff
Captif mené comme beste mastine	animal, by the people of Bi-
Par Begourdans amenee pres de Tarbe.	gorre brought near to Tarbes.

St Paul de Mausole is just outside Nostradamus' birthplace of St Rémy. The quatrain seems to describe the capture of a goat, or goatboy, who is taken to Bigorre in Navarre.

30

Nepueu & sang du sainct nou-veau venu,	Nephew and of the blood of the newly created saint,
Par le surnom soustient arcs & couvert	through his surname he will sustain the arches and the
Seront chassez mis à mort chassez nu,	roof. They will be driven out naked and chased to their
En rouge & noir convertiront leur vert.	deaths, their green will be converted to red and black.

[1]caprine—Latin adjective = appertaining to goats.

31

Le saint Empire viendra en Germanie
Ismaelites[1] trouveront lieux ouverts.
Anes vouldront aussi la Carmanie,[2]
Les soustenens de terre tous couverts.

The Holy Empire will come to Germany, the Arabs will find open places; the asses will also want Carmania, the supporters completely covered with earth.

32

Le grand empire chacun an devoir estre
Un sur les autres le viendra obtenir,
Mais peu de temps sera son regne & estre,
Deux ans aux naves se pourra soustenir.

The empire each year should become great. One will come to hold (power) over all the others. But his kingdom and life will last a short time. In two years he will be able to maintain himself in his ships.

33

La faction cruelle à robbe longue,
Viendra cacher souz les pointus poignars
Saisir Florence le duc & lieu diphlongue[3]
Sa descouverte par immeaurs & flangnards.[4]

The cruel party with long robes will hide sharp daggers underneath. The Duke to seize Florence and the place of two words. Its discovery through young ones and flatterers.

---

[1]*Ismaelites*—Not Jews but Arabs, who claim descent from Ishmaël, son of Abraham.

[2]*Carmanie*—Either the Persian province at the entrance to the Persian Gulf, or an unsolved anagram.

[3]*diphlongue*—Erratum for *diphtongue* = double word.

[4]*flangnards*—Provençal = flatterer or wheedler.

34

Gaulois qu'empire par guerre oc- *cupera* *Par son beau frere mineur sera* *trahi,* *Par cheval rude voltigiant trai-* *nera,* *Du fait le frere long temps sera* *haï.*	The Gaul who gains his em- pire through war will be be- trayed by his younger brother- in-law. He will be dragged by an untrained nervous horse, for the act the brother will be hated for a long time.

NAPOLEON AND THE KING OF NAPLES

The King of Naples, Joachim Murat, married Napoleon's younger sister Caroline. He first betrayed Napoleon in 1814, but sided with him in 1815. He was also a renowned cavalry leader. Apparently, according to Robb (1942) this quatrain converted the eminent Professor Jacques Barzun of Columbia University, and Professor Siceloff, who stated that the chances of this quatrain being fulfilled were 'about zero'.

35

Puisnay royal flagrand d'ardent *libide,* *Pour se jouir de cousine ger-* *maine,* *Habit de femme au temple* *d'Arthemide:* *Allant murdri par incognu du* *Marne.*	The younger son of a king flagrant with burning lust to enjoy his first cousin. Women's attire in the temple of Diana going to be murdered by the unknown man from Marne.

The last line suggests that a Duke of Mayenne or Maine will be involved in a royal scandal but unfortunately, though a probable situation, it does not seem to tie in with anything specific.

36

Apres le Roi du soucq guerres parlant,	After the king (of the stump?) speaks of wars, the United Island will despise him. For several years the good one gnaws and pillages, through tyranny on the island its values change.
L'isle Harmotique[1] le tiendra à mespris,	
Quelques ans bons rongeant un & pillant	
Par tyrranie à l'isle changeant pris.[2]	

The United Island may well be the British Isles, bringing the date to after 1603. Line 3 probably describes the privateers of the late 16th Century and early 17th Century, such as Drake, Hawkins and Raleigh. But it is difficult to interpret the adjective *'de soucq'* as applying to James I, he did not limp.

37

L'assemblee grande pres du lac de Borget,	The great crowd near to the lake of Le Bourget, they will rally near to Montmelian, going further ahead the thoughtful ones draw up a plan, Chambery, St Julian de Maurienne, fight.
Se ralieront pres de Montmelian,	
Marchans plus oultre pensifz feront proget	
Chambry, Moraine combat sainct Julian.	

38

Amour alegre non loing pose le siege,	'Light of love' will not hold the siege for long, for the converted barbarian will be all the garrisons; the Ursins and Adria give security for the French, for fear of the army being handed over to the Grisons.
Au sainct barbar seront les garnisons,	
Ursins[1] Hadrie pour Galois feront plaige,	
Pour peur rendus de l'armee du Grisons.[3]	

[1]*Harmotique*—Dubious probably from Greek, *armoskitos* = joined together, fitting together?

[2]*pris*—Mod. French, *prix.* = prize, worth.

[3]*Grisons* = The people of South-east Switzerland.

HENRI OF NAVARRE

Henri's usual nickname among his contemporaries was 'Vert Galant', which is very close to Nostradamus' *'armour allegre'*. During the Siege of Paris, 1590, Henri could not hold the siege for longer than four complete months, because of the advance of the Duke of Parma from Flanders. Nostradamus describes the city garrison as devoted to things converted and barbarous, by which he means the clerical revolutionaries. Henri also changed his religion to get the French throne. The last two lines are unclear.

39

Premier fils veufve malheureux mariage,	The first son, a widow, an unfortunate marriage without any children: two Islands thrown into discord. Before eighteen years of age, a minor: of the other even lower will be the betrothal.
Sans nuls enfans deux Isles en discorde,	
Avant dixhuict incompetant eage,	
De l'autre pres plus bas sera l'accord.	

MARY QUEEN OF SCOTS AND FRANCIS II

This is one of Nostradamus' notoriously successful quatrains, and appears to have been understood by the French Court of the time. Francis II, the eldest son of the widowed Catherine de' Medici, married Mary Stuart, an unfortunate marriage which was childless. Because of Mary's return to Scotland she caused discord between England and her own country. Francis was still not quite eighteen years old when he died (seventeen years, ten months, fifteen days). His younger brother Charles IX was betrothed to Elizabeth of Austria when only eleven years old. This quatrain is quite astonishingly accurate. See I. 86, X. 55.

40

Le jeune nay au regne Britannique,	The young born to the realm of Britain, which his dying father had commended to him. Once he is dead, London will dispute with him, and the kingdom will be demanded back from the son.
Qu'aura le pere mourant recommandé,	
Icelui mort LONOLE¹ donra topique,	
Et à son fils le regne demandé.	

¹*Lonole*—Probably erratum for *Londres* = London.

ABDICATION OF EDWARD VIII, 1936

This refers back to X. 22. Edward VIII is the true heir to the British throne which was left to him by his dying father. But he will cause scandal (*topique*) in London by his behaviour with Mrs. Simpson, and public hostility towards her earlier divorce caused the King to abdicate, the kingdom taken back from him by the people and given to his brother.

41

En la frontiere de Caussade & *Charlus,*	On the boundary of Caussade and Caylus, not very far from
Non guieres loing du fonds de la *vallee,*	the depths of the valley, music from Villefranche to the sound
De ville Franche musique à son *de luths;*	of lutes, surrounded by cymbals and a great (deal) of
Environnez combouls[1] *& grand* *mytee.*[2]	stringed (instruments).

All the places mentioned are small villages within fifty miles of Agen where Nostradamus once lived. Perhaps here he is just describing a festival he witnessed?

42

Le regne humain d'Anglique gen- *iture,*	The human reign of English offspring will cause the king-
Fera son regne paix union tenir,	dom to remain united in peace. Half captured in his
Captive guerre demi de sa clos- *ture,*	enclosure in the war, for a long time peace will be main-
Long temps la paix leur fera *maintenir.*	tained by them.

PAX BRITANNICA

This is a general but very apt quatrain, which describes Britain and the Pax Britannica of the 19th Century, or possibly the long peace England enjoyed under Walpole and the early Georges. The first is more acceptable because of England's vast influence in the 19th Century.

---

[1]*combouls*—Greek, *kumbalon* = cymbal.
[2]*mytee*—Dubious, possibly from *mitos* = a stringed instrument?

43

Le trop bon temps trop de bonté royalle:	Too much of good times and too much royal bounty, made
Fais & deffais prompt subit negligence,	and quickly undone by sudden negligence. He will lightly
Legier croira faux despouse loyalle,	believe false his loyal wife whom in his benevolence he
Lui mis à mort par sa benevolence.	puts to death.

LOUIS XVI

Louis XVI was put to death because he did not bother to apply himself properly to affairs of state. The weakness and irresolution of character that he displayed, and the great ease with which he believed reports that his wife, Marie Antoinette was involved, other than thoughtless, in the affair of the Diamond Necklace, all these, plus his kindness, left him defenceless before the Revolutionaries.

44

Par lors qu'un Roi sera contre les siens,	Where a king is (chosen) against his people a native of
Natif de Blois subjugera Ligures:	Blois will subdue the League.
Mammel,[1] Cordube & les Dalmatiens,	Mammel, Cordoba and the Dalmatians; of the seven then
Des sept puis l'ombre à Roi estrennes[2] & lemurs.[3]	a shadow to the King, new money and dead ghosts.

HENRI III

See VIII. 38 and 52 which also discuss a king from Blois. It probably refers to Henri III of France who will subjugate the League (line 2). He was descended from the Court of Blois and Nostradamus elsewhere calls him *'le grand du Blois'*. The seven in the final line is yet another reference to the seven children of Catherine de' Medici.

[1]*Mammel*—Unsolved place name; perhaps Mamel, in the Baltic?
[2]*estrennes* = Handsel, earned money.
[3]*lemurs*—Latin, *lemures* = spirits of the dead.

45

L'ombre du Regne de Navarre non vrai, *Fera la vie de fort illegitime:* *La veu promis incertain de Cambrai* *Roi Orleans donra mur legitime.*	The shadow of the kingdom of Navarre is not true, it will make the life of a strong man illegal. The uncertain vow promised at Cambrai,[1] the king at Orléans will give a lawful boundary (wall).

HENRI IV OF NAVARRE

Henri of Navarre has still only a shadow of a kingdom since he has not yet gained true possession of France. He did lead an irregular life with many mistresses, including the wife of Balagny, the governor of Cambrai, to whom Henri gave in return the hereditary possession of the town (line 3). Orléans may represent here either the family or the town.

46

Vie sort mort de L'OR vilaine indigne, *Sera de Saxe non nouveau electeur:* *De Brunsuic mandra d'amour signe,* *Faux le rendant aux peuple seducteur.*	Because of the GOLD, the life, fate and death of an unworthy, sordid man: he will not be the new Elector of Saxony. From Brunswick he will send for a sign of love, the false seducer giving it to the people.

This quatrain appears to be set in Germany, and to state that Saxony will not have a new Elector. Maurice did not enter the fight against Charles V until 1552 while the Duchy of Brunswick played no significant role in the 16th Century, so maybe this quatrain is reasonably accurate.

---

[1]*Cambrai*—A reference to the Peace of Cambrai 1529 when the French gave up their claims to Flanders.

47

De Bourze ville à la dame Guir-
lande,
L'on mettra¹ sus par la trahison
faicte,
Le grand prelat de Leon par For-
mande,²
Faux pellerins & ravisseurs de-
faicte.

In the town of Burgos, to the Garland lady they will give the verdict on the treason committed; the great prelate of Leon through Formande, undone by false pilgrims and thieves.

48

Du plus profound de l'Espaigne
enseigne,
Sortant du bout & des fins de
l'Europe,
Troubles passant aupres du pont
de Laigne,
Sera deffaicte par bandes sa grand
troppe.

Banners from the furthest corners of Spain, coming from the ends and borders of Europe. Trouble passing near the bridge of Laigne, its great army will be routed by bands (of men).

SPANISH CIVIL WAR FOLLOWED BY WORLD WAR II

The first lines describe well enough the Spanish Civil War and the involvement of the Germans and Italians. Nostradamus sees this trouble growing, i.e. the Second World War, until it is stretched all over Europe. Laignes a town forty odd miles north-west of Dijon was occupied by the Germans. It is interesting to note that Nostradamus sees the occupying army as being routed by its enemies, the Allied Forces, as it was in 1944 and 1945.

49

Jardin du monde au pres de cité
neufve,
Dans le chemin des montaignes
cavees,
Sera saisi & plongé dans la
Cuve,
Beauvant par force eaux soulfre
envenimees.

Garden of the world near the New City, in the road of the hollow mountains. It will be seized and plunged in the tank, forced to drink water poisoned with sulphur.

¹*mettra*—Literally, impose a verdict, place.
²*Formande*—Formentera, the Balearic island?

THREE MILE ISLAND. 1979

This is a fascinating quatrain containing the idea of a water supply being poisoned. The *cité neufve* is New York, as usual. Harrisburg, Pennsylvania, where the disastrous leak of nuclear water occurred in 1979 is only 180 miles away, 'The garden of the world near New City'. The road of hollow mountains is interesting. Could that be the nearest Nostradamus could get to describing a city of skyscrapers? The tank is obviously the poisoned water at Harrisburg. See I. 87, IX. 92.

50

La Meuse au jour terre de Luxembourg,
Descouvrira Saturn & trois en lurne,
Montaigne & pleine ville, cité & bourg,
Lorraine deluge trahison par grand hurne.

By day, the Meuse in the land of Luxembourg, will find Saturn and three in Aquarius; mountain and plain, town, city and borough; flood in Lorraine betrayed by the great urn.

51

Des lieux plus bas du pays de Lorraine,
Seront des basses Allemaignes unis,
Par ceux du siege Picards, Normans, du Maisne,
Et aux cantons ce seront reunis.

Some of the lowest places in the county of Lorraine will be united with the lower Germanies. Through the people of the seats of Picardy, Normandy and Maine, they will be reunited to the cantons.

FRANCE AND GERMANY, 1871

Lorraine and the regions to the South (*plus bas*) such as Alsace, were united to Lower Germany with the consent of those defeated in the Siege of Paris in 1871, the people of France, Picards, Normans and from Maine. All those areas suffered German occupation. Lorraine was not returned to France until 1919.

52

Au Lieu[1] où LAYE & Scelde se
  marient,
Seront les nopces de longtemps
  maniees,
Au lieu d'Anvers où la crappe[2]
  charient[3]
Jeune viellesse consorte intami-
  nee.

At the place where the LAYE
and the Scheldt join the marriage will be arranged a long
time ago. At the place in Antwerp where the chaff is carried a young undefiled wife,
and old age.

An obscure marriage between a very young girl and an old
suitor which takes place at Ghent.

53

Les trois pellices de loing
  s'entrebatron,
La plus grand moindgre demeu-
  rera à l'escoute:
Le grand Selin n'en fera plus
  patron,
Le nommera feu pelte blanche
  routte.

Three prostitutes will quarrel
for a long time; the greatest
will remain to hear the least.
The great Selin will no longer
be her patron, she will call
him fire, shield, a white rout.

If Selim does refer to Henri II here this would describe his
many royal mistresses, presumably rivals to Diane de Poitiers,
such as Gabrielle d'Estrées. I imagine 'white rout' is intended
to mean a lily-livered coward!

54

Nee en ce monde par concubine
  fertive,
A deux hault mise par les tristes
  nouvelles,
Entre ennemis sera prinse captive,
Et amené à Malings & Bruxelles.

Born into this world of a furtive concubine, at two raised
high by the bad news. She will
be taken captive among enemies and brought to Malines
and Brussels.

[1]lieu—Ghent.
[2]crappe—O.F. = chaff.
[3]charier—O.F. = to carry, to cast about.

55

Les malheureuses nopces celebreront,	The unfortunate marriage will be celebrated with great joy, but the end is unhappy. The mother will despise the daughter-in-law Mary, the Apollo dead and the daughter-in-law more pitiful.
En grand joye, mais la fin malheureuse:	
Mary & mere nore desdaigneront,	
Le Phybe mort & nore plus piteuse.	

FRANCIS II AND MARY QUEEN OF SCOTS, 1558–60

The word Mary is spelt with a *y* in the original, and this makes it likely to refer to Mary Queen of Scots and her unhappy wedding, see X. 39. Catherine de' Medici disliked Mary intensely and the latter called the Queen Mother 'a merchant's daughter'. The strange word Phybe may well mean Francis II, Mary's husband, if one takes the first syllable (*Phy*) (*phi*) for F. and the *be* for beta, second letter of the alphabet, thus F II, Francis II. They married in 1558 and Francis died in 1560. See I. 86, X. 39.

56

Prelat royal son baissant trop tiré,	The royal priest bowing too low, a great flow of blood will come out of his mouth. The Anglican reign, a realm breathing, for a long time dead as a stump, living in Tunis.
Grand fleux de sang sortira par sa bouche,	
Le reign Anglique par regne respiré,	
Long temps mort vif en Tunis comme souche.	

57

Le soublevé ne cognoistra son sceptre,	The uplifted one will not know his sceptre, he will disgrace the young children of the greatest ones. There was never so filthy and cruel a being, for their wives, the king will banish them to death.
Les enfants jeunes des plus grands honnira:	
Oncques ne fut un plus ord[1] cruel estre,	
Pour leurs espouses à mort noir[2] bannira.	

---

[1]*ord*—O.F. = filth.
[2]*noir*—Usual Nostradamus anagram for king.

58

Au temps du dueil que le felin monarque,	At a time of mourning the feline monarch will make war

Au temps du dueil que le felin
    monarque,
Guerroiera le jeune Aemathien:
Gaule bansler perecliter la bar-
    que¹
Tenter Phossens² au Ponant en-
    tretien.

At a time of mourning the feline monarch will make war with the young Aemathien. France to shake, the bark will be in danger, Marseilles to be tried, a talk in the West.

LOUIS XIV

Aemathien, the child of the dawn, that is the sun, must refer here to Louis XIV who adopted the sun as his device and was also called the Sun King. When there is a time of mourning for Louis XIII, the wily monarch, Philip IV of Spain, will go to war against Aemathien. France is shaken by the civil war of the Fronde, and the bark of the Papacy is threatened by the development of Jansenism. Phossen is Marseilles, which Louis XIV entered by breaching the walls in 1660. A year earlier he went to the West of France (Ponant means Occident) and on the island of Bidussoa concluded the peace of the Pyrenees and his marriage with the Infanta Maria Theresa. The island is still called l'Isle de la Conférence.

59

Dedans Lyons vingt cinq d'une
    alaine,
Cinq citoyens Germains, Bres-
    sans, Latins,
Par dessous noble conduiront
    longue traine,
Et descouverts par abbois les ma-
    stins.

In Lyons, twenty-five of the same breath, five citizens, Germans, Bressans, Latins, under a noble they will lead a long train and are discovered by the barking of the mastiffs.

1560

In September 1560 five citizens from Lyons and twenty others, including some German Protestants, entered into a conspiracy to hand over the city to the Huguenots. It was suspected at the time that the main people behind the plot were the Prince de Condé and the Vidame de Chartres. It was discovered in time by the guards.

¹la barque—the Papacy, bark of St. Peter.
²Phossens = Phoceans, founders of Marseilles.

60

Je pleure Nisse, Mannego, Pize,
    Gennes,
Savone, Sienne, Capue, Modene,
    Malte:
Le dessus sang & glaive par es-
    trennes,
Feu, tremblera terre, eau, mal-
    heureuse nolte.[1]

I weep for Nice, Monaco,
Pisa, Genoa, Savona, Siena,
Capua, Modena and Malta.
The blood and sword above
for a gift, fire, the earth will
tremble, water, an unhappy
reluctance.

61

Betta,[2] Vienne, Emorre,[3] Sacarb-
    ance,[4]
Voudront livrer au Barbares
    Pannone:
Par picque & feu, enorme viol-
    ance,
Les conjurez descouvers par ma-
    trone.

Betta, Vienna, Emorre, Sapron, they will want to deliver
Hungary to the Barbarians;
great violence through pike
and fire, the conspirators discovered by a matron.

This quatrain appears to be linked with the following ones, X.
62 and 63, but they are all very obscure.

62

Pres de Sorbin pour affaillir On-
    grie,
L'herault de Bude les viendra
    advertir:
Chef Bizantin, Sallon de Sclav-
    onie,
A loi d'Arabes les viendra con-
    vertir.

Near Sorbia in order to assail
Hungary, the herald of Brudes
will come to warn them. The
Byzantine chief, Salona of
Slavonia, he will come to con-
vert them to Arab law.

---

[1]nolte—Probably from Latin, nonvoluntas = unwilling.
[2]Betta—Possibly Baetis, the Guadalquivir River?
[3]Emorre—Uncertain place name.
[4]Sacarbance—Latin, Scarbantia = modern Sapron.

63

Cydron,[1] *Raguse,*[2] *la cité au sainct Hieron.*[3]	Cydonia, Ragusa, the city holy to Hieron, the healing help
Reverdira le medicant succours,	will make it green again, the
Mort fils de Roi par mort de deux heron,[4]	king's son dead because of the death of two heroes, Arabia
L'Arabe Ongrie feront un mesme cours.	and Hungary will take the same steps.

64

Pleure Milan, pleure Luques, Florance,	Weep Milan, weep Lucca and Florence, when your great
Que ton grand Duc sur le char montera,	Duke climbs into the chariot. To change the seat it ad-
Changer le siege pres de Venise s'advance,	vances close to Venice when at Rome the Colonnas will
Lors que Colomne[5] *à Rome changera:*	change.

ITALY 19th CENTURY

When the Grand Duke left Italy, Austria abandoned the province of Venetia to Napoleon III, who gave it in turn to Victor Emmanuel. Florence became the latter's new capital until the seat of all Italian government was moved to Rome, when the temporal powers of the Papacy declined.

65

O vaste Romone ta ruine s'approche,	O great Rome your ruin draws near, not of your walls but of
Non de tes murs de ton sang & substance;	your blood and substance; the harsh one in letters will make
L'aspre par lettres fera si horrible coche,	so horrid a notch, pointed steel wounding all up to the
Fer poinctu mis à tous jusques au manche.	sleeve.

[1]*Cydron*—Now modern Canea.
[2]*Raguse*—Now Dubrovnik.
[3]*Hieron*—Dubious personal name?
[4]*heron*—Mostly regarded as a false rhyme for heroes.
[5]*Colonne*—A great Roman family, the Colonnas.

66

Le chef de Londres par regne l'Americh,	The London premier through American power will burden
L'isle de l'Escosse tempiera par gellee:	the island of Scotland with a cold thing. Reb the King will
Roi Reb auront un si faux antechrist	have so dreadful an antichrist who will bring them all into
Que les mettra trestous dans la meslee.	the troubles.

POLARIS IN SCOTLAND AND USA

A most interesting quatrain. The Premier of London at the time specified was Harold Macmillan who had a good relationship with America. It was during his office that Scotland was burdened with the cold thing (the Polaris submarines). Roi Reb sounds strange but links this even firmly with another antichrist to come who will lead all of them, i.e. Britain and USA into trouble. It has been suggested to me by various interested parties that Reb stands for Nixon. This would make a great deal of sense of the Watergate affair.

67

Le tremblement si fort au mois de May,	A very great trembling in the month of May, Saturn in Ca-
Saturne, Caper, Jupiter, Mercure au beuf:	pricorn, Jupiter and Mercury in Taurus. Venus also in Can-
Venus aussi Cancer, Mars, en Nonnay,[1]	cer, Mars in Virgo, then hail will fall greater than an egg.
Tombera gresse lors plus grosse qu'un euf.	

The accumulation of planets in the zodiac here referred to is apparently very rare, but all it predicts here is an earthquake in May and a great fall of hail. The dates are April 1929 or May 3755.

[1]*Nonnay* = Virgo, as *nonnay* comes from *Noone,* or *Nonnain* a nun, or virgin.

68

L'armee de mer devant cité tiendra
Puis partir sans faire longue alee,
Citoyens grande proie en terre prendra,
Retourner classe,[1] reprendre grand emblee.[2]

The army of the sea will stand before the city then depart without making a long passage. A great prey of citizens will be taken on land, the fleet returns to seize (by) great robbery.

69

Le fait luisant de neuf vieux esleué
Seront si grand par midi aquilon,
De sa seur propre grande alles[3] levé.
Fuyant meurdri au buisson d'ambellon.[4]

The shining deed of the new old one exalted, will be so great in the south and north. Raised by his own sister great crowds arise, fleeing is murdered in the bushes at Ambellon.

70

L'oeil par object ferra telle excroissance,
Tant & ardente que tumbera la neige,
Champ arrousé viendra en descroissance,
Que le primat succumbera à Rege.

Because of an object the eye will swell so much, burning so greatly that the snow will fall. The watered fields will start to shrink when the Primate dies at Reggio.

71

La terre & l'air gelleront si grand eau,
Lors qu'on viendra pour jeudi venerer,
Ce qui sera jamais ne feut si beau,
Des quatre pars le viendront honnorer.

The earth and air will freeze so much water when they come to venerate on Thursdays. He who will come will never be as fair as the few partners who come to honour him.

---

[1]*classe*—Latin, *classis* = a fleet.
[2]*emblee*—O.F. = robbery or thieving.
[3]*alles*—O.F. = trip, speed, crowd.
[4]*ambellon*—Dubious, possibly village of Ambel?

USA?

This is interesting in that the Christian Sabbath is Sunday, for Jews it is Saturday, and for Muslims, Friday. Could Thursday possibly refer to the United States unique tradition of Thanksgiving, which is held on a Thursday? See I. 50 who had *Jeudi pour sa feste* . . . ? An unknown quantity.

72

L'an mil neuf cens nonante neuf sept mois,	In the year 1999, and seven months, from the sky will
Du ciel viendra un grand Roi deffraieur.	come the great King of Terror. He will bring back to life
Resusciter le grand Roi d'Angolmois.[1]	the great king of the Mongols.
Avant que Mars regner par bon heur.	Before and after War reigns happily.

WAR IN 1999—THIRD ANTICHRIST

In this gloomy prediction Nostradamus seems to foresee the end of the world at the Millennium, the year 2000. He was greatly influenced in this by medieval thinking which held all millenniums in great dread. From the verse it appears that first we must suffer the Asian antichrist 'the King of Mongols' before the advent of this new and terrifying figure. Note that Nostradamus expects war both before and after his coming. Professor Hideo Itokawa of Japan who runs a team of computer experts was quoted in an article in the *Guardian* newspaper on 26 February, 1980, saying that until he had seen my documentary film on Nostradamus he had never heard of him, but that their conclusions came to the same thing. It adds up to a nagging sense of insecurity about the closing years of this century. The Third Antichrist will be rampant at this time. Nostradamus expects war both before and after this period. See V. 50, VI. 33, X. 74, 75.

73

Le temps present avecques le passé	The present time together
Sera jugé par grand Jovialiste,	with the past will be judged
Le monde tard lui sera lassé,	by the great man of Jupiter.
Et desloyal par le clergé juriste.	Too late will the world be tired of him and disloyal through the oathtaking clergy.

[1]*Angolmois*—Not Angoumois in Western France but the anagram of the O.F., *Mongolois*.

By *Jovialiste* Nostradamus means a follower of Jupiter, and, by extension, a pagan. The quatrain has been applied to both Rabelais and Voltaire, but was probably intended as a dig at Calvin, Nostradamus' arch enemy.

74

An revolu du grand nombre septiesme	The year of the great seventh number accomplished, it will appear at the time of the games of slaughter, not far from the age of the great millennium, when the dead will come out of their graves.
Apparoistra au temps Jeux d'Hecatombe,	
Non esloigné du grand eage milliesme	
Que les entres sortiront de leur tombe.	

OLYMPIC GAMES

This is a slightly ambiguous quatrain. It could refer to the last Olympic Games and the slaughter of the Israeli athletes in 1976, or the 'year of the great seventh number being accomplished', could mean 1984—in which case great troubles and slaughter will occur. 1984 is certainly not far from the age of the Great Millennium. Nostradamus does specifically refer to games which makes the Olympics seem the most likely target. They are already causing a great deal of international dissension.

75

Tant attendu ne reviendra jamais	Long awaited he will never return in Europe, he will appear in Asia; One of the league issued from great Hermes, he will grow above all other powers in the Orient.
Dedans l'Europe, en Asie apparoistra	
Un de la ligue islu du grand Hermes,	
Et sur tous rois des orientz croistra.	

RULE OF ISLAM 1980s

In Hermetic terms Hermes stands for Mercury and Jupiter which equals Islam. Christ was technically an European but the new Antichrist who rules all the Orient will come from Asia. Is this the man in the blue turban who will overturn the Ayatollah? See II. 2, V. 27, VI. 80, IX. 73, X. 72.

76

Le grand senat discernera la pompe	The great Senate will see the parade for one who afterwards will be driven out, vanquished. His adherents will be there at the sound of a trumpet, their possessions for sale, the enemies driven out.
A l'un qu'apres sera vaincu chassé,	
Ses adherans seront à son de trompe,	
Biens publiez ennemis deschassez.	

NIXON

This seems a quite specific description of Nixon and the Watergate bandwagon. The Senate will dismiss him, as indeed they did, and many of his ex-colleagues sold their memoirs to great profit, 'possessions for sale'. Nixon has now almost reaccomplished social acceptability, 'his enemies driven out'.

77

Trente adherens de l'ordre des quiretres[1]	Thirty members of the order of Quirities, banished, their belongings given to their bold adversaries. All their good actions will be taken as wrong, the fleet scattered, delivered up to the Corsairs.
Bannis leurs biens donnez ses adversaires,	
Tous leurs bienfais seront pour desmerites	
Classe[2] *espargie*[3] *delivrez aux corsaires.*	

ITALY/RUSSIA, 1945

This is usually accepted as referring to post-Fascist Italy, and the corsairs are then understood to be the Russians, who received a large part of the Italian navy.

78

Subite joie en subite tristesse	Sudden joy into sudden sadness will beat Rome for the graces embraced; Mourning, cries, tears, weeping, blood, excellent rejoicing, contrary bands surprised and trussed up.
Sera à Romme aux graces embrassees.	
Deuil, cris, pleurs, larm, sang excellant liesse	
Contraires bandes surprinses & troussees.	

[1] *quiretres* = (*a*) Roman citizens in their civil capacity. (*b*) Low Latin, renowned warriors.
[2] *classe*—Latin, *classis* = a fleet.
[3] *espargie*—O.F., *espargier* = to sprinkle, dispense.

79

Les vieux chemins seront tous embelis,	The old roads will all be improved, they will go to (a place) similar (to) Memphis. The great Mercury of Hercules' fleur de lis, will cause land, sea and country to tremble.
Lon passera à Memphis somentrée,[1]	
Le grand Mercure d'Hercules fleur de lis	
Faisant trembler terre, mer & contree.	

80

Au regne grand du grand regne regnant	In the kingdom of the great one reigning with a great rule by force of arms he will cause to be opened the great gates of brass; the king and duke allied the port demolished, the ship (sunk) to the bottom and a serene day.
Par force d'armes les grands portes d'airain	
Fera ouvrir le roi & duc joignant,	
Port demoli nef à fons jour serain.	

81

Mis tresor temple citadins Hesperiques	Treasure is placed in a temple by Western citizens withdrawn therein to a secret place, the temple to open by hungry bonds, recaptured, ravished, a terrible prey in the midst.
Dans icelui retiré en secret lieu,	
Le temple ouvrir les liens fameliques.	
Reprens ravis proie horrible au milieu.	

AMERICAN OR SPANISH WEALTH?

During the 16th Century gold poured into Spain from her possessions in the New World. Could Nostradamus be taken literally in this case, that a great amount of treasure is hidden in some Spanish Cathedral? However, problems arise with line 3. How can a bond be hungry? It has been suggested that this is an imaginative description of economic crisis in the United States (Hesperiques' other meaning) to be followed by a riot at Fort Knox, the greatest gold hoard in the world.

[1]*somentrée*—From Greek, *symmetros* = like, resembling.

82

Cris, pleurs, larmes viendront avec coteaux	With the knives will come cries, tears and weeping, seeming to flee they will make a final assault around the parks they will set up high platforms, the living pushed back and murdered instantly.
Semblant fouir donront dernier assault.	
Lentour parques planter profons plateaux,	
Vifs repoulsez & meurdris de prinsault.[1]	

83

De batailler ne sera donné signe,	The signal will not be given to fight, they will be obliged to go out of the park; the banner around Ghent will be recognized, he who will put all his followers to death.
Du parc seront contraint de sortir hors,	
De Gand lentour sera cogneu l'ensigne,	
Qui fera mettre de tous les siens à mors.	

84

La naturelle à si hault hault non bas	The illegitimate girl so high, high not low, the late return will make the grieved ones contented. The Reconciled one will not be without disputes by employing and wasting all his time.
Le tard retour fera martis contens,	
Le Recloing[2] ne sera sans debatz	
En empliant & pendant tous son temps.	

ELIZABETH I

Some people regard line 1 as describing Elizabeth Tudor whom Pope Paul IV declared to be a bastard through the illegality of her mother's marriage. She was considered to be one also by most English Catholics.

---

[1] de prinsault—O.F. = firstly, at once, immediately, etc.

[2] Recloing—Dubious. Possibly derived from Latin, recolligo = to regain, be reconciled?

85

Le vieil tribung au point de la trehemide	The old tribune on the point of trembling will be pressed
Sera pressee captif ne deslivrer,	not to give up the captive.
Le vieil tribung au point de la trehemide	The old, not old speaking timidly of the evil to free his
Par legitime à ses amis livrer.	friends in a lawful manner.

FRANCE, 1940–3

This quatrain has been mentioned as a general description of France around 1940–1 when Marshal Pétain was negotiating with the Germans about prisoners of war who were being used as slave labour.

86

Comme un griphon viendra le roi d'Europe	The king of Europe will come like a griffon, accompanied
Accompaigné de ceux d'Aquilon,	by those of the North; he will
De rouges & blancz conduira grand troppe	lead a great troop of red and white, they will go against the
Et iront contre le roi de Babilon.[1]	king of Babylon.

ALLIED FORCES, 1815

The King of Europe was the Allied Forces which marched against Napoleon, the king of Egypt, before he was made first Consul. The great army of red and white uniforms are the tunics of the English and the Austrians. The English may well be described as from the North, as also Russia.

87

Grand roi viendra prendre port pres de Nisse	A great king will come to anchor near Nice, the death of
Le grand empire de la mort si enfera	the great empire is thus accomplished. He will place his
Aux Antipolles posera son genisse,	heifer in Antibes, plunder at sea, all will vanish.
Par mer la Pille tout esvanoira.	

[1]*Babylon*—In medieval texts the King of Egypt is often called the King of Babylon.

88

Piedz & Cheval à la seconde veille	Foot and horse at the second watch, they will make an entry laying waste all at sea. He will enter the port of Marseilles, tears, cries and blood, never a time so bitter.
Feront entree vastient tour par la mer,	
Dedans la poil¹ entrera de Marseille,	
Pleurs, cris, & sang onc nul temps si amer.	

89

De brique en marbre seront les murs reduits	The walls will change from brick to marble, seventy-five peaceful years. Joy to people, the aqueduct reopened, health, abundant fruit, joy and mellifluous times.
Sept & cinquante annees pacifiques,	
Joie aux humains renoué Laqueduict,	
Santé, grandz fruict joye & temps melifique.²	

LOUIS XIV

This general quatrain seems to describe the prosperity of France under her great King Louis XIV.

90

Cent foix mourra le tyran inhumain.	A hundred times the inhuman tyrant will die and a wise and carefree man put in his place. He will have the whole senate in his hands, he will be troubled by a wretched scoundrel.
Mis à son lieu scavant & debonnaire,	
Tout le senat sera dessoubz sa main,	
Faché sera par malin themeraire.	

NAPOLEON IN ST HELENA

Napoleon is dying a hundred deaths through his enforced captivity; in his place is elected Louis XVIII, often called '*le debonnaire*'. Both houses of Parliament, the Senate, will profess

¹*poil*—Usually regarded as erratum for port.
²*melifique*—From Latin, *mellificus* = honey making. Nostradamus probably meant to write *mellifluus*.

devotion to their new king down to the last man. The trouble referred to in the final line was the assassination of the Duke de Berry in line for the throne through his father, Charles X.

91

Clergé Romain l'an mil six cens
& neuf,
Au chef de l'an feras election
D'un gris & noir de la Compagne
issu,
Qui onc ne feut si maling.

In the year 1609, the Roman Clergy at the head of the year will have an election; one of grey and black come forth from Campania, never was there one as wicked as he.

Pope Paul V reigned from 1605 to 1621 as Pope. But in the year 1609 he fell ill, and according to contemporary reports, there was a great deal of intriguing going on in the Courts of France and Rome should the Pope die an opportune death. See VIII. 71.

92

Devant le pere l'enfant sera tué:
Le pere apres entre cordes de jonc,
Genevois peuple sera esvertué
Gisant le chief au milieu comme
un tronc.

In front of the father the child will be killed, the father afterwards between ropes of rushes. The people of Geneva will be exerted, the chief lying in their midst like a trunk.

93

La barque neufve recevra les voyages,
Là & aupres transferont l'empire,
Beaucaire, Arles retiendront les
hostages
Pres deux colomnes trouvees de
porphire.

The new Bark will go on voyages, there and nearer they will transfer the empire. Beaucaire & Arles will retain the hostages near where two columns of porphyry are found.

PIUS VI, 1799

This quatrain implies that the Papacy will be moved as in I. 32, and V. 45 etc. Both Beaucaire and Arles are near the Rhône river which borders Valence where Pope Pius VI died in captivity in 1799.

94

De Nismes, d'Arles, & Vienne
    contemner,
N'obei tant à l'edict Hespericque:[1]
Aux labouriez[2] pour le grand
    condamner,
Six eschappez en habit seraph-
    icque.[3]

Scorn from Nîmes, Arles and
Vienne, not to obey at all the
Western edict; in order that
the great may condemn the
tormented, six escape in
Franciscan garb.

95

Dans les Espaignes viendra Roi
    trespuissant,
Par mer & terre subjugant or
    midi,
Ce mal fera rabaissant le crois-
    sant,
Baisser les aesles à ceux du vend-
    redi.[4]

Into Spain will come a very
powerful king, he will subjugate the south by land and
sea. This evil will cause a lowering of the crescent again, a
lowering of the wings of the
people of Friday.

PHILIP II OF SPAIN

The nearest this appears to come to fulfilment is Philip II
of Spain who persecuted the Moors, made several futile ex-
peditions to North Africa and was involved in the Battle of
Lepanto 1571.

96

Religion du nom des mers vain-
    cra,
Contre le secte fils Adaluncatif,[5]
Secte obstinee deploree craindra,
Des deux blessez par Aleph &
    Aleph.

The religion called after the
seas will overcome, against
the sect of the son Adaluncatif; the stubborn lamentable
sect will fear the two men
wounded by A & A.[6]

[1]*Hespericque*—Western? American? Spanish?
[2]*labouriez*—O.F. = to be tormented.
[3]*seraphicque*—The true name of the Franciscan order is the Order
of Seraphim.
[4]The Mahometans celebrate their Sabbath on a Friday.
[5]*Adaluncatif*—Unsolved name, possibly containing Calif among the
anagram?
[6]A & A—Aleph, letter A in Hebrew. Alif in Arabic.

This quatrain should be easy to solve but is not. The anagram for Adaluncatif is still unbroken. The Λ's in line 4 are not much help since a great number of Arab names begin with A.

97

Triremes pleines tout aage captif,
Temps bon à mal, le doux pour amertume;
Proie à Barbares trop tost seront hastifs,
Cupid de veoir plaindre au vent la plume.

Triremes full of captives of all ages good times for bad, sweet ones for the bitter; hasty they will be too quickly prey for the Barbarians anxious to see the plume (of smoke) wail in the wind.

98

La splendeur claire à pucelle joyeuse,
Ne luira plus long temps sera sans sel:
Avec marchans,[1] ruffiens loups odieuse,
Tous pesle mesle monstre universel.

For the joyful maiden the bright splendour will shine no more, for a long time she will lack salt. With merchants, bullies, odious wolves all confusion the universal monster.

FRENCH THIRD REPUBLIC

The Third Republic in France was typified as Marianne, and so might refer in a general way to France between 1940–4, lacking wisdom 'salt' in her behaviour. The confusion and beasts refer to the Nazi invasion.

99

La fin le loup, le lyon, beuf, & l'asne,
Timide dama[2] seront avec mastins,
Plus ne cherra à eux la douce manne,
Plus vigilance & custode aux mastins.

The end of the wolf, the lion, ox and the ass, the timid deer will be with the mastiffs. No longer will the sweet manna fall upon them; more vigilance and guarding for the mastiffs.

---

[1]*marchans*—May mean mercenaries here?
[2]*dama*—Latin = a deer.

100

Le grand empire sera par Angle-
terre,
Le pempotam¹ des ans plus de
trois cens:
Grandes copies² passer par mer
& terre,
Les Lusitains³ n'en seront pas
contens.

A great empire will be for
England, the all powerful for
more than 300 years. Great
forces cross by land and sea.
The Portuguese will not be
content.

GREAT BRITAIN

In this interesting quatrain Nostradamus foresees a great
future for Britain lasting for three hundred years. Most people
take it from the reign of Elizabeth to that of Victoria, fifty
years longer than prophesied. It is unclear what the Portuguese have to do with this, and line 3 is also tricky, does it
refer to English forces, or to the forces that will end Britain's
greatness? A good ambiguous twist with which to end in the
typical Nostradamus tradition. See III. 57.

STIRLING
DISTRICT
LIBRARY

¹*pempotam*—From the Greek, *pan* = all, and the Latin, *potens* =
powerful.
²*copies*—Latin, *copia* = troops.
³*Lusitains*—Classical name for Portuguese.

THE FURTHER PROPHECIES OF NOSTRADAMUS

BY ERIKA CHEETHAM

Many of the prophecies contained in *The Centuries* of 16th Century astrologer and seer Michel de Nostredame have already come true . . .

In this fascinating and deeply-reseached sequel to her international bestseller, THE PROPHECIES OF NOSTRADAMUS, Erika Cheetham focuses attention on Nostradamus' view of our present world and what is to come:

WAR IN THE MIDDLE EAST

THE GROWTH IN MILITARY MIGHT OF
THE THREE GREAT POWERS

THE RISE OF THE THIRD ANTI-CHRIST
FROM THE EAST

THE END OF THE PAPACY

A VAST EARTHQUAKE IN THE U.S.A.

THE END OF THE BRITISH MONARCHY

0 552 12299 8

A SELECTED LIST OF NON-FICTION TITLES AVAILABLE FROM CORGI BOOKS

THE PRICES SHOWN BELOW WERE CORRECT AT THE TIME OF GOING TO PRESS. HOWEVER TRANSWORLD PUBLISHERS RESERVE THE RIGHT TO SHOW NEW RETAIL PRICES ON COVERS WHICH MAY DIFFER FROM THOSE PREVIOUSLY ADVERTISED IN THE TEXT OR ELSEWHERE.

All Corgi/Bantam Books are available at your bookshop or newsagent, or can be ordered from the following address:
Corgi/Bantam Books,
Cash Sales Department,
P.O. Box 11, Falmouth, Cornwall TR10 9EN

UK and B.F.P.O. customers please send a cheque or postal order (no currency) and allow £1.00 for postage and packing for the first book plus 50p for the second book and 30p for each additional book to a maximum charge of £3.00 (7 books plus).

Overseas customers, including Eire, please allow £2.00 for postage and packing for the first book plus £1.00 for the second book and 50p for each subsequent title ordered.

NAME (Block Letters) ....

ADDRESS ....

....